NEUROBIOLOGY OF CENTRAL D_1-DOPAMINE RECEPTORS

ADVANCES IN EXPERIMENTAL MEDICINE AND BIOLOGY

Recent Volumes in this Series

A Continuation Order Plan is available for this series. A continuation order will bring delivery of each new volume immediately upon publication. Volumes are billed only upon actual shipment. For further information please contact the publisher.

NEUROBIOLOGY OF CENTRAL D_1-DOPAMINE RECEPTORS

Edited by

George R. Breese
University of North Carolina at Chapel Hill
Chapel Hill, North Carolina

and

Ian Creese
University of California, San Diego
La Jolla, California

PLENUM PRESS • NEW YORK AND LONDON

Library of Congress Cataloging in Publication Data

Neurobiology of central D_1-dopamine receptors.

(Advances in experimental medicine and biology; v. 204)
Includes bibliographies and index.
1. Dopamine — Receptors. I. Breese, George R. II. Creese, Ian. III. Series. [DNLM:
1. Neurobiology. 2. Receptors, Dopamine — drug effects. 3. Receptors, Dopamine —
physiology. W1 AD559 v. 204 / WL 102.8 N49408]
QP563.D66N47   1986   599′.01′88   86-18716

ISBN-13: 978-1-4684-5193-1   e-ISBN-13: 978-1-4684-5191-7
DOI: 10.1007/978-1-4684-5191-7

© 1986 Plenum Press, New York
Softcover reprint of the hardcover 1st edition 1986
A Division of Plenum Publishing Corporation
233 Spring Street, New York, N.Y. 10013

PREFACE

    Our understanding of the functional mechanisms relating
dopamine activity to normal and abnormal behavior has been
turned "upside-down" by the recent developments described in
the chapters of this volume. Heretofore, it was generally
agreed that all of the pharmacological and behavioral
properties ascribed to dopamine systems were mediated via
activation or inhibition of the subtype of dopamine receptors
termed D_2. The properties of these receptors were first
characterized in 1975 following their identification by
receptor binding techniques utilizing ^{3}H-butyrophenones,
potent antipsychotic drugs, used in the treatment of
schizophrenia. Although another subtype of dopamine receptor
had already been identified a few years earlier, now termed
the D_1 receptor, its functional properties were unknown -
other than the fact that it was associated with the activation
of the enzyme adenylate cyclase. Our absence of knowledge of
the behavioral functions of this receptor stemmed primarily
from the lack of selective agonist and antagonists for D_1
receptors - drugs which did not also interact with D_2
receptors. Selective agents for D_2 receptors did exist and
hence the behavioral roles of D_2 receptors were easily
ascribed.

    The work described in this text is primarily stimulated
by the development of two selective D_1 receptor drugs - the
antagonist SCH 23390 and the agonist SKF 38393. The studies
described herein clearly show that D_1 receptors do indeed have
many behavioral functions, on the surface often similar to
those responses mediated by D_2 receptors. These observations
hold hope for the development of new dopaminergic agents for
use in the treatment of psychiatric and neurologic diseases
that may be more selective in their actions and lack some of
the side effects of the presently used mixed or D_2 receptor
selective agents. These studies are the beginning of an
active period of new research strategies that will provide a
greater understanding of the role of dopamine systems in
behavior.

    We should like to thank Schering Corporation for
financial support in the preparation of this volume. We
should also like to thank Carolyn Reams for manuscript
preparation.

                                        George R. Breese
                                        Ian Creese
                                        April, 1986

                                                              v

CONTENTS

BENZAZEPINES: STRUCTURE-ACTIVITY RELATIONSHIPS BETWEEN D_1 RECEPTOR BLOCKADE AND SELECTED PHARMACOLOGICAL EFFECTS

Louis C. Iorio, Allen Barnett, William Billard
and Elijah H. Gold

Schering Research
Bloomfield, N.J.   07003

SCH 23390 is (R)-(+)-7-chloro-8-hydroxy-3-methyl-1-phenyl-2,3,4,5-tetrahydro-1-H-3-benzazepine. Its synthesis was based on the benzazepine series synthesized more than 15 years ago by Dr. Lewis Walter and Mr. Wei Chang at Schering Research Laboratories, and highlighted by the work done with the 7,8-dimethoxy analog of SCH 23390, SCH 12679. This earlier-described drug (Barnett et al., 1974) manifested potent inhibition of aggression invoked in animals by such diverse methods as social isolation, septal and olfactory bulb lesions and electrical stimulation, and aggression occurring spontaneously in monkeys (attack phenomena) and rats (muricide). With respect to antipsychotic potential, SCH 12679 did differ from the standards in that it did not block conditioned avoidance responding (CAR) in rats, an effect which we consider an important index of antipsychotic potential. In fact, these effects of SCH 12679 seen in animals were carried over in clinical trials with acute and chronic schizophrenics, severely retarded people, and hyperkinetic adolescents: namely, antiaggressive effects were observed but not antipsychotic activity (Keskiner et al., 1971; Itil et al., 1972; Park et al., 1972; Albert et al., 1977).

Dopamine antagonist properties and the ability to block CAR in rats was built into the benzazepine series through the additional efforts at Schering of Dr. Eli Gold and Mr. Wei Chang. These efforts culminated in the synthesis of SCH 23390.

The pharmacologic characterization of SCH 23390 (Iorio et al., 1981, 1983) revealed that this drug, among other effects, blocked CAR in rats, as do standard antipsychotics. However, SCH 23390 differed from the standards in blocking dopamine-sensitive adenylate cyclase at very low concentrations (11 nM), not blocking ^{3}H-spiperone binding, not causing hyperprolactinemia and not blocking apomorphine-induced emesis in dogs. Since the latter three properties are identified as D_2 receptor events, SCH 23390 was identified as a specific D_1 receptor antagonist. This conclusion was soon confirmed by Hyttel (1983) showing that SCH 23390 displaced ^{3}H-piflutixol

1

Table 1. Displacement of ^{3}H-23390 and ^{3}H-Spiperone Binding by Dopamine Receptor Agonists and Antagonists

Drugs	D-1 ^{3}H-SCH 23390 Displacement K_i(nM)	D-2 ^{3}H-Spiperone Displacement K_i (nM)	Relative Concs. Needed for 50% Displacement
ANTAGONISTS:			
SCH 23390	0.3	760	1:2533
cis(Z)Flupentixol	4.3	0.8	5.4:1
trans(E)Flupentixol	907	94	9.6:1
cis(Z)Piflutixol	2.9	1.0	2.9:1
trans(E)Piflutixol	95	73	1.3:1
(+)Butaclamol	14.6	1.8	9.1:1
(-)Butaclamol	25,500	131,000	1:5
Chlorpromazine	74	8.2	9:1
Fluphenazine	11.2	1.2	9.3:1
Perphenazine	29.9	1.3	23:1
Thioridazine	59	9.1	6.5:1
Spiperone	8,400	0.12	70,000:1
Haloperidol	835	1.8	418:1
Sulpiride (R)	30,000	1,102	27:1
Sulpiride (S)	>100,000	10	10,000:1
AGONISTS:			
SK&F 82526	1	1209	1:93
SK&F 38393	57	6700	1:117
Apomorphine	432	590	1:13
LY 171555	55,000	698	78:1

from D_1 binding sites at concentrations much lower than those that displaced ^{3}H-spiperone from D_2 sites.

Prior to the disclosure of SCH 23390 as a specific D_1 receptor antagonist, research on dopaminergic function, including the concept of two dopamine receptors (the D_1 but not the D_2 associated with adenylate cyclase) proposed by Kebabian and Calne (1979), relied on the use of the selective D_2 agonists and antagonists and selective D_1 agonists. It is clear that the identification of SCH 23390 as the missing link in the quartet of tools needed to fully investigate dopaminergic function has rekindled universal interest and research in this area.

A major advance in this area of research was the synthesis and description of the binding properties of tritiated (N-methyl-^{3}H) SCH 23390 (Billard et al., 1984). This near-ideal ligand, with a specific activity of 72 Ci/mmole, manifested saturable stereospecific binding to a single binding site with very low non-specific binding. Moreover, its binding capacity (69 pmoles/g tissue) approximated values published using ^{3}H-piflutixol and ^{3}H-flupentixol as ligands for D_1 receptor binding sites (Hyttel, 1978).

As measured in rat striatal homogenates (Table 1), none of the standard neuroleptics demonstrated selective displacement of ^{3}H-SCH 23390 binding (the exception being

2

Table 2. Structure-Activity Relationships of
SCH 23390 Analogs: 7-Position Substituents

| SCH No. | X | Receptor Displacement K_i (nM) | | D_2/D_1 Ratio |
		D_1	D_2	
23390	Cl	0.3	760	2533
24543	Br	0.3	765	2550
25873	F	10.5	5,441	518
23389	CH_3	1.1	1,062	965
23982	H	5.7	1,666	292
25688	i-propyl	17	424	24
25523	t-butyl	1000	>10,000	>10
15198	OCH_3	2.4	3,770	1570
26457	OCH_2CF_3	223	9,288	40
15379	OH	52	1,339	26
25819	CH_2OH	53	1,849	35
26713	CN	35.1	26,000	740
24905	$(CH_3)_2NCH_2$	132	12,000	91
26057	$CONH_2$	52	184	3.5

(-) butaclamol which was very weak (μM range) against ^{3}H-SCH
23390).   Only cis(Z)piflutixol and trans(E)piflutixol
approached equipotent displacement of both ligands. The
others showed specificities for D_2 binding sites,i.e.,
specific displacement of ^{3}H-spiperone, ranging over many log
units. As previously reported in experiments using [3]H-
piflutixol and ^{3}H-spiperone as ligands (Leff et al., 1984), we
also showed that sulpiride had marked specificity for [3]H-
spiperone sites over ^{3}H-SCH 23390 sites and that the isomers
showed reverse specificity, i.e. S>R at D_2 sites and R>S at D_1
sites. Of the agonists tested, SK&F 82526 and SK&F 38393
showed about 100 fold specificity for ^{3}H-SCH 23390 binding
sites, apomorphine was approximately equipotent at both sites,
and LY171555 showed about 80-fold specificity for D_2 sites.

     The first series of studies we undertook was to evaluate
the ability of selected analogs of SCH 23390 to displace [3]H-
SCH 23390 and ^{3}H-spiperone. Of the compounds in which the
moiety at the 7-position was changed (Table 2), it is clear
that SCH 23390 (chloro) and the bromo-analog are the most
potent displacers of ^{3}H-SCH 23390, both being about 20-fold
more potent than the H-analog. The methyl>methoxy>fluoro
analogues are also extremely potent (K_i's <11 nM). These
compounds are also the most specific for D_1 binding sites,
with differential blockade ranging from 290-2500 fold. The

Table 3. Structure-Activity Relationship of SCH 23390
Analogs: 8-Position Substituents

		Receptor Displacement K_i (nM)		
SCH No.	X	D_1	D_2	D_2/D_1 Ratio
23390	OH	0.3	760	2533
26418	SH	249	36,101	145
37718	CH_2OH	148	4,296	29
23985	OCH_3	181	709	4
37193	$CONH_2$	324	27,000	83
37372	CO_2H	10,000	2,300	0.3
25076	$OCON(CH_3)_2$	127	7,521	60
37149	CN	144	31,585	221
26430	$NHSO_2CH_3$	213	1,800	8

cyano-analog is the only other specific D_1 antagonist in this range (740 fold) but it is much weaker at the D_1 site (K_i = 53 nM) than SCH 23390. In general, this table shows that benzazepines with a variety of substituents in the 7-position retain their selectivity for D_1 sites, albeit over a large potency range.

On retention of the chloro moiety in the 7-position and altering substituents at the 8-position (Table 3), much less tolerance with respect to potency is observed. None of the analogs approaches the potency of SCH 23390, the closest being less than 1/400th as potent. Despite this, specificity seems to be retained (except for the 8-COOH analog), but only the 8-SH and 8-CN analogs have greater than 100-fold specificity.

With respect to substitution at the 3-N position (Table 4), the methyl moiety was optimal for affinity at both D_1 and D_2 receptor sites. The N-desmethyl analog was 1/20th as potent as SCH 23390. Addition of larger alkyl groups reduced potency more than 100 fold, either because of a direct steric effect or because the nitrogen lone electron pair is directed to a non-equatorial position relative to the azo ring, instead of the preferred equatorial position as has been shown for D_1 agonists (Kaiser and Jain, 1985).

Our next step was to determine the correlation between displacement of ^{3}H-SCH 23390 and blockade of dopamine-sensitive adenylate cyclase (DSAC). Our results (Table 5), although obtained with a limited number of SCH 23390 analogs, show a high correlation (r = 0.95). The results in

Table 4. Structure-Activity Relationship of SCH 23390
Analogs: N-Position Substituents

| SCH No. | R | Receptor Displacement K_i (nM) | | D_2/D_1 Ratio |
		D_1	D_2	
24518	H	6	1838	306
23390	CH_3	0.3	760	2533
25013	CH_3CH_2	41	15,919	388
24219	$CH_3CH_2CH_2$	3,600	400,000	111

Table 5. Displacement by Selected Benzazepines of ^{3}H-SCH
23390 Binding and Inhibition of Rat Striatal
DA-Sensitive Adenylate Cyclase

SCH No.	(R/S)	X	Y	^{3}H-SCH 23390 Displacement K_i (nM)	Rat Striatal DSAC Inhibition K_i (nM)
23390	R	Cl	OH	0.3	0.8
23388	S	Cl	OH	192	>10,000
24543	R	Br	OH	0.3	0.4
25873	R	F	OH	10.5	0.6
26418	R	Cl	SH	249	56.0
23389	R	CH_3	OH	1	2.4
23391	S	CH_3	OH	831	253
12679	R	OCH_3	OCH_3	491	183
15198	R	OCH_3	OH	2.4	0.4
15199	R	OH	OCH_3	294	19.7
15379	R	OH	OH	52	6.7

this table also illustrate stereospecificity for the SCH
23390-SCH 23388 and SCH 23398-SCH 23391 enantiomer pairs: for
each pair, the R-isomer has much greater affinity for D_1
binding sites and for inhibiting DSAC than the S-isomer.

These data strongly support the concept of a direct connection between D_1 receptors and adenylate cyclase, as proposed by Kebabian and Calne (1979).

Having shown the strong relationship between affinity for D_1 binding sites and blockade of DSAC, we turned our attention toward evaluating the relationship between these effects and inhibition of conditioned avoidance responding (CAR) in rats. For these studies, we administered the drug subcutaneously to minimize the additional variables that oral administration might impose on the results. Our results (Table 6) with a number of analogs of SCH 23390 indicate that the correlation between D_1 receptor affinity and CAR inhibition is also very high ($r = 0.93$). Moreover, inhibition of CAR by the more potent analogs appeared to occur at doses too low for D_2 receptor effects. Table 6 also illustrates another very important point. As we have previously reported (Billard et al, 1984), SCH 23390 ($K_i = 760$ nM) and its S-enantiomer SCH 23388 ($K_i = 988$ nM) are nearly equipotent in displacing ^{3}H-spiperone from D_2 receptor binding sites, yet this study shows that the anti-CAR potency of SCH 23390 is about 3000 times more potent than those of SCH 23388. Since there is no reason to suspect radical differences in absorption, metabolism, or excretion of these optical isomers especially by the s.c. route, it seems highly unlikely that the anti-CAR effects of SCH 23390 is mediated via D_2 receptor blockade. Thus, it seems reasonable to conclude that selective blockade of D_1 receptor sites can evoke a behavior that heretofore has been attributed to D_2 receptor block. The apparent paradox that the same behavior can occur by blockade of two apparently biochemically and functionally distinct receptors (Stoof and Kebabian, 1981) remains the subject of much research in our own as well as other laboratories. However, this subject will be discussed in ensuing chapters and will not be further addressed in this communication. Instead, we will direct our attention to two aspects of the pharmacology of SCH 23390 that need clarification: 1) its cataleptogenic effects as related to block of CAR and 2) its duration of action.

We had reported (Iorio et al., 1981, 1983) that SCH 23390 did not cause catalepsy in rats at oral doses several times greater than anti-CAR doses. For that evaluation, we used the raised parallel bar test, in which a rat's forepaws are placed on a suspended bar ten cm off the floor and the time that the rat remained immobile on the bar was equated to catalepsy. Others (Christensen et al., 1984) have since reported cataleptogenic effects in rats after parenteral administration of SCH 23390. These investigators used the vertical screen test, in which immobility of a rat placed in the center of a wire mesh screen is equated to catalepsy. These reports prompted us to re-examine the effects of SCH 23390 after parenteral administration. We again used the CAR to evaluate behavior, but we switched to the inclined screen (60°) test because we subsequently found it to be much more sensitive to drug effects than the parallel bar test, i.e. rats tend to remain immobile for longer periods of time. In this test, a 10 x 20" wire mesh screen (1 cm squares) is set at 60° from the horizontal position. Rats are placed in the center of this screen and the time to the first movement of any kind (head or limbs) is recorded, with a cut off time of 60 seconds. Throughout the balance of this report, the term

Table 6. D_1 Receptor Displacement and Blockade of
Conditioned Avoidance Responding in Rats

SCH No.	X	D_1 Receptor Displacement K_i (nM)	CAR (rats) MED, mg/kg, sc
23390	Cl (R)	0.3	0.01
23388	Cl (S)	192	30
24543	Br	0.3	0.03
25873	F	10.5	0.3
23389	CH_3	1.1	0.1
23982	H	5.7	0.1
25688	i-propyl	17	10
25523	t-butyl	1000	>10
15198	OCH_3	2.4	0.1
26457	OCH_2CF_3	223	>30
15379	OH	52	>10
25819	CH_2OH	53	>30
26713	CN	35.1	10
24905	$(CH_3)_2NCH_2$	132	10
26057	$CONH_2$	52	3

immobility will be used instead of catalepsy because we do in fact measure inhibition of spontaneous movement of rats placed on the screen.

For this study, we compared the time-course relationships between effects in the CAR test and the inclined screen test for comparable doses of SCH 23390 and haloperidol. SCH 23390 was administered at 0.2 mg/kg sc, a dose 20 times its anti-CAR MED (0.01 mg/kg, sc) determined 30 min after injection, and haloperidol was administered at 2 mg/kg (sc), a dose 20 times its anti-CAR MED (0.1 mg/kg, sc) obtained 30 min after injection.

The results of these studies are best understood by looking at the apparatus and paradigm used for the CAR test (Figure 1). A rat placed on the 8 x 10" electrified grid undergoes 20 consecutive trials. Each trial consists of 3 periods. The first period lasts 5 seconds: at its start the plunger recedes and a tone is sounded. If the rat climbs to the platform in this period, the response is considered an avoidance response. During the succeeding 10-second period, the tone is continued and a scrambled 10 mV shock is delivered to the grid. Climbing to the platform during this period constitutes an escape. If the rat does not climb to the platform in either of these first two periods, a failure is recorded. The tone and shock are then ended, the platform returns to its starting position and an intertrial period lasting 45 seconds ensues. After two sessions on two consecutive days, rats usually register avoidance responses on more than 90% of the trials. Performances of vehicle- and drug-treated groups of 6 rats are compared on the third day to evaluate drug effects.

APPARATUS

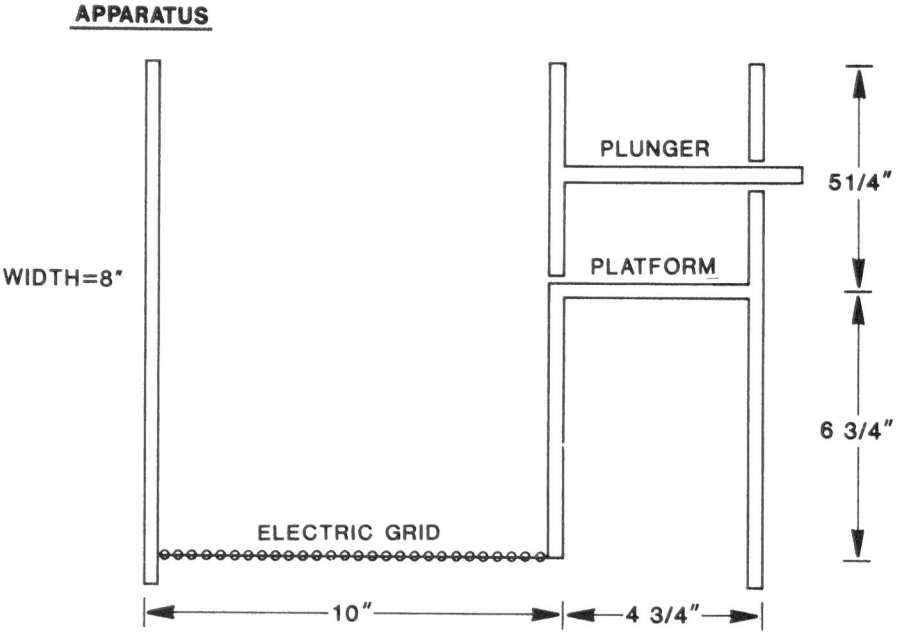

PARADIGM

PERIODS		
AVOID	ESCAPE	INTERTRIAL
PLUNGER RECEDES + TONE	TONE + SHOCK	TONE + SHOCK OFF PLUNGER PUSHES RAT ONTO GRID

(x 20)

|◄—5 sec—►|◄———10 sec———►|◄—ʃ 45 sec ʃ—►|

Fig. 1. Details of the apparatus and paradigm used in the conditioned avoidance test in rats.

The results with SCH 23390 (Figure 2) show that at this high parenteral dose (0.2 mg/kg, sc), rats failed to respond in the CAR test when tested 30 min after dosing. Responding begins at 1 hour, and at 2 hours failures and escapes occur about 25% and 50% of the time, respectively. At 3 hours, the rats respond all the time, including escaping about 25% of the time. At 4 hours, the effects of SCH 23390 are completely gone and the animals' behavior is normal. A comparison with the immobility effects on the inclined screen shows that failures and immobility appear to be correlated. For example, at 30 min after dosing, rats placed on the inclined screen remained immobile an average of about 50% (30 min) of the test period (60 min) and rats tested at the same time after dosing failed to respond at all in the CAR test. With time, both immobility and failures seemed to decrease in parallel.

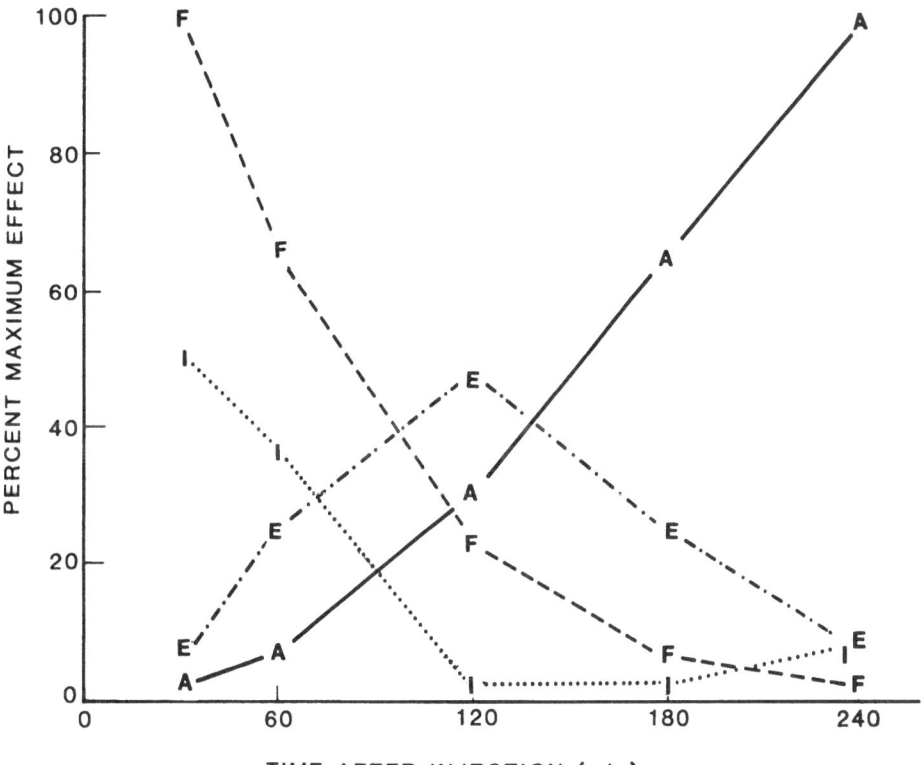

Fig. 2. Effects of SCH 23390, 0.2 mg/kg (sc), in the CAR and Inclined Screen (60°) tests in rats. A represents avoidance, E represents escapes, and F represents failures in the CAR test. I represents immobility time (failure to move) on the inclined screen.

While it is tempting to speculate that the failures seen in the CAR test were somehow caused by the drug-evoked immobility as measured in the inclined screen test, the results obtained with haloperidol, in contrast, suggest lack of a cause-effect relationship. For example, at 30 min after administration of haloperidol at the high dose of 2 mg/kg (sc), almost 2/3 of treated animals failed to respond in the CAR test, yet no immobility was observed in the Inclined Screen test at this time (Figure 3). Similarly, at later time points, failures ranged from 40-60% of responses while immobility was maximal. Thus, these data suggest that these two effects can be dissociated and may be mediated via different mechanisms. A further example of this is shown in Figure 4, which shows a comparison of the anti-CAR and immobility effects of SCH 23390 and its S-isomer, SCH 23388. Here, it is clear that SCH 23390 at low parenteral doses has

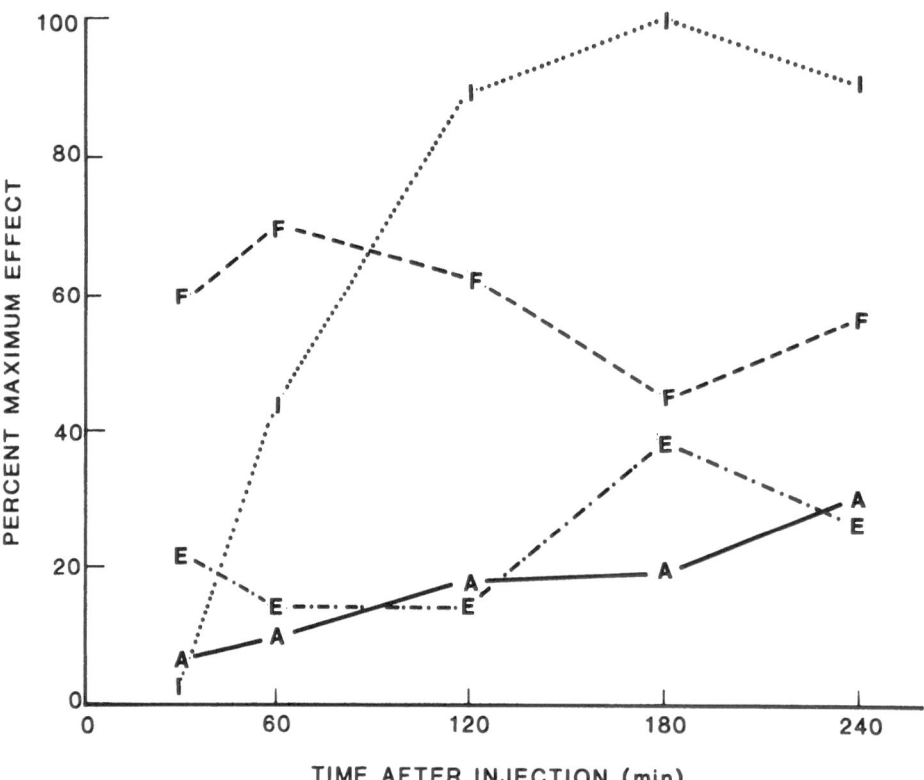

Fig. 3. Effects of haloperidol, 2 mg/kg (sc), in the CAR and Inclined Screen (60°) tests in rats. This dose of this drug is about 20 times the MED obtained in the CAR test at 30 min after injection to rats. See figure 2 legend for A,E,F & I designations.

anti-CAR effects without causing immobility. In contrast, SCH 23388 (the S-isomer) does not cause immobility at any dose tested but significant anti-CAR effects are seen at the higher doses tested.

With respect to the duration of action of SCH 23390, we reported (Iorio et al., 1981, 1983) a short duration based on blockade of CAR in rats after oral administration and blockade of aggression or hypermobility in monkeys after parenteral administration. As shown above (Fig. 2) for blockade of CAR in rats, SCH 23390, administered subcutaneously at a dose (0.2 mg/kg, sc) 20 times its anti-CAR MED obtained 30 minutes after dosing, has a duration of action less than 4 hours. This confirms our initial findings. However, a recent report (Schulz et al., 1985) shows that SCH 23390 administered

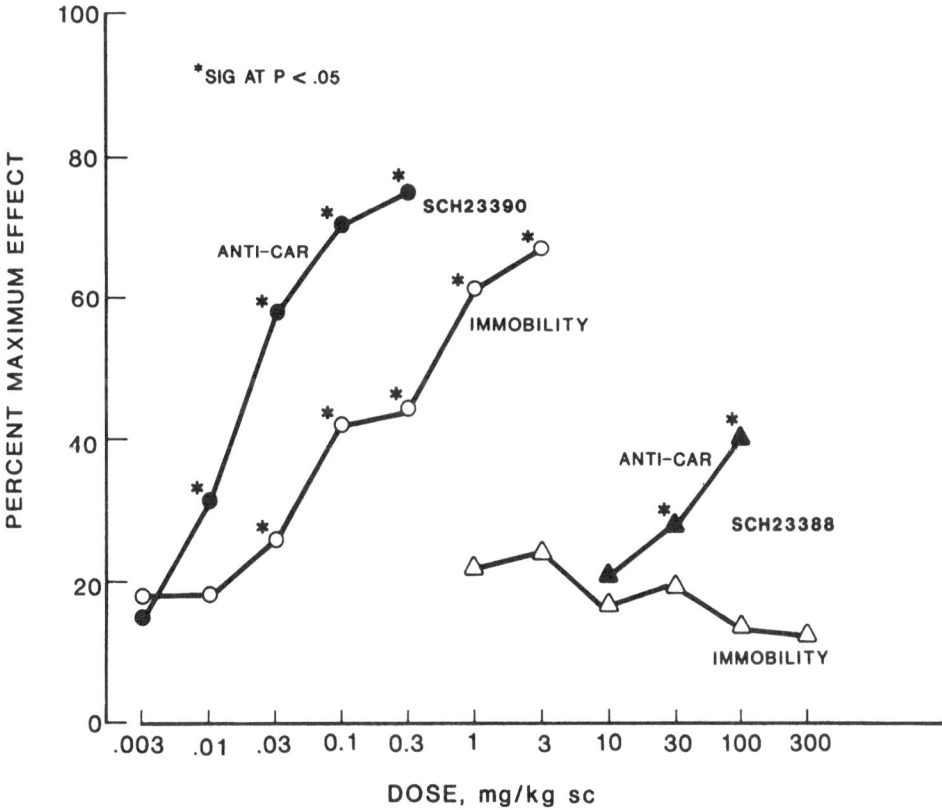

Fig. 4.   Effects of SCH 23390 and SCH 23388 (its S-isomer) in the CAR and Inclined Screen (60°) test in rats.

intraperitoneally to rats at a dose of 0.1 mg/kg had a significant effect 8 hours after administration, as measured by <u>in vivo</u> blockade of DSAC and blockade of amphetamine-induced hypermobility. We then undertook studies to help reconcile our different results. We re-evaluated the duration of action of SCH 23390 for blocking both apomorphine and d-amphetamine-induced stereotypy in rats after subcutaneous administration. Figure 5 shows that SCH 23390 blocks apomorphine-induced stereotypy with an ED_{50} obtained at 30 minutes after dosing of about 0.02 mg/kg sc. This is the same ED_{50} we reported previously (Iorio et al., 1981; 1983) for blockade of CAR obtained 30 min after dosing. Note that the blockade decreases with time (eg., the dose of 0.1 mg/kg sc which completely blocked apomorphine at 30 min after dosing was inactive at 4 hours after dosing). In contrast, SCH 23390

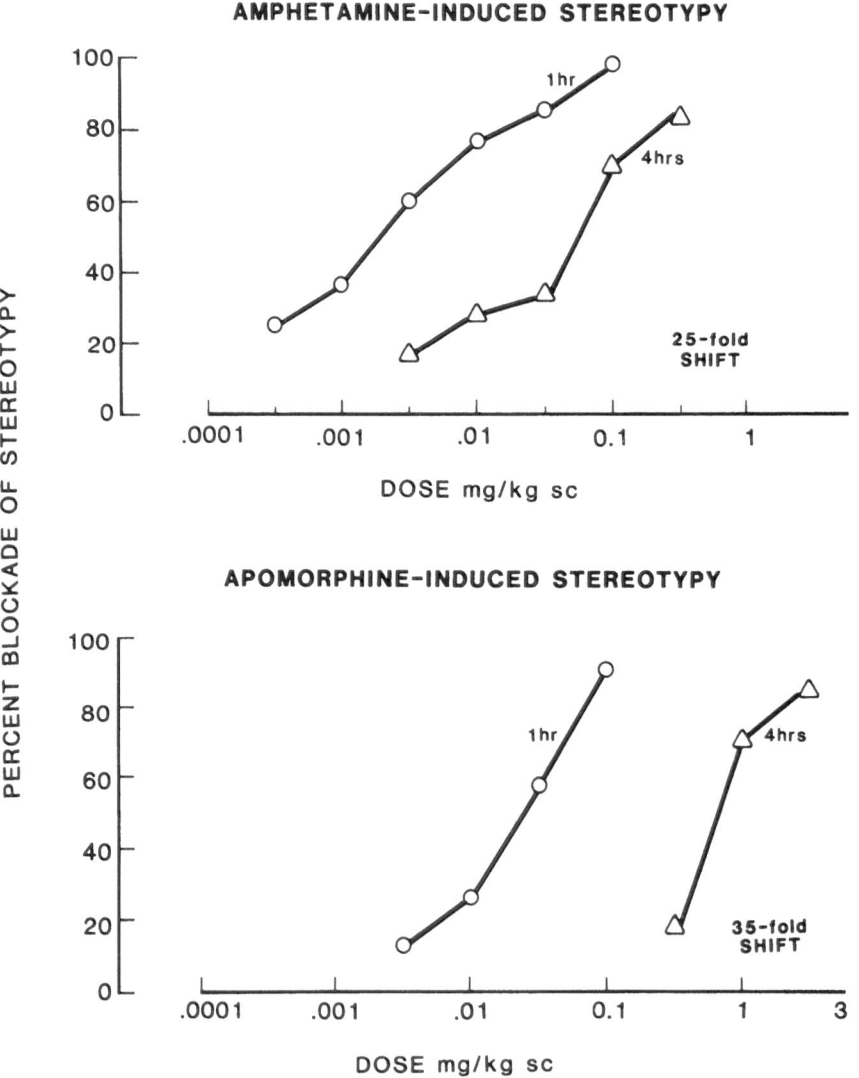

Fig. 5.   Duration of action of SCH 23390 for blockade off amphetamine- and apomorphine-induced stereotypy in rats.

at 30 minutes after dosing blocked d-amphetamine at lower doses: the ED_{50} is about 0.003 mg/kg (sc), about 10 times more potent than in blocking apomorphine-induced stereotypy. Moreover, although the blockade decreases with time, it is only slightly decreased at 4 hours after dosing of the high dose used (0.1 mg/kg, sc). These results suggest a unique interaction between SCH 23390 and d-amphetamine, which we are currently investigating in our laboratories.

In summary, we have reviewed the historical origins of SCH 23390 and its unique pharmacologic profile as a potential antipsychotic drug which differs from all known standards in that it is a specific D_1 receptor antagonist. This latter point is strongly supported in studies with SCH 23390 analogs by the high correlation between displacement of ^{3}H-SCH 23390 from rat striatal homogenates, blockade of dopamine-sensitive adenylate cyclase from rat striata and inhibition of conditioned avoidance responding (CAR) in rats. The possibility that the CAR inhibition was mediated via D_2 receptor blockade appears to be ruled out, because SCH 23390 and its S-isomer, SCH 23388, which have approximately equal affinities for D_2 receptors, have markedly different potencies in blocking CAR. In addition, a detailed evaluation of the effects of SCH 23390 and haloperidol in the Inclined Screen and CAR tests suggests that the immobility caused by these drugs and the incidence of failures, (i.e., the lack of responding during the electric shock period) are not related and hence greater dissociation of these effects might be achieved in novel compounds.

ACKNOWLEDGEMENTS

We are indebted to Drs. J. Berger, A. Elliott and K. Petrakis for the synthesis of several of the benzazepines in Tables 2 and 3.

REFERENCES

Albert, J.M., Elie, R., Cooper, S.F., Clermont, A. and Langlois, Y., 1977, Efficacy of SCH 12679 in the management of aggressive mental retardates, Curr. Therap. Res., 21:786.

Barnett, A., Taber, R.I. and Steiner, S.R., 1974, The behavioral pharmacology of SCH 12679, a new psychoactive agent, Psychopharmacol., 36:281.

Billard, W., Ruperto, V., Crosby, G., Iorio, L.C. and Barnett, A., 1974, Characterization of the binding of ^{3}H-SCH 23390, a selective D_1 receptor antagonist ligand, in rat striatum, Life Sci., 35:1885.

Christensen, A.V., Arnt, J., Hyttel, J., Larsen, J.-J. and Svendsen, O., 1984, Pharmacological effects of a specific D_2 antagonist SCH 23390 in comparison with neuroleptics, Life Sciences, 34:1529.

Hyttel, J., 1978, Effects of neuroleptics on ^{3}H-haloperidol and ^{3}H-flupentixol binding and on adenylate cyclase activity in vitro, Life Sciences, 1978, 23:551.

Hyttel, J., 1983, SCH 23390-the first selective dopamine D_1 antagonist, Europ J. Pharmacol, 91:153.

Iorio, L.C., Hoser, V., Korduba, C.A., Leitz, F. and Barnett, A., 1981, SCH 23390, a benzazepine with atypical effects on dopaminergic systems, Pharmacologist, 23:137.

Iorio, L.C., Barnett, A., Leitz, F., Houser, V.P. and Korduba, C.A., 1983, SCH 23390, a potential benzazepine antipsychotic with unique interactions on dopaminergic systems, J. Pharmacol. Exp. Therap., 226:462.

Itil, J.M., Stock, M.J., Duffy, A.D., Esquenazi, A., Saletu B. and Han, T.H., 1972, Therapeutic trials and EEG investigations with SCH 12679 in behaviorally disturbed adolescents, Curr. Therap. Res., 14:136.

Kaiser, C. and Jain, J., 1985, Dopamine receptors: functions subtypes and emerging concepts, Med. Res. Rev., 5:145.

Kebabian, J. and Calne, D.B., 1979, Multiple receptors for dopamine, Nature (Lond.) 277:93.

Keskiner, A., Itil, J.M., Han, T.H., Saletu, B. and Hsu, W., 1971, Clinical, toxicological and electroencephalographic study with SCH 12679 in chronic schizophrenics, Curr. Therap. Res., 13:714.

Leff, S.E., Chen, A. and Creese, I., 1984, Sulpiride isomers exhibit reversed stereospecificity for D_1 and D_2 dopamine receptors in the CNS, Neuropharmacol., 23:589.

Park, S., Gershon, S. and Floyd, A., 1972, A clinical trial of a benzazepine (SCH 12679) in acute schizophrenic patients, Curr. Therapy. Res., 14:298.

Schulz, D.W., Staples, L. and Mailman, R.B., 1985, SCH 23390 causes persistent antidopaminergic effects in vivo: evidence for long term occupation of receptors, Life Sci., 36:1941.

Stoof, J.C. and Kebabian, J.W., 1981, Opposing roles for D_1 and D_2 dopamine receptors in efflux of cyclic AMP from rat neostriatum, Nature, 294:366.

CHARACTERIZATION OF DOPAMINE D-1 AND D-2 RECEPTORS

John Hyttel and Jørn Arnt

Department of Pharmacology and Toxicology. H. Lundbeck A/S, Ottiliavej 7-9, DK-2500 Copenhagen-Valby, Denmark

CHARACTERIZATION WITH RECEPTOR-BINDING TECHNIQUE

DA receptors can be classified into two types, D-1 and D-2 (Kebabian and Calne, 1979). The D-1 receptors are coupled to a DA-dependent adenylate cyclase (AC) in a stimulatory manner, whereas D-2 receptors are independent of AC or coupled in an inhibitory manner (Stoof and Kebabian, 1982).

Tritium labelled haloperidol (^{3}H-HAL), ^{3}H-spiperone (^{3}H-SPI) and ^{3}H-domperidone (Snyder et al., 1975; Seeman et al., 1975; Leysen et al., 1978; Laduron and Leysen, 1979) are butyrophenone ligands which label D-2 receptors (see below). For labelling of D-1 receptors two thioxanthene ligands ^{3}H-cis(Z)-flupentixol (^{3}H-FPT) and ^{3}H-piflutixol (^{3}H-PIF) were introduced by Hyttel (1978a,b, 1980, 1981, 1982). Recently, the selective D-1 antagonist SCH 23390 (Hyttel, 1983, 1984; Iorio et al., 1983; Cross et al., 1983; Christensen et al., 1984; O'Boyle and Waddington, 1984; Schultz et al., 1985) has been shown to be a most useful, reliable and specific ligand (^{3}H-SCH) for D-1 receptors (Billard et al., 1984; Andersen et al., 1985; Andersen and Grønvald, 1985; Hyttel and Arnt, 1986; Hyttel, 1986).

In displacement experiments with neuroleptics (to be commented on below) quite different results were obtained dependent on whether a butyrophenone ligand or a thioxanthene ligand was used. These observations together with other (also to be commented on below) resulted in the postulation that ^{3}H-FPT and ^{3}H-PIF label the AC coupled D-1 receptors, whereas butyrophenone ligands label D-2 receptors.

Since cis(Z)-flupentixol and piflutixol have high affinity for both D-1 and D-2 receptors these thioxanthene ligands might be expected to bind to both populations of DA receptors. Cross and Owen (1980) showed that ^{3}H-FPT in fact binds to both D-1 and D-2 sites in calf striatal membranes. Approximately 20% of the specific binding was displaced by butyrophenones at low concentrations (D-2 site), whereas the remaining 80% required high butyrophenone concentrations for displacement. Similar results were later published for ^{3}H-PIF binding to rat striatal membranes (Hyttel, 1982). Here the D-1 and D-2 components consisted of 75% and 25%, respectively. Today suitable concentrations of D-2 antagonists, spiperone or sulpiride, are included in the ^{3}H-PIF assay to exclude binding to D-2 receptors (Hyttel, 1982; Fleminger et al., 1983). In contrast ^{3}H-SCH selectively labels D-1 receptors. This ligand has a half-life of 11-23 min (Billard et al., 1984; Andersen et al., 1985; Hyttel and Arnt, 1986) on the receptors, has a high affinity (K_D 0.15-0.60 nM, loc.cit.), low unspecific binding and is rather insensitive to pH-changes (loc.cit.).

This introduction has mainly focussed on D-1 receptor ligands. Butyrophenone ligand binding has been extensively reviewed in the past (for references see Seeman, 1980; Leysen, 1984).

The statement that thioxanthene and SCH 23390 on the one hand and butyrophenone ligands on the other label different receptors comes from a variety of experiments where these ligands show differences.

First of all, the number of binding sites for these ligands differ. Two to six times as many D-1 sites as D-2 sites are found in corpus striatum of rat, calf and man (table 1). In mouse the same ratio is found (Hyttel and Arnt, 1986). Also in other brain structures rich in DA the number of D-1 sites is greater than that of D-2 sites (Hyttel, 1978 a,b; Hyttel and Arnt, 1986). In olfactory tubercles the ratio D-1/D-2 receptor number is even greater than in corpus striatum (Hyttel, 1978 a). In a recent study the distribution of the binding of ^{3}H-PIF and ^{3}H-SPI as well as DA stimulated AC activity was measured in corpus striatum, nucleus accumbens and olfactory tubercles. More D-1 than D-2 receptors were found in all three structures but the ratio D-1/D-2 increased from corpus striatum, via nucleus accumbens to olfactory tubercles (Hyttel, 1985). The activity of DA-stimulated AC was almost equal in the three structures and in this respect the distribution of AC resembled that of ^{3}H-PIF binding to D-1 receptors.

The distribution of D-1 and D-2 receptors within the rat corpus striatum provides another basis of distinction between these receptor types. By lesion of striatal cell bodies with the neurotoxin kainic acid (KA) (Schwarcz et al. 1978) a clear dissociation between AC activity and ^{3}H-HAL binding sites in striatum could be seen. The nearly complete loss of the AC activity indicates that it is largely confined to neurones intrinsic to the striatum and to striatal output neurones, while the persistence of 65% of ^{3}H-HAL binding in the same striatum suggests that a majority of the binding sites are contained on other tissue elements. An additional depletion of ^{3}H-HAL binding after cortical ablation favours the localization to axons or terminals of the cortico-striatal projection. Similar results were obtained by Leff et al. (1981) who found that ^{3}H-FPT binding was diminished 70-80% in contrast to a 50% reduction in ^{3}H-butyrophenone binding (^{3}H-SPI, ^{3}H-domperidone) after kainate lesion of the corpus striatum. Almost identical results were obtained by Hyttel and Arnt (1986) using ^{3}H-SCH and ^{3}H-SPI as ligands.

Cross and Waddington (1981) also found that ^{3}H-FPT binding was depleted to a greater extent than ^{3}H-SPI binding. Reductions in binding of both ligands were significantly correlated with reduction in glutamic acid decarboxylase (GAD) activity. After extrapolation to complete loss of GAD activity, 30-40% of ^{3}H-SPI binding sites remained in the lesioned striata, whereas all ^{3}H-FPT binding sites were destroyed, suggesting that the majority of ^{3}H-FPT binding sites are located on those striatal cell bodies destroyed by KA. These results thus show that ^{3}H-FPT and ^{3}H-SCH predominantly label D-1 receptors, located on striatal KA-sensitive cell bodies. The binding of ^{3}H-HAL and ^{3}H-SPI to D-2 receptors is divided between striatal KA-sensitive cell bodies and striatal KA-insensitive elements, possibly terminals of cortical efferent fibres and the nigro-striatal projection.

Results from Davies et al. (1982) suggest that there is no such clear distinction. They showed that after cortical ablation B_{max} for ^{3}H-FPT binding decreased approximately 40%, indicating that some ^{3}H-FPT binding sites share the same distribution pattern as ^{3}H-SPI.

Another feature which differentiates D-1 and D-2 receptors is the molecular size. By the irradiation inactivation technique using 10 MeV electrons Nielsen et al. (1984) measured the target size of binding of ^{3}H-PIF and ^{3}H-SPI as well as the DA-stimulated AC. The estimated molecular sizes were deduced by reference to proteins with known molecular weights which were irradiated in the same tissue. The molecular weights of D-1 and D-2 receptors were 79,500 and 136,700 daltons, respectively. The size of the DA-stimulated AC was 202,000 daltons. The size

Table 1

Dopamine D-1 and D-2 receptor number

Species		Ligand D-1	Ligand D-2	Receptor number D-1	(n)	Receptor number D-2	(n)	References
				pmol/g tissue				
Rat	Striatum	3H-FPT	3H-HAL	78.0 ± 13.4	(4)	26.1 ± 1.9	(3)	Hyttel 1978 a,b
		3H-PIF	-	76		-		Hyttel 1981
		3H-PIF	3H-SPI	38.9 ± 7.6	(3)	17.5 ± 1.0	(3)	Hyttel et al. 1983
		3H-PIF	3H-SPI	70 ± 5		17.8 ± 0.2		Fleminger et al. 1982
		3H-PIF	3H-SPI	88 ± 5		13.8 ± 1.2		Fleminger et al. 1984
		3H-PIF	3H-SPI	122		20.6 ± 1.6		Jenner et al. 1984
		3H-SCH	-	85.6 ± 6.0	(2)	-		Andersen et al. 1985
		3H-SCH	-	73.9; 69.0		-		Billard et al. 1984
		3H-SCH	3H-SPI	98 ± 3.9	(6)	45 ± 2.7	(6)	Hyttel and Arnt 1986
Rat	Nucl. acc.	3H-SCH	-	58 ± 4.0	(2)			Hyttel and Arnt 1986
Rat	Frontal cortex	3H-SCH	-	6.9 ± 2.5	(3)			Hyttel and Arnt 1986
		3H-SCH	-	13.4 ± 2.1	(4)			Andersen et al. 1985
Mouse	Striatum	3H-SCH	3H-SPI	106 ± 16	(16)	45 ± 8.4	(6)	Hyttel and Arnt 1986
				fmol/mg protein				
Rat	Striatum	3H-FPT	3H-SPI	605	(2)	329	(2)	Cross and Waddington 1981
		3H-FPT	3H-SPI	2020 ± 1150		494 ± 62		Murrin 1983
		3H-FPT	-	1007		-		Davies et al. 1982
		3H-SCH	-	1421 ± 138	(5)	-		Porceddu et al. 1985
		3H-SCH	3H-SPI	1260 ± 85	(6)	560 ± 37	(6)	Hyttel and Arnt 1986
Mouse	Striatum	3H-SCH	3H-SPI	1440 ± 190	(16)	540 ± 43	(6)	Hyttel and Arnt 1986
Calf	Striatum	3H-FPT	-	860 ± 210	(4)			Cross and Owen 1980
Human	Putamen	3H-FPT	3H-SPI	335 ± 46	(3)	110 ± 5	(3)	Cross et al. 1983
		3H-PIF	3H-SPI	734 ± 58		331 ± 54		Cross and Rossor 1983

obtained for the D-2 receptor is similar to that described for ^{3}H-SPI binding in canine and human brain (123,000 daltons) estimated by the irradiation inactivation technique (Lilly et al., 1983), and in solubilized calf caudate (150,000-200,000) estimated by gel filtration (Lerner et al., 1981). It is too early to conclude much from these results, although a factor of approximately 2 between D-1 and D-2 sites is apparent. However, the 202,000 dalton size of AC can accommodate the 79,500 dalton size of the D-1 receptor. Recent studies using the same technique but with ^{3}H-SCH as a ligand showed a similar molecular weight (79,000 dalton) (Gredal et al., 1986).

With advanced age (22 months as compared to 4 months) there is a selective decrease (25%) in rat striatal D-2 receptor number (^{3}H-SPI binding) with no significant change in D-1 receptor number (^{3}H-PIF) (O'Boyle and Waddington, 1984). In a study using 1 year old rats lesioned unilaterally with 6-OHDA 9 months previously it was found that the ^{3}H-SCH binding in the control side was diminished to approximately 60% as compared to 1.5-2.5 months old rats (Hyttel and Arnt, 1986). Whether this diminuation is due to the age of the rats, to the contralateral lesion or to the different drugs tested during the last 8 months is still unsolved.

After prolonged treatment of rats with haloperidol an increase in D-2 receptor number is observed (Burt et al., 1977; Owen et al., 1980; Christensen and Hyttel, 1981). However, no change in D-1 receptor number (^{3}H-FPT) is seen (Christensen and Hyttel 1981). This has been confirmed in many experiments with different neuroleptic treatments. Administration of cis(Z)-flupentixol to rats for 18 months increased the number of ^{3}H-SPI binding sites in striatum and potentiated DA-stimulated AC, but did not alter specific ^{3}H-PIF binding (Murugaiah et al. 1983). In a study where neuroleptics were administered for 21 days, haloperidol, cis(Z)-flupentixol and sulpiride all increased striatal and mesolimbic ^{3}H-SPI binding. ^{3}H-PIF binding was unaltered after haloperidol and sulpiride treatment but increased in striatum after cis(Z)-flupentixol treatment (Fleminger et al., 1982, 1983). Creese and Chen (1985) showed that the D-1-receptor number (^{3}H-FPT) increased whereas the D-2 receptor-number (^{3}H-SPI) remained unchanged after 4 weeks treatment of rats with the D-1 selective SCH 23390. This has been confirmed by Porceddu et al. (1985) and Hyttel (1986) using ^{3}H-SCH as a ligand for D-1 receptors. Interestingly, the last author found that a reciprocal effect took place since D-2 receptor number decreased when D-1 receptor number increased and visa versa after spiperone pretreatment. The mixed D-1/D-2 antagonist zuclopenthixol induced only a slight increase in D-2 receptor number (loc.cit.).

A similar difference was seen after unilateral lesions of rat medial forebrain bundle by 6-OHDA. Whereas a 22% increase in B_{max} for ^{3}H-SPI binding was seen in the lesioned side no change was seen in ^{3}H-PIF binding. No changes were seen in Kd for either ligand (Hyttel et al., 1983). The lack of change in D-1-receptor number and K_D has been confirmed using ^{3}H-SCH as a ligand (Hyttel and Arnt, 1986).

In man the number of D-1 and D-2 receptors is different (table 1) and influenced differently by diseases. In post-mortem brain from schizophrenic patients the D-2 receptor number (measured by 1.2 nM ^{3}H-SPI) was increased by comparison with controls. However, in schizophrenic patients with movement disorder ^{3}H-SPI binding was not increased in comparison with those without such disorder. D-1 receptors (measured as ^{3}H-FPT binding) were found to be similar in controls and schizophrenic patients, with and without movement disorders (Crow et al., 1981, 1982). Using domperidone to differentiate ^{3}H-FPT binding between D-1 and D-2 sites, it was found that only D-2 sites were increased in drug-free schizophrenics (Cross et al., 1981; Owen et al., 1981). In post mortem brains from Huntington's disease patients, both D-1 and D-2 receptor number was decreased 45-50% in putamen as compared to controls. A selective loss (48%) of D-1 receptors was observed in substantia nigra pars reticulata of patients with Huntington's disease, but not in pars compacta. No differences in D-2 receptor number were observed between the groups in either region of substantia nigra (Cross and Rossor, 1983). Pimoule et al. (1985) found ^{3}H-SCH binding in post-mortem human putamen

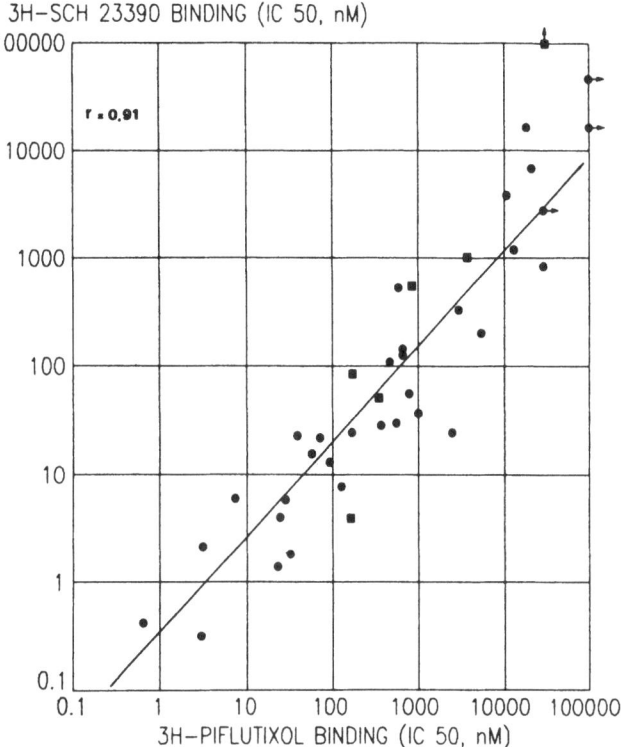

3H–SCH 23390 BINDING (IC 50, nM)

3H–PIFLUTIXOL BINDING (IC 50, nM)

Fig. 1
Correlation between affinities in the ^{3}H-piflutixol- and ^{3}H-SCH 23390-binding tests. Squares represent agonists, circles antagonists.

unmodified in either schizophrenia or Parkinson's disease, whereas Raisman et al. (1985) found ^{3}H-SCH binding increased in putamen of Parkinsonian patients not treated with L-DOPA from 5 days to 4 years before death but similar to control values in patients in L-DOPA therapy until death.

All this information points to the conclusion that thioxanthene ligands/SCH 23390 and butyrophenone ligands - under controlled conditions - label two distinct DA-receptor populations, D-1 and D-2, respectively.

One of the first clues to a difference between binding of thioxanthenes and butyrophenones was the difference in the order of potency of neuroleptics tested for displacement of the binding (Hyttel, 1978a,b, 1981, 1982; Hyttel and Christensen. 1983; Hyttel et al., 1983; Cross and Owen, 1980). Thioxanthenes are potent displacers at both D-1 and D-2 receptors. Phenothiazines and piperazino-6-7-6-tricyclics are more potent displacers at D-2 than at D-1 receptors, whereas butyrophenones, diphenylbutylpiperidines and benzamides have almost no activity at D-1 receptors but are potent displacers of D-2 binding (table 2). This difference in effect of neuroleptics is comparable to the difference in their ability to inhibit DA-stimulated AC activity (Miller et al., 1974; Clement-Cormier et al., 1974; Laduron, 1976). The inability of benzamides to inhibit DA-stimulated AC (Jenner et al., 1978; Portaleone et al., 1978) was confirmed by Hyttel (1980), who also showed that these compounds had extremely low affinity for ^{3}H-FPT binding sites. Thus, these results - like the kainic acid lesion experiments - point to a close linkage between ^{3}H-FPT binding sites and the DA stimulated AC. The results obtained using ^{3}H-SCH as a ligand are highly correlated to those obtained using either ^{3}H-FPT, ^{3}H-PIF or AC (Andersen et al., 1985; Hyttel and Arnt, 1986) (fig. 1).

Table 2   Inhibition by neuroleptics of DA-receptor binding and DA-stimulated adenylate cyclase in rat striatal tissue in vitro

Compound	D-1 receptors			AC	D-2 receptors	
	³H-SCH	³H-FPT	³H-PIF		³H-HAL	³H-SPI
THIOXANTHENES						
Cis(Z)-clopenthixol	1.4	12	23	26	2.6	6.4
Trans(E)-clopenthixol	110	480	480	440	39	110
Cis(Z)-flupentixol	2.2	3.0	3.2	18	3.1	3.2
Trans(E)-flupentixol	130	820	670	170	73	500
Cis(Z)-piflutixol	0.41	0.56	0.66	34	1.5	2.8
Trans(E)-piflutixol	23	110	40	1100	120	500
Teflutixol	5.8	13	28	77	6.9	19
Cis-thiothixene	13	34	94	260	0.71	6.2
PHENOTHIAZINES						
Chlorpromazine	29	48	380	400	12	24
Perphenazine	22	27	72	130	1.3	9.0
Trifluoperazine	7.8	23	130	210	3.4	5.3
BUTYROPHENONES + ANALOGUES						
Bromperidol	25	140	2500	160	1.7	6.4
Domperidone	3900	2800	11000	>100000	1.0	7.0
Droperidol	860	1100	28000	3600	3.0	2.1
Halopemide	6800	9000	21000	43000	7.3	99
Haloperidol	36	230	1000	220	3.0	8.2
Spiperone	210	1300	5400	1200	0.17	0.74
DIPHENYLBUTYLPIPERIDINES						
Fluspiriline	57	290	780	1100	3.1	11
Penfluridol	30	200	570	990	28	8.6
Pimozide	530	300	610	1900	1.3	1.2

cont.

Compound	D-1 receptors			AC	D-2 receptors	
	3H-SCH	3H-FPT	3H-PIF		3H-HAL	3H-SPI
BENZAMIDES						
Clebopride	16000	29000	18000	>100000	8.7	17
(±) Sulpiride	48000	32000	>100000	560000	160	820
YM 09151-2	2800	–	>30000	11000	1.7	0.49
PIPERAZINO-6-7-6-TRICYCLICS						
Clothiapine	16	36	56	80	31	46
Clozapine	140	220	680	1400	210	420
Methiothepin	6.0	16	7.4	37	1.2	2.6
MISCELLANEOUS						
(+) Butaclamol	3.9	6.8	25	310	1.5	12
SCH 23390	0.32	–	3.0	61	4500	3800
Tefludazine	24	49	170	260	8.8	19

Each drug was tested in five concentrations in triplicate. The IC50-values are expressed in nM. At least two separate determinations have been performed with each drug.
Concentrations of ligands and DA were: ^{3}H-SCH, 0.5 nM; ^{3}H-FPT, 2 nM; ^{3}H-PIF, 0.5 nM; DA, 40 µM; ^{3}H-HAL, 2 nM; ^{3}H-SPI, 0.5 nM.

Table 3　　　　　　Effect of DA agonists on D-1 and D-2 receptors

| | D-1 | | D-2 |
	^{3}H-SCH	^{3}H-PIF	^{3}H-SPI
SK & F 38393	85	170	48000
Metergoline	3.9	160	61
Transdihydrolisuride	51	360	8.9
Apomorphine	550	850	98
Quinpirole (LY 171555)	>100000	30000	2900
Pergolide	1000	3700	26

Ic50 values in nM. Each drug was tested in five concentrations in triplicate. At least two separate determinations have been performed with each drug.

In table 2, values for standard neuroleptics have been tabulated. The above stated differentiation of neuroleptics is clear. Thioxanthenes have a ratio D-1/D-2 close to 1, indicating affinity for both D-1 and D-2 receptors. This is also found for the piperazino-substituted neuroleptics with a 6-7-6 tricyclic ring system (clozapine, clotiapine etc.). For phenothiazines the ratio is higher, indicating that the D-2 component becomes more prominent in this series. Butyrophenones, diphenylbutyl-piperidines and benzamides all have much higher affinity for D-2. YM 09151-2 must be considered the most selective D-2 antagonist whereas SCH 23390 is the most selective D-1 receptor antagonist.

There is a very high correlation between results obtained with the different D-1 ligands or with the adenylate cyclase assay e.g.: ^{3}H-SCH vs. ^{3}H-PIF, r = 0.91 (n = 35) and ^{3}H-SCH vs. adenylate cyclase, r = 0.92 (n = 28). This is true when al tested compounds are included and when DA agonists and DA antagonists are compared separately, e.g.: ^{3}H-SCH vs. ^{3}H-PIF, agonists r = 0.84 (n = 5), antagonists r = 0.91 (n = 28).

The effects of DA agonists on D-1 and D-2 receptors are shown in table 3. It appears that they can be differentiated into selective D-1, selective D-2 and mixed D-1/D-2 agonists. SK & F 38393 is the most selective DA D-1 agonist. Apomorphine is a mixed D-1/D-2 agonist. Pergolide is the most selective D-2 agonist. In these binding tests quinpirole is less selective, although in functional tests it is extremely selective (Hyttel, 1984).

The present results have clearly shown that DA D-1 and D-2 receptors can be distinguished by the use of ^{3}H-thioxanthene/^{3}H-SCH 23390 and ^{3}H-butyrophenone ligands, respectively. The receptors show a different distribution and number in brain, have different neuronal localization and have different molecular size. In addition their number changes with age, after long-term neuroleptic treatment and after 6-OHDA lesions. The affinity of both neuroleptics and agonists for these receptors are very different. Finally, only the D-1 receptor is coupled in a stimulatory manner to the enzyme AC.

BEHAVIOURAL CHARACTERIZATION

Previously, results obtained in behavioural tests for neuroleptics have been related to the effect on D-2 receptors (Creese et al. 1976). However, several newer experiments point to an involvement of D-1 receptors in these behaviours and possibly also in the clinical effect.

The methylphenidate antagonistic effect of butyrophenones and diphenylbutyl-piperidines (D-2 blockers) is markedly attenuated by concomitant treatment with an anticholinergic agent, a GABA agonist or diazepam. The effect of thioxanthenes (D-

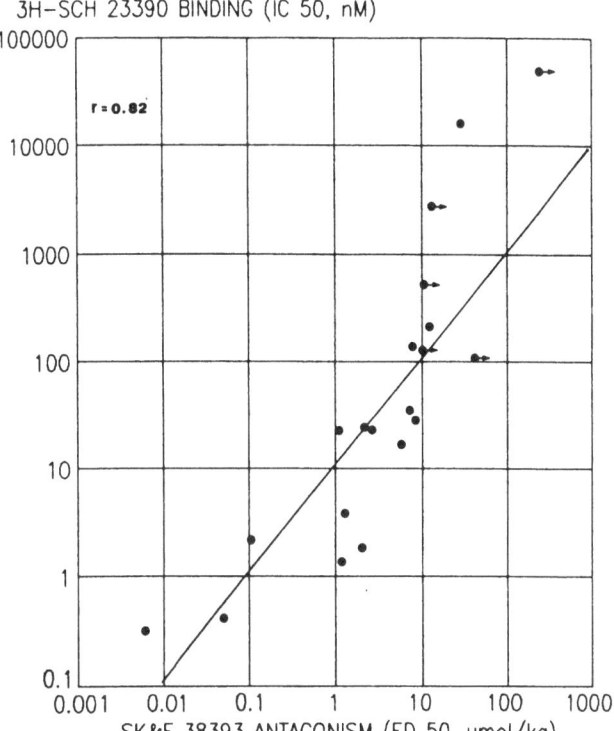

Fig. 2

Correlation between the antagonism of the SK & F 38393-induced rotation in unilaterally 6-OHDA lesioned rats and the affinity in the ^{3}H-SCH 23390-binding test.

1/D-2 blockers) and SCH 23390 (D-1 blocker) is almost unchanged (Christensen et al., 1979, 1980, 1984). This classification of neuroleptics is the same as shown above in binding experiments.

The difference between thioxanthenes and butyrophenones in combination with scopolamine is also seen in conditioned avoidance experiments, amphetamine-induced turning in 6-OHDA lesioned rats, 6,7-ADTN-induced hyperactivity and in catalepsy (Arnt et al., 1981).

During prolonged treatment with neuroleptics, supersensitivity to DA agonist and tolerance to neuroleptics develop. In mice, however, supersensitivity, tolerance and cross-tolerance do not develop after thioxanthenes or SCH 23390 but certainly after butyrophenones, diphenylbutylpiperidines and benzamides (Christensen and Hyttel, 1982; Hyttel et al., 1983; Hyttel and Christensen, 1983). The D-1 component of the thioxanthenes could be responsible for the absence of supersensitivity development as shown in combination experiments. Tolerance to the effect of haloperidol was not seen when the mice were concomitantly treated with either SCH 23390 or cis(Z)-clopenthixol (Christensen et al., 1985; Hyttel and Christensen, 1984). In line with the behavioural effects haloperidol incrased D-2-receptor number (^{3}H-SPI-binding), whereas SCH 23390 and zuclopenthixol were without effect, in mice treated for 12 days. Neither drugs induced changes in D-1-receptor number (Hyttel, 1986).

A more direct involvement of D-1 receptors was shown by Arnt and Hyttel (1984). In rats with unilateral 6-OHDA lesions the D-1 agonist SK & F 38393 and the

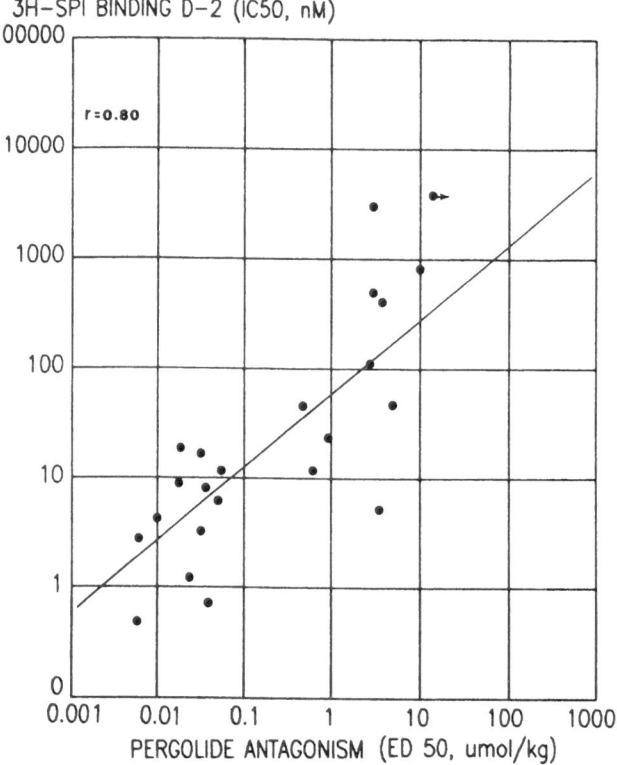

Fig. 3
Correlation between the antagonism of the pergolide-induced rotation in unilaterally 6-OHDA lesioned rats and the affinity in the ^{3}H-spiperone binding test.

D-2 agonist pergolide both induced strong contralateral circling behaviour. The circling induced by SK & F 38393 was blocked by SCH 23390 (ED50 0.006 µmol/kg s.c.), but SCH 23390 in doses up to 14 µmol/kg did not antagonize pergolide-induced circling. In contrast, selective D-2 antagonists, such as clebopride and spiperone had the reverse selectivity, whereas thioxanthenes (mixed D-1/D-2 blockers) antagonized the circling induced by both agonists. These results have been extended to a larger series of DA antagonist (Figs. 2 and 3). It was found that the ED50 values for inhibition of SK & F 38393-induced circling correlated significantly to the affinities for ^{3}H-SCH 23390 binding sites in vitro (r = 0.82), whereas ED50 values in the pergolide model correlated to affinities to ^{3}H-spiperone binding sites (r = 0.80). No correlation was found between SK & F 38393 antagonism and ^{3}H-SPI binding and between pergolide antagonism and ^{3}H-SCH binding (not shown). Thus, these experiments indicate that SK & F 38393 and pergolide induce circling by stimulation of separate D-1 and D-2 receptor sites, and indicate that these two test models can be used for evaluation of D-1/D-2 receptor selectivity in vivo.

In order to evaluate the possible importance of the unlesioned hemisphere (where D-1/D-2 interactions are different) for the results in the circling behaviour models (cf. Costall et al., 1983) additional experiments were made using rats with bilateral 6-OHDA lesions (Arnt, 1985 a). These experiments confirmed the selectivity observed in the circling experiments, since hyperactivity/stereotypy induced by SK & F 38393 was blocked by SCH 23390, but not by spiperone or clebopride, whereas the effect of pergolide was blocked by spiperone and clebopride but untouched by SCH 23390.

A similar differentiation between D-1 and D-2 sites was also found in rats treated for four days with reserpine (Arnt, 1985 b).

As a spin-off from the above-mentioned experiments it has been demonstrated that the circling/hyperactivity induced by apomorphine in rats with unilateral/bilateral 6-OHDA lesions involved simultaneous stimulation of D-1 and D-2 receptors, since only mixed D-1/D-2 antagonists completely blocked the effect of apomorphine. Selective antagonists (D-1 or D-2) were only partially effective (Arnt, 1985 a; Arnt and Hyttel, 1985; Herrera-Marschitz and Ungerstedt, 1985).

References

Andersen, P.H. and Grønvald, F.C., 1985, A comparison between dopamine-stimulated adenylate cyclase and ^{3}H-SCH 23390 binding in rat striatum, Acta Neurol. Scand., 72:225.

Andersen, P.H., Grønvald, F.C. and Aas Jansen, J., 1985, A comparison between dopamine-stimulated adenylate cyclase and ^{3}H-SCH 23390 binding in rat striatum, Life Sci., 37:1971.

Andersen, P.H. and Grønvald, F.C., 1986, Specific binding of ^{3}H-SCH 23390 to dopamine D1 receptors in vivo, Life Sci., in press.

Arnt, J., Christensen, A.V. and Hyttel, J., 1981, Differential reversal by scopolamine of effects of neuroleptics in rats. Relevance for evaluation of therapeutic and extrapyramidal side-effect potential, Neuropharmacology, 20:1331.

Arnt, J. and Hyttel, J., 1985, Differential involvement of dopamine D-1 and D-2 receptors in the circling behaviour induced by apomorphine, SK & F 38393, pergolide and LY 171555 in 6-hydroxydopamine-lesioned rats. Psychopharmacology, 85:346.

Arnt, J., 1985 a, Hyperactivity induced by stimulation of separate dopamine D-1 and D-2 receptors in rats with bilateral 6-OHDA lesions, Life Sci., 37:717.

Arnt, J., 1985 b, Behavioural stimulation is induced by separate dopamine D-1 and D-2 receptor sites in reserpine-pretreated but not in normal rats, Eur. J. Pharmacol., 113:79.

Billard, W., Ruperto, V., Crosby, G., Iorio, L.C. and Barnett, A., 1984, Characterization of the binding of ^{3}H-SCH 23390, a selective D-1 receptor antagonist ligand, in rat striatum, Life Sci., 35:1885.

Burt, D.R., Creese, I. and S.H. Snyder, 1977, Antischizophrenic drugs: Chronic treatment elevates dopamine receptor binding in brain, Science, 196:326.

Christensen, A.V., Arnt, J. and Svendsen, O., 1985, Pharmacological differentiation of dopamine D-1 and D-2 antagonists after single and repeated administration, in: Dyskinesia - Research & Treatment, Casey, D., Chase, T.N., Christensen, A.V. and Gerlach, J., eds., Springer Verlag, Heidelberg.

Christensen, A.V., Arnt, J., Hyttel, J., Larsen, J.-J. and Svendsen, O., 1984, Pharmacological effects of a specific dopamine D-1 antagonist SCH 23390 in comparison with neuroleptics, Life Sci., 34:1529.

Christensen, A.V., Arnt, J. and Scheel-Krüger, J., 1979, Decreased antistereotypic effect of neuroleptics after additional treatment with a benzodiazepine, a GABA agonist and an anticholinergic compound. Life Sci., 24: 1395.

Christensen, A.V., Arnt, J. and Scheel-Krüger, J., 1980, GABA-dopamine/neuroleptic interaction after systemic administration, Brain Res. Bull., 5, suppl.2:885.

Christensen, A.V. and Hyttel, J., 1981, Prolonged treatment with the GABA agonist THIP increases dopamine receptor binding more than it changes dopaminergic behaviour in mice, Drug Develop. Res., 1:255.

Christensen, A.V. and Hyttel, J., 1982, Neuroleptics and the clinical implications of adaptation of dopamine neurons, Pharmacy International, 3:329.

Clement-Cormier, Y.C., Kebabian, J.W., Petzold, G.L. and Greengard, P., 1974, Dopamine-sensitive adenylate cyclase in mammalian brain: A possible site of action of antipsychotic drugs, Proc. Nat. Acad. Sci. U.S.A., 71:1113.

Costall, B., Kelly, M.E. and Naylor, R.J., 1983, Does contralateral circling involve action of drugs on hyposensive striatal dopamine receptors in the hemisphere contralateral to denervation?, Neuropharmacology, 22:295.

Creese, I., Burt, D.R. and Snyder, S.H.. 1976, Dopamine receptor binding predicts clinical and pharmacological potencies of antischizophrenic drugs, Science, 192:481.

Cross, A.J., Crow, T.J. and Owen, F., 1981, ^{3}H-flupenthixol binding in post-mortem brains of schizophrenics: Evidence for a selective increase in D 2 receptors, Psychopharmacology, 74:122.

Cross, A.J., Marshal, R.D., Johnson, J.A. and Owen, F., 1983, Preferential inhibition of ligand binding to calf striatal dopamine D-1 receptors by SCH 23390, Neuropharmacology, 22:1327.

Cross, A.J. and Owen, F., 1980, Characteristics of ^{3}H-cis-flupenthixol binding to calf brain membranes, Eur. J. Pharmacol., 65:341.

Cross, A.J. and Rossor, M., 1983, Dopamine D-1 and D-2 receptors in Huntington's disease, Eur. J. Pharmacol., 88:223.

Cross, A.J. and Waddington, J.L., 1981, Kainic acid lesions dissociate (^{3}H)spiperone and (^{3}H)cis-flupenthixol binding sites in rat striatum, Eur. J. Pharmacol., 71:327.

Crow, T.J., Cross, A.J., Johnstone, E.C., Owen, F., Owens, D.G.C. and Waddington, J.L., 1981, Tardive dyskinesia - Disease process or drug effect? in: Biological Psychiatry, C. Perris, G. Stuwe and B. Jansson, eds., Elsevier/North-Holland Biomedical Press.

Crow, T.J., Cross, A.J., Johnstone, E.C., Owen, F., Owens, D.G:C. and Waddington, J.L., 1982, Abnormal involuntary movements in schizophrenia: Are they related to the disease process or its treatment? Are they associated with changes in dopamine receptors? J. Clin. Psychopharmacol., 2:336.

Davies, S.W., Templeton, W.W. and Woodruff, G.N., 1982, Reduction of specific (^{3}H)cis-flupenthixol binding sites in rat striatum following decortication, Br. J. Pharmacol., 77:358P.

Fleminger, S., Hall, M.D., Jenner, P., Kilpatrick, G., Mann, S., Marsden, C.D. and Rupniak, N.M.J., 1984, Differential effects of administration of haloperidol, sulpiride or clozapine for 12 months on rat striatal function, Br. J. Pharmacol., 82:288P.

Fleminger, S., Jenner, P., Marsden, C.D. and Rupniak, N.M.J., 1982, Dopamine receptor supersensitivity produced by repeated neuroleptic administration correlates with increased D-2 receptors, Br. J. Pharmacol., 77:456P.

Fleminger, S., Rupniak, N.M.J., Hall, M.D., Jenner, P. and Marsden, C.D., 1983, Changes in apomorphine-induced stereotypy as a result of subacute neuroleptic treatment correlates with increased D-2 receptors, but not with increases in D-1 receptors, Biochem. Pharmacol., 19:2921.

Gredal, O., Nielsen, M. and Hyttel, J., 1986, Target size of dopamine D-1 receptors in rat corpus striatum estimated by ^{3}H-SCH 23390 binding. Eur. J. Pharmacol., submitted.

Herrera-Marschitz, M. , and Ungerstedt, U., 1985, Effect of the dopamine D-1 antagonist SCH 23390 on rotational behaviour induced by apomorphine and pergolide in 6-hydroxy-dopamine denervated rats, Eur. J. Pharmacol., 109:349.

Hyttel, J., 1978 a, Effects of neuroleptics on ^{3}H-haloperidol and ^{3}H-cis(Z)-flupenthixol binding and on adenylate cyclase activity in vitro, Life Sci., 23:551.

Hyttel, J., 1978 b, A comparison of the effect of neuroleptic drugs on the binding of ^{3}H-haloperidol and ^{3}H-cis(Z)-flupenthixol and on adenylate cyclase activity in rat striatal tissue in vitro, Prog. Neuro-Psychopharmacol., 2:329.

Hyttel, J., 1980, Further evidence that ^{3}H-cis(Z)-flupenthixol binds to the adenylate cyclase-associated dopamine receptor (D-1) in rat corpus striatum, Psychopharmacology, 67:107.

Hyttel, J., 1981, Similarities between the binding of ^{3}H-piflutixol and ^{3}H-flupentixol to rat striatal dopamine receptors in vitro, Life Sci., 28:563.

Hyttel, J., 1982, Preferential labelling of adenylate cyclase coupled dopamine receptors with thioxanthene neuroleptics, in: Advances in dopamine research, M. Kohsaka, T. Shomori, Y. Tsukada and G.N. Woodruff, eds., Advances in the biosciences, 37:147. Pergamon Press, Oxford.

Hyttel, J., 1983, SCH 23390 - The first selective dopamine D-1 antagonist, Eur. J. Pharmacol., 91:153.

Hyttel, J., 1984, Functional evidence for selective dopamine D-1 receptor blockade by SCH 23390, Neuropharmacology, 23:1395.

Hyttel, J., 1985, Dopamine D-1 and D-2 receptors. Characterization and differential effects of neuroleptics, Proceedings of the VIIIth International Symposium on Medicinal Chemistry, Dahlbom, R. and Nilsson, J.L.G., eds., Acta Pharmaceutica Suecica, suppl. 1:426.

Hyttel, J., 1986, Effect of prolonged treatment with neuroleptics on dopamine D-1 and D-2 receptor number in corpus striatum of rat and mouse, J. Neural. Transmission, in press.

Hyttel, J. and Arnt, J., 1986, Characterization of binding of ^{3}H-SCH 23390 to dopamine D-1 receptors. Correlation to other D-1 and D-2 measures and effect of selective lesions, J. Neural. Transmission, in press.

Hyttel, J. and Christensen, A.V., 1983, Biochemical and pharmacological differentiation of neuroleptic effect on dopamine D-1 and D-2 receptors, J.Neural.Transmiss., supp. 18:157.

Hyttel, J. and Christensen, A.V., 1984, Do dopamine D-1 receptors contribute to the antipsychotic effects and side effects of neuroleptic drugs ?. Clin. Neuropharmacol. 7, suppl. 1:546.

Hyttel, J., Christensen, A.V. and Arnt, J., 1983, Neuroleptic classification: Implications for tardive dyskinesia, Mod.Probl. Pharmacopsychiat., 21:49.

Iorio, L.C., Barnett, A., Leitz, F.H., Houser, V.P. and Korduba, C.A., 1983, SCH 23390, a potential benzazepine antipsychotic with unique interactions on dopaminergic systems, J.Pharmacol. exp. Ther., 226:462.

Jenner, P., Elliott, P.N.C., Clow, A., Reavill, C. and Marsden, C.D., 1978, A comparison of in vitro and in vivo dopamine receptor antagonism produced by substituted benzamide drugs, J. Pharm. Pharmacol., 30:46.

Jenner, P., Kilpatrick, G.J. and Marsden, C.D., 1984, CHAPS solubilises D_2 but not D_1-binding sites from rat striatal preparations, Br. J. Pharmacol., 81:52P.

Kebabian, J.W. and Calne, D.B., 1979, Multiple receptors for dopamine, Nature, 277:93.

Laduron, P., 1976, Limiting factors in the antagonism of neuroleptics on dopamine-sensitive adenylate cyclase, J.Pharm. Pharmacol., 28:250.

Laduron, P.M. and Leysen, J.E., 1979, Domperidone, a specific in vitro dopamine antagonist, devoid of in vivo central dopaminergic activity, Biochem. Pharmacol., 28:2161.

Leff, S., Lynne, A., Hyttel, J. and Creese, I., 1981, Kainate lesion dissociates striatal dopamine receptor radioligand binding sites, Eur. J. Pharmacol., 70:71.

Lerner, M.H., Rosengarten, H. and Friedhoff, A.J., 1981, Solubilization and characterization of ^{3}H-spiroperidol binding sites of calf caudate, Life Sci., 29:2367.

Leysen, J.E., 1984, Receptors for neuroleptic drugs, Advances in Human Psychopharmacology, 3:315.

Leysen, J.E., Gommeren, W. and Laduron, P.M., 1978, Spiperone: A ligand of choice for neuroleptic receptors. 1. Kinetics and characteristics of in vitro binding, Biochem.Pharmacol., 27:307.

Lilly, L., Frazer, C.M., Jung, C.Y., Seeman, P. and Venter, J.C., 1983, Molecular size of the canine and human brain D_2 dopamine receptor as determined by radiation inactivation, Mol. Pharmacol., 24:10.

Miller, R.J., Horn, A.S. and Iversen, L.L., 1974, The action of neuroleptic drugs on dopamine-stimulated adenosine cyclic 3',5'-monophosphate production in rat neostriatum and limbic forebrain, Mol.Pharmacol., 10:759.

Murrin, L.C., 1983, Characteristics of ^{3}H-cis-flupenthixol binding in rat striatum, Life Sci., 33:2179.

Murugaiah, K., Fleminger, J., Theodorou, A., Jenner, P., Marsden, C.D., 1983, Persistant increase in striatal dopamine stimulated adenylate cyclase activity persists for more than 6 months but disappears after 1 year following withdrawal from 18 months cis-flupenthixol intake, Biochem. Pharmacol., 32:2495.

Nielsen, M., Klimek, V. and Hyttel, J., 1984, Distinct target size of dopamine D-1 and D-2 receptors in rat striatum, Life Sci., 35:325.

O'Boyle, K.M. and Waddington, J.L., 1984, Selective and stereospecific interactions of R-SK & F 38393 with (^{3}H)piflutixol but not (^{3}H)spiperone binding to striatal D_1 and D_2 dopamine receptors: Comparison with SCH 23390, Eur.J.Pharmacol., 98:433.

O'Boyle, K.M. and Waddington, J.L., 1984, Loss of rat striatal dopamine receptors with agening is selective for D-2 but not D-1 sites: Association with increased non-specific binding of the D-1 ligand (^{3}H) piflutixol. Eur. J. Pharmacol., 105:171.

Owen, F., Cross, A.J., Crow, T.J., Poulter, M. & Waddington, J.L., 1981, Increased dopamine receptors in schizophrenia: Specificity and relationship to drugs and symptomtology, in: Biological psychiatry. C. Perris, G. Stuwe and B. Jansson, eds., Elsevier/North-Holland Biomedical Press.

Owen, F., Cross, A.J., Waddington, J.L., Poulter, M., Gamble, S.J. and Crow T.J., 1980, Dopamine-mediated behaviour and ^{3}H-spiperone binding to striatal membranes in rats after nine months haloperidol administration, Life Sci., 26:55.

Pimoule, C., Schoemaker, H., Reynolds, G.P. and Langer, S.Z., 1985, (^{3}H) SCH 23390 labeled D_1 dopamine receptors are unchanged in schizophrenia and parkinson's disease, Eur. J. Pharmacol., 114:235.

Porceddu, M.L., Ongini, E. and Biggio, G., 1985, (^{3}H) SCH 23390 binding sites increase after chronic blockade of D-1 dopamine receptors. Eur. J. Pharmacol., 118:367.

Portaleone, P., Crispino, A. and DiCarlo, R., 1978, Effect of substituted benzamides on the cAMP system in the hypothalamus and striatum of the rat, Neurosci.lett., 9:233.

Raisman, R., Cash, R., Ruberg, M. Javoy-Agid, F. and Agid, Y., 1985, Binding of (^{3}H) SCH 23390 to D-1 receptors in the putamen of control and parkinsonian subjects, Eur. J. Pharmacol., 113:467.

Schultz, D.W., Stanford, E.J., Wyrick, S.W. and Mailman, R.B., 1985, Binding of (^{3}H) SCH 23390 in rat brain: Regional distribution and effects of assay conditions and GTP suggest interaction of a D_1-like dopamine receptor. J. Neurochem., 45:1601.

Schwarcz, R., Creese, I., Coyle, J.T. and Snyder, S.H., 1978, Dopamine receptors localized on cerebral cortical afferents to rat corpus striatum, Nature, 271:766.

Seeman, P., 1980, Brain dopamine receptors, Pharmacol.Rev., 32:229.

Snyder, S.H., Creese, I. and Burt, D.R., 1975, The brain's dopamine receptor: Labelling with (^{3}H) dopamine and (^{3}H) haloperidol, Psychopharmacol. Commun., 1: 663.

Stoof, J.C. and Kebabian, J.W., 1982, Independent in vitro regulation by the D-2 dopamine receptor of dopamine-stimulated efflux of cyclic AMP and K$^+$-stimulated release of acetylcholine from rat neostriatum, Brain Res., 250:263.

BIOCHEMICAL AND BEHAVIORAL STUDIES OF D_1 DOPAMINE RECEPTORS

UTILIZING SCH 23390

Ellen J. Hess and Ian Creese

Department of Neurosciences
University of California, San Diego
La Jolla, California 92093

INTRODUCTION

Previous research has demonstrated the existence of two distinct dopamine receptor subtypes (Kebabian & Calne, 1979; Creese et al., 1983), possessing unique pharmacologic and biochemical properties. D_1 dopamine receptors stimulate adenylate cyclase activity (Hyttel, 1978), while D_2 dopamine receptors inhibit this enzyme (Stoof and Kebabian, 1981; Onali et al., 1984; Battaglia et al., 1985). However, both receptor subtypes co-exist in many tissues making the determination of their respective physiological and behavioral roles difficult. All neuroleptics, commonly used drugs in the treatment of schizophrenia, have been shown to be either mixed D_1/D_2 dopamine receptor antagonists or selective D_2 dopamine receptor antagonists. Thus, D_2 dopamine receptors have been implicated as the site mediating the antipsychotic and antidopaminergic activity of neuroleptics (Creese et al., 1976; Seeman et al., 1976). By inference, D_2 dopamine receptors have been considered to mediate dopaminergic agonists' behavioral effects as well (Seeman, 1981).

The functional role of D_1 dopamine receptors has not been clearly defined due to the lack of selective, high affinity D_1 dopamine receptor ligands. To date, the thioxanthenes, $[^3H]$cis-flupentixol and $[^3H]$cis-piflutixol, have been the only suitable radioligands available for labeling D_1 dopamine receptors. Since these ligands exhibit similar affinities for both D_1 and D_2 dopamine receptors, as well as high non-specific binding (30-50% of total binding) (Hyttel, 1981; Leff et al., 1985a), they have not been ideal tools for investigating D_1 dopamine receptor pharmacology, molecular mechanisms or behavioral function. Recently, a D_1 selective antagonist, SCH 23390, was developed (Iorio et al., 1983) which crosses the blood/brain barrier allowing its use in behavioral experiments. SCH 23390 has since been tritiated, making detailed D_1 dopamine receptor characterization possible. This novel benza-zepine exhibits nanomolar potency in inhibiting dopamine stimulation of striatal adenylate cyclase activity (Onali et al., 1984; Plantje et al., 1984; Hyttel, 1984; Battaglia et

al., 1985), exhibiting a K_i value of approximately 0.5 nM for
the striatal D_1 dopamine receptor (Billard et al., 1985;
Schulz et al., 1985) In contrast, its affinity for D_2 dopamine
receptors is orders of magnitude lower ($2 \times 10^{-7}M$) indicating
that, unlike flupentixol and piflutixol, SCH 23390 is selective for D_1 dopamine receptors. Hence, the advent of this
first truly selective D_1 dopamine receptor antagonist has
provided the tool for research into the functional correlates
of D_1 dopamine receptor activation and antagonism.

CHARACTERIZATION OF [^{3}H]SCH 23390 BINDING TO D_1 DOPAMINE
RECEPTORS

This laboratory had recently extensively characterized
the binding properties of [^{3}H]flupentixol to D_1 dopamine
receptors by using unlabeled spiperone or domperidone to
block [^{3}H]flupentixol binding to D_2 receptors (Leff et al.,
1985a; 1985b). It was shown that while antagonist inhibition
of [^{3}H]flupentixol-labeled D_1 dopamine receptors exhibited
homogeneous binding characteristics, agonists compete with
both high and low affinity binding components. Additionally,
these studies demonstrated that in the presence of guanine
nucleotides, the high affinity agonist binding component was
reduced or abolished, suggesting that there was interconver-
sion of high affinity to low affinity agonist-binding states
of the receptor. This phenomenon is similar to that observed
for D_2 dopamine receptors (Sibley et al.,1982), β-adrenoceptors
(Heidenrich et al., 1980) and α-2 adrenoceptors (Hoffman et
al., 1982), and is thought to reflect receptor interaction
with a guanine nucleotide regulatory subunit (N) involved, in
this case, with linkage to adenylate cyclase.

In turn, we have undertaken a detailed investigation of
antagonist and agonist interactions with D_1 dopamine receptors
labeled by [^{3}H]SCH 23390 and the effect of guanine nucleotides
on the regulation of agonist interactions with this receptor
(Hess et al., in press). In rat striatum, [^{3}H]SCH 23390
appears to be selective for the D_1 dopamine receptor. [^{3}H]SCH
23390 binding is saturable, monophasic and exhibits high
affinity (Kd = 0.49 nM). Scatchard analyses of saturation data
indicate that the site density in striatum, 64 ± 12.9 pmol/g
wet weight tissue, corresponds well with densities reported
for D_1 dopamine receptors labeled by [^{3}H]flupentixol (Hyttel,
1978; Leff et al., 1985b). Additionally, greater than 90% of
striatal [^{3}H]SCH 23390 binding is D_1 dopamine receptor
specific. Antagonist competitions for [^{3}H]SCH 23390 binding
are monophasic, suggesting that [^{3}H]SCH 23390 labels a
homogeneous population of sites. That the affinities of
antagonist inhibition of [^{3}H]SCH 23390 correlate well with
their respective affinities in both inhibiting D_1 receptor
binding of [^{3}H]flupentixol (Figure 1) or antagonizing
dopamine-stimulated adenylate cyclase activity indicates that
SCH 23390 is D_1 receptor selective. These findings corroborate
and extend the earlier reports by Billard et al. (1984).

In contrast to the monophasic competitions by antagonists, agonist interactions with [^{3}H]SCH 23390 binding
were complex, yielding shallow competition curves, consistent
with the preliminary report of Seeman et al. (1985). Agonist
competitions consistently modeled best to two sites composed

of a high affinity component (R_H) comprising 30-40% of the
total number of specific binding sites and a low affinity site
(R_L) comprising the remaining 60-70% of specific binding
sites.

In many adenylate cyclase-coupled receptor systems,
including D_2 dopamine receptors, α-$_2$ and β-adrenoceptors,
guanine nucleotides regulate agonist interactions with
[^{3}H]antagonist-labeled receptors. The effect of guanine
nucleotides, such as GTP, is primarily to reduce the overall
affinity of agonists for these receptors (i.e. shift curves to
the right) by reducing the percent of agonist high affinity
binding (%R_H). Consistent with these systems, we have found
that in the presence of 0.3 mM GTP, agonist competition for
[^{3}H]SCH 23390 binding was shifted to the right and steepened
(Figure 2), resulting in an approximate 50% reduction in the
high affinity agonist binding site density. No significant
change in K_H for any of the agonists was observed nor was any
difference in the %R_H reductions apparent between partial and
full agonists. That guanine nucleotides can promote an
apparent shift in agonist competition curves, decreasing the
%R_H without affecting [^{3}H]SCH 23390 binding suggests that the

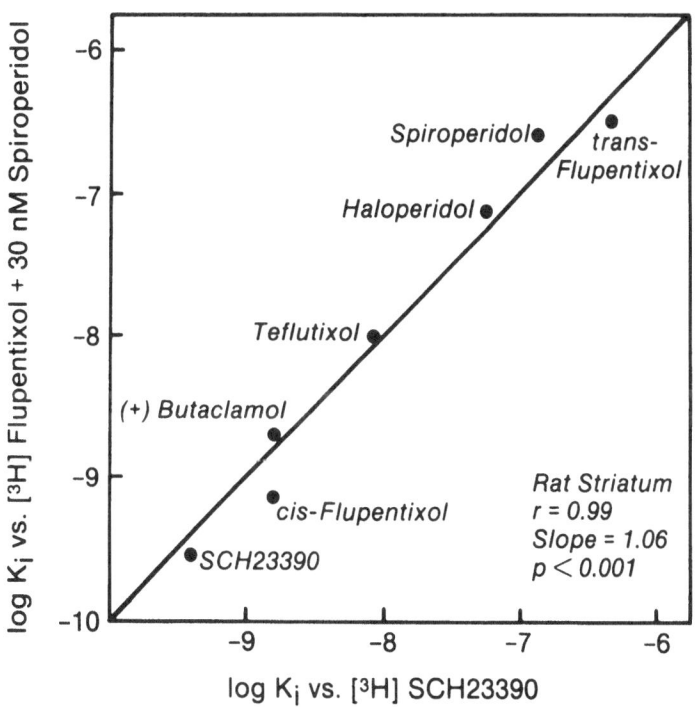

Figure 1. Correlation between antagonist inhibition of
[^{3}H]SCH 23390 and [^{3}H]flupentixol binding in
rat striatal homogenates. Log K_i values for
[^{3}H] SCH 23390 binding and [^{3}H]flupentixol
binding were derived from data obtained in this
laboratory (Hess et al., in press; Leff et al.,
1985a).

high and low affinity agonist components of binding represent partially interconvertible states of a single receptor population.

This observation is consistent with the proposed two state model, modified from the original ternary complex model (Boeynaems, and Dumont, 1975; Jacobs and Cuatrecasas, 1976), for the D_1 dopamine receptor selectively labeled by [^{3}H]flupentixol (Leff et al., 1985a,b). Briefly, this model hypothesizes that both agonists (A) and antagonists bind to

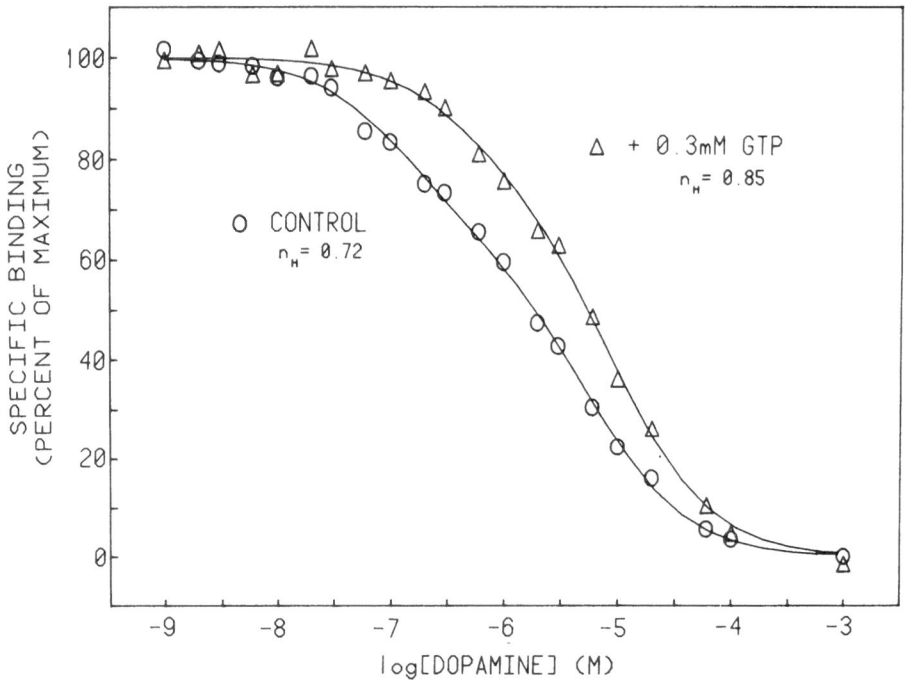

Figure 2. Curves are described by computer-fitted curves for dopamine inhibition of [^{3}H]SCH 23390 binding in the presence and absence of 0.3 mM GTP. Experimentally determined points are from representative experiments consisting of duplicate determinations of 21 concentrations of dopamine using 0.25 nM [^{3}H]SCH 23390 where 100% specific binding represents 1300 cpm in both the presence and absence of 0.3 mM GTP. Competition curves were fit best by a two-site computer derived model where the affinity of [^{3}H]SCH 23390 was constrained to be equal (K_D = 0.5 nM) at both high (R_H) and low (R_L) affinity sites. Computer-fitted parameters were derived for dopamine competitions in the absence of 0.3 mM GTP (n=4): K_H = 197 $\pm$ 112 nM, K_L = 3971 $\pm$ 1034 nM, %R_H = 37 $\pm$ 6; and in the presence of 0.3 mM GTP (n=4): K_H = 303 $\pm$ 29, K_L = 5222 $\pm$ 29, %R_H = 18 $\pm$ 5.

the receptor (R) recognition site, but only agonists promote or stabilize the interaction between R and the guanine nucleotide regulatory subunit (N). Thus, a ternary complex is formed (ARN) which has high affinity for agonists, representing the R_H state of the receptor. In this model, the addition of guanine nucleotides promotes the dissociation of N and R which then exhibits low affinity for agonists, representing the R_L agonist binding state (for review see Limbird, 1981).

Unfortunately, in frontal cortex, [^{3}H]SCH 23390 can also label S_2 serotonin receptors. SCH 23390 has an affinity of 7.0 nM for [^{3}H]ketanserin binding to S_2 serotonin receptors in frontal cortex. Thus, if nanomolar concentrations of [^{3}H]SCH 23390 are used, significant numbers of S_2 serotonin

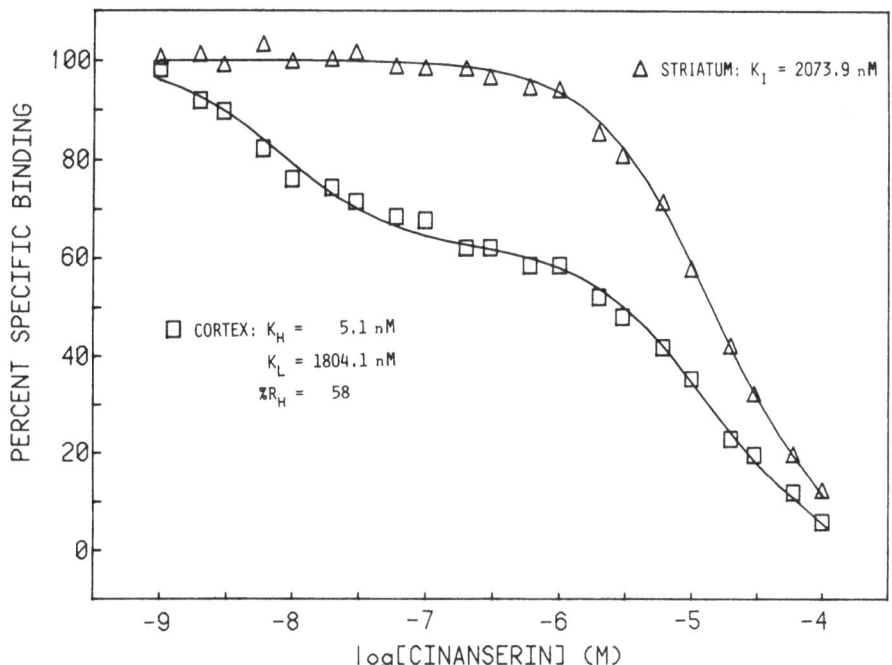

Figure 3. Competition of cinanserin for 3 nM [^{3}H]SCH 23390 binding in rat striatum and frontal cortex. Representative competition curves consisted of duplicate determinations for each concentration of inhibitor. Competition curves in striatal homogenates were fit best by a one-site computer model where the affinity of [^{3}H]SCH 23390 was constrained to be 0.49 nM, its affinity at D_1 receptor sites. Conversely, competition curves in homogenates of rat frontal cortex were fit best by a two-site computer derived model where the affinity of [^{3}H]SCH 23390 was constrained to be 7 nM at the high affinity cinanserin binding site, as defined by the affinity of SCH 23390 for S_2 serotonin receptors, and 0.49 nM at the lower affinity cinanserin binding site.

receptors will be labeled. This is shown in Figure 3 where 3 nM [^{3}H]SCH 23390 binding to frontal cortex membranes is partially displaced with high affinity by the selective S_2 serotonin receptor antagonist cinanserin. Cinanserin has an affinity of approximately 5 nM for this high affinity component of [^{3}H]SCH 23390 displacement, corresponding to the affinity of cinanserin previously reported for the S_2 serotonin receptor (Battaglia et al., 1984). In striatum, however, there is no evidence for significant S_2 serotonin receptor labeling by [^{3}H]SCH 23390; cinanserin competes for [^{3}H]SCH 23390 binding in the striatum monophasically and with low affinity (Figure 3). Furthermore, [^{3}H]SCH 23390 saturation analyses in striatum in the presence and absence of 40 nM ketanserin to block any possible S_2 serotonin receptor labeling were identical (data not shown). Although S_2 serotonin receptors are present in the striatum (Leysen et al., 1983), they may not be detected using [^{3}H]SCH23390 as a radiolabel due to the relatively small S_2 serotonin receptor population compared to the much larger population of D_1 dopamine receptors. In addition, the concentrations of [^{3}H]SCH 23390 employed in our studies of striatal binding were much less than the K_D of [^{3}H]SCH 23390 at S_2 serotonin receptors. Consequently, less than half of this already small population would be labeled. Conversely, there is a large population of S_2 serotonin receptors in frontal cortex where the density of D_1 dopamine receptors is low, facilitating detection of S_2 serotonin receptors labeled by [^{3}H]SCH 23390. Interestingly, cinanserin competition for [^{3}H]SCH 23390 binding in frontal cortex is biphasic, with the low affinity component corresponding to the affinity of cinanserin at D_1 dopamine receptors as determined in the striatum. This suggests that a small population of D_1 dopamine receptors is present in rat frontal cortex and can be studied with [^{3}H]SCH 23390.

POTENTIAL CLINICAL UTILITY OF SCH 23390

Neuroleptics, administered to rodents in vivo, induce catalepsy, suppress conditioned avoidance responses, and antagonize the hyperactivity and stereotypy responses elicited by dopamine agonists. These behaviors are elicited by both D_2 dopamine receptor antagonists or mixed D_1/D_2 receptor antagonists and are generally predictive of antipsychotic activity. Consequently, these behavioral effects have been used by the pharmaceutical industry as screens for potential new antipsychotic drugs (Janssen & Van Brever, 1978). Neuroleptics are also generally antiemetic and have been shown to induce hyperprolactinemia by blocking dopamine receptors in the anterior pituitary. Since this tissue lacks D_1 dopamine receptors, it is clear that hyperprolactinemia is a pure D_2 receptor mediated response. While SCH 23390 is a selective D_1 dopamine receptor antagonist, this benzazepine suprisingly mimics some of the behavioral effects previously associated with D_2 dopamine receptor antagonists - such as blocking agonist-induced stereotypy and hyperactivity, as well as inducing catalepsy (Iorio et al., 1983; Christensen et al., 1984; Mailman et al., 1984; Hoffman and Beninger, 1985). However, SCH 23390 neither antagonizes emesis nor produces hyperprolactinemia - indicating that SCH 23390 administered in vivo is probably not acting as an antagonist at D_2 dopamine receptors.

That SCH 23390 can induce these neuroleptic behavioral effects without blockade of D_2 dopamine receptors suggests that it may be an effective antipsychotic agent. Why might this be important? Certainly more than enough neuroleptics already exist. A major side effect of the chronic neuroleptic administration used in treating schizophrenia is tardive dyskinesia, characterized by uncontrollable movements of the mouth, tongue and extremities. The chronic treatment of animals with neuroleptics does not usually result in such obvious dyskinetic movements but it does produce an enhanced sensitivity to the motoric effects of dopamine agonists (Tarsy and Baldessarini, 1974). An increase in the number of D_2 dopamine receptors is concomitantly produced (Creese et al., 1983). Since chronic treatment with either D_2 receptor-selective or mixed D_1/D_2 receptor-selective antagonists produces identical behavioral supersensitivity but D_2 receptor-selective antagonists cause a selective D_2 receptor up regulation, it has been concluded that the increase in D_2 receptors is both necessary and sufficient for the production of the enhanced behavioral sensitivity to dopamine agonists (Fleminger et al., 1983). It has therefore been suggested that the side effect of tardive dyskinesia may result from a selective D_2 dopamine receptor up-regulation, although this has not yet been directly shown in biochemical studies of drug treated schizophrenic brains (Cross et al., 1983). If chronic treatment with the D_1 receptor selective antagonist SCH 23390 does not increase D_2 receptor number, it may therefore lack the liability to produce tardive dyskinesia.

BIOCHEMICAL EFFECTS OF CHRONIC SCH 23390 ADMINISTRATION

Indeed, in a preliminary investigation of this hypothesis we found that after treating rats chronically with SCH 23390 (0.5 mg/kg/day for 21 days), striatal D_1 dopamine receptors were significantly increased while no change was observed in the D_2 dopamine receptor population (Creese and Chen, 1985) (Table 1).

In order to investigate this hypothesis further, we have examined the selectivity of SCH 23390 administered in vivo for D_1 receptors, the effect of chronic SCH 23390 treatment on adenylate cyclase activity as well as on dopamine receptor binding, and tested rats for their locomotor activity and stereotypy responses to selective D_1 and D_2 dopamine receptor agonists following chronic treatment with SCH 23390.

Receptor Selectivity of SCH 23390

After chronic treatment with SCH 23390, an increase in D_1 dopamine receptors, as determined by [^{3}H]SCH 23390 binding, was observed. These results are consistent with the previous study by this laboratory in which [^{3}H]flupentixol was employed to measure D_1 dopamine receptor binding after chronic SCH 23390 treatment (Creese and Chen, 1985). That no increase in D_2 dopamine receptors was observed indicates that this effect is D_1 dopamine receptor selective; thus, SCH 23390 maintains its D_1 dopamine receptor specificity in vivo even after chronic treatment. This conclusion is supported by studies utilizing in vivo N-ethoxycarbonyl-2-ethoxy-1,2-dihydroquinoline (EEDQ) treatment.

TABLE 1. Effect of 21 Day Treatment with 0.5mg/kg/day
          SCH 23390 on Rat Striatal D_1 and D_2 Receptor
          Parameters

D_1 [^{3}H]flupentixol binding

	CONTROL	CHRONIC SCH 23390
B_{max} (pmol/g) wet wt.	56.6 ± 1.5	70.3* ± 3.5
K_D (nM)	0.27 ± 0.013	0.30 ± 0.025

D_2 [^{3}H]spiperone binding

	CONTROL	CHRONIC SCH 23390
Bmax (pmol/g) wet wt.	26.4 ± 0.8	26.9 ± 0.5
K_D (nM)	0.10 ± 0.007	0.12 ± 0.009

*$p = 0.005$ (2 tailed t-test). All other comparisons were
not significant ($p > 0.05$). Data expressed as mean ±
S.E.M., n=6 in all cases.

EEDQ has been shown to be an irreversible pharmacologic
antagonist at a variety of neurotransmitter receptors including α-adrenergic, muscarinic, and serotonergic receptors
(Belleau et al., 1969; Chang et al., 1970; Battaglia et al.,
in press). We recently demonstrated that peripheral administration of EEDQ results in a dose-dependent reduction in both
D_1 and D_2 dopamine receptor binding (Hamblin & Creese, 1983).
That EEDQ acts as an irreversible antagonist at dopamine
receptors is suggested by the continued significant reduction
in receptor density even after extensive wash procedures. The
mechanism of action of EEDQ is thought to be due to its
ability to activate carboxyl groups. EEDQ induces the creation
of highly reactive mixed carbonic anhydrides from carboxyl
groups which, in turn, interact with nucleophillic groups such
as free α-amino groups (Belleau et al., 1969). To date, it is
unclear whether, with respect to the D_1 dopamine receptor,
EEDQ itself irreversibly binds to the receptor recognition
site or whether EEDQ simply acts in a non-receptor site
directed manner to catalyze internal irreversible alterations
at the recognition site.

Significantly, treatment with SCH 23390 (0.5 mg/kg,
s.c.) prior to peripheral administration of EEDQ protects D_1
dopamine receptors from irreversible blockade by EEDQ, but
neither D_2 dopamine nor S_2 serotonin receptors are protected
from EEDQ-induced modifications by the SCH 23390 pretreatment.
This indicates that SCH 23390, in all probability, interacts
in vivo exclusively with D_1 dopamine receptors at the dose
which was chronically administered to rats in our study.

Additionally, this refutes the suggestion that SCH 23390 administered in vivo may be converted to a D_2 dopamine receptor selective compound upon metabolism (Christensen et al., 1984). These data have been supported by Meller et al. (1985) using a similar paradigm to examine the specificity of neuroleptics administered in vivo. That peripherally administered SCH 23390 demonstrates selectivity for D_1 dopamine receptors suggests that the behavioral data reported herein are not confounded by any obvious non-specific effects of this drug.

D_1 Receptor Binding and Adenylate Cyclase Coupling After Chronic SCH 23390 Administration

Interestingly, although the D_1 dopamine receptor B_{max} was increased by the chronic SCH 23390 treatment, no change was observed in agonist competition for [^{3}H]SCH 23390 binding (Figure 4). Nor was any change observed in the rightward shift

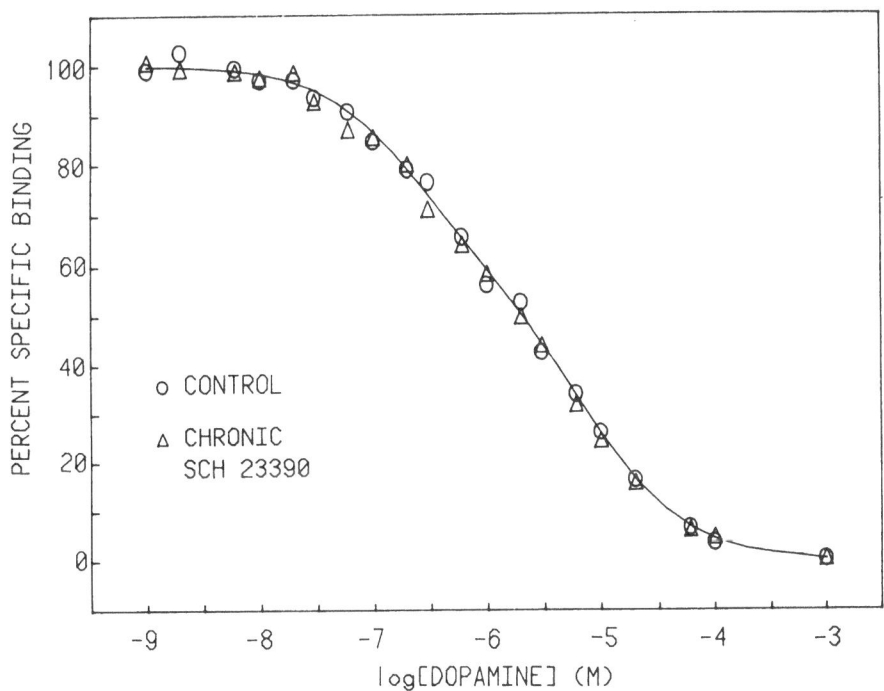

Figure 4. Computer-fitted curves for dopamine inhibition of [^{3}H]SCH 23390 binding in control and chronic SCH 23390 treated tissue. Experimentally determined points are from representative experiments using 0.25 nM [^{3}H]SCH 23390. Competition curves were fit best by a two-site computer derived model where the affinity of [^{3}H]SCH 23390 was constrained to be equal (K_D = 0.5 nM) at both high (R_H) and low (R_L) affinity sites. The dissociation constants for high (K_H) and low (K_L) affinity agonist-binding sites were determined while constraining the non-specific binding parameter defined by 100 nM cis-flupentixol.

of these agonist competition curves induced by guanine nucleo-tides. These data indicate that the coupling of the D_1 dopamine receptor to the guanine nucleotide regulatory protein (N) does not appear to be perturbed following chronic SCH 23390 treatment. That the R_H/R_L ratio remains constant between control and treated animals, also suggests that there must exist some mechanism by which this ratio is maintained after receptor up-regulation. Theoretically, if the population of N is stoichiometrically-limiting (which is likely as 100% R_H is never induced by agonists) and R increases, the percent of high affinity agonist binding sites (R_H) should be reduced due to the percent decrease in potential R to N coupling. An excess or spare pool of N, however, would maintain the R_H/R_L ratio after receptor upregulation. Alternatively, if N is stoichiometrically-limiting (as we have previously suggested - see below and Battaglia et al., submitted), it may also undergo concomitant upregulation with D_1 dopamine receptors, maintaining a constant R_H/R_L ratio. This may occur either through an increase in the actual population of N subunits or through an increase in the efficacy of the R/N coupling mechanism.

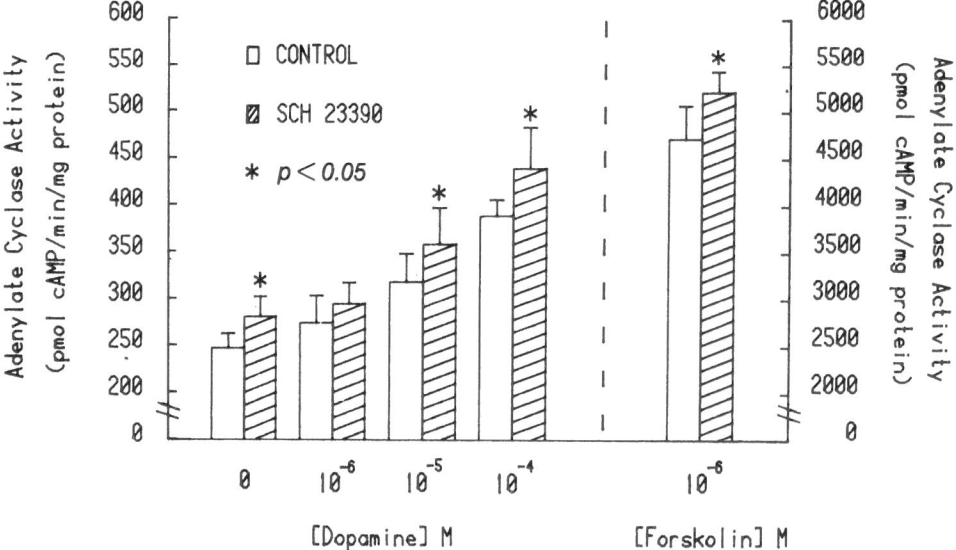

Figure 5. Adenylate cyclase activity in control and chronic SCH 23390 treated tissue. Bars represent mean + S.E.M. of dopamine and forskolin-stimulated cAMP production in the presence of 100 μM GTP. Asterisks denote adenylate cyclase stimulation in chronic SCH 23390 treated tissue significantly greater than control tissue, $p < 0.05$.

After chronic SCH 23390 treatment, in addition to the increased D_1 receptor binding, adenylate cyclase activity was enhanced by a small (9 - 13%) but significant amount. However, not only did dopamine-stimulated cAMP production increase, but guanine nucleotide and forskolin-stimulated adenylate cyclase activity also increased (Figure 5). It is important to note that dopamine-stimulated adenylate cyclase activity was increased by only the same percent as guanine nucleotide-stimulated adenylate cyclase activity. Furthermore, dopamine EC_{50}'s in control and tissue from chronically SCH 23390 treated rats was identical. This indicates that dopamine-stimulated cAMP production was not detectably potentiated by the increase in receptor number over the more general, less specific, increase in adenylate cyclase activity. Rather, the increase observed in dopamine-stimulated adenylate cyclase activity most probably reflects the overall increase observed in guanine nucleotide-stimulated enzyme activity. The results of the agonist competition curves plus the adenylate cyclase data suggest that the guanine nucleotide regulatory protein, rather than the adenylate cyclase itself, is in some manner "upregulated" with the receptor.

D_1 Dopamine Receptor/Adenylate Cyclase Stoichiometry

That no percentage increase is observed in dopamine-stimulated adenylate cyclase activity after D_1 dopamine receptor upregulation is, at first sight, surprising. However, in other experiments we have demonstrated the existence of spare D_1 dopamine receptors in the striatum of normal control rats, explaining this observation (Hess et al., submitted).

In these experiments, we again utilized peripheral administration of the irreversible protein-modifying reagent, EEDQ, as a tool for investigating D_1 dopamine receptor/effector interactions. Since striatal adenylate cyclase stimulation may be elicited by a number of reagents such as dopamine, GTP and forskolin which act specifically via receptor, N or at the catalytic subunit, respectively, these reagents may be used as "biochemical markers" in adenylate cyclase assays to determine the functional integrity of each subunit. After in vivo EEDQ treatment, no change in adenylate cyclase stimulation above basal activity is observed in the presence of the putative Ns effectors: GTP, Gpp(NH)p, and NaF (Figure 6). Likewise, stimulation by forskolin, thought to act directly at the catalytic subunit (Seamon et al., 1981), is unaltered by EEDQ administration (Figure 7). However, we have found that both the D_1 dopamine receptor binding of [^{3}H]SCH 23390 and adenylate cyclase stimulation by dopamine are markedly reduced after in vivo EEDQ treatment in a dose-dependent manner (Figure 8). Thus, peripherally administered EEDQ acts in a receptor-specific manner, but leaves Ns and the catalytic subunit of adenylate cyclase functionally intact.

Because the Ns and catalytic moieties are not functionally modified, peripheral EEDQ administration may be used as a tool to assess the stoichiometry of D_1 dopamine receptor/effector interactions. That is, by progressively blocking increasing numbers of receptors and monitoring adenylate cyclase activity, the loss of D_1 dopamine receptors may be correlated with a decrease in D_1 dopamine receptor-mediated stimulation of adenylate cyclase activity. Interestingly, we have found that the loss in D_1 dopamine receptor binding does not correlate directly with observed reductions in dopamine-stimulated adenylate cyclase activity; approximately 40% of D_1 dopamine receptor binding may be lost with no significant reduction in the Vmax of dopamine-stimulated adenylate cyclase activity. That is, only approximately 60% of the original D_1 dopamine receptor population is necessary for full <u>in vitro</u> agonist-stimulation of adenylate cyclase activity. Thus, these data suggest that the D_1 dopamine receptor population is not a stoichiometrically-limiting factor in agonist-stimulation of adenylate cyclase.

This finding has important neurophysiologic implications. Receptor occupancy is determined by transmitter (or drug) concentration. Since only ~60% occupancy of the normal D_1 dopamine receptor population is required for maximal effector stimulation, the transmitter concentration necessary to elicit full stimulation (~2 x K_D) is considerably less than that concentration necessary for 100% receptor occupancy(100 x K_D). The existence of these "spare" receptors, then, potentially

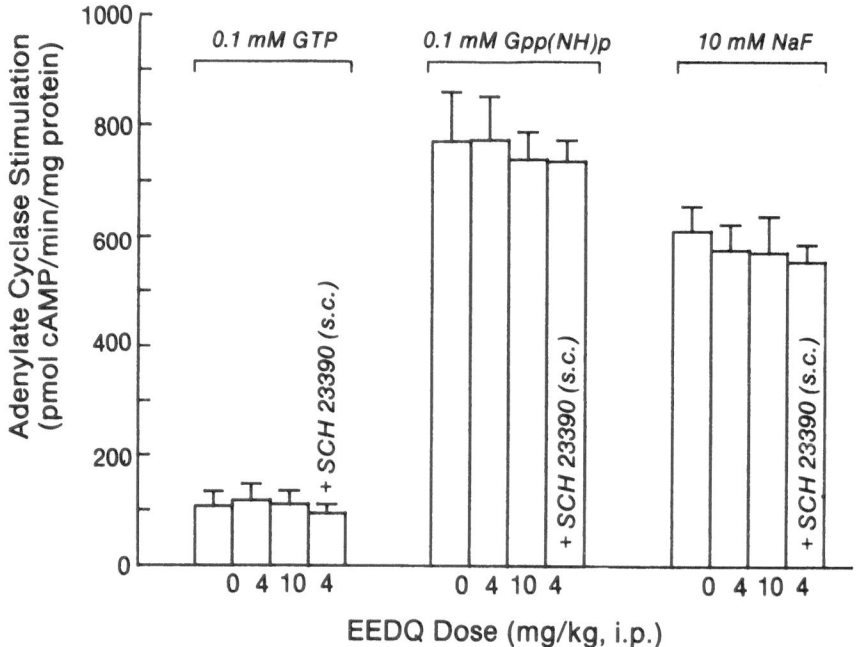

Figure 6.   Effect of <u>in vivo</u> EEDQ administration on adenylate cyclase activity stimulated via the guanine nucleotide regulatory protein. Bars represent the mean + S.E.M. of stimulation by 0.1 mM GTP, 0.1 mM Gpp(NH)p and 10 mM NaF above basal activity (n=4-6). 4 mg/kg + SCH 23390 (s.c.) bars denote treatment with 0.5 mg/kg (s.c.) SCH 23390 prior to 4 mg/kg EEDQ treatment. No significant differences were observed between control and EEDQ treated tissue.

enhances neurotransmission by reducing the effective concentration of dopamine required to diffuse across the synaptic cleft to achieve a full response.

In light of this finding, it is not surprising that a ~20% increase in D1 dopamine receptors after chronic SCH 23390 treatment did not increase the receptor-stimulated adenylate cyclase activity since ~40% of the normosensitive D_1 dopamine receptor population may be considered "spare". Receptor upregulation, then, probably does not act directly to increase cAMP production but rather supersensitivity is manifested by reducing the effective transmitter (or drug) concentration necessary to induce a maximal response. That is, by increasing receptor number, the percent receptor occupancy necessary to activate a full effector response is reduced. Thus, after receptor upregulation a leftward shift in the dopamine EC_{50} might be expected. The data presented here do not reflect such a shift, probably due to the lack of an adenylate cyclase assay sensitive enough to detect

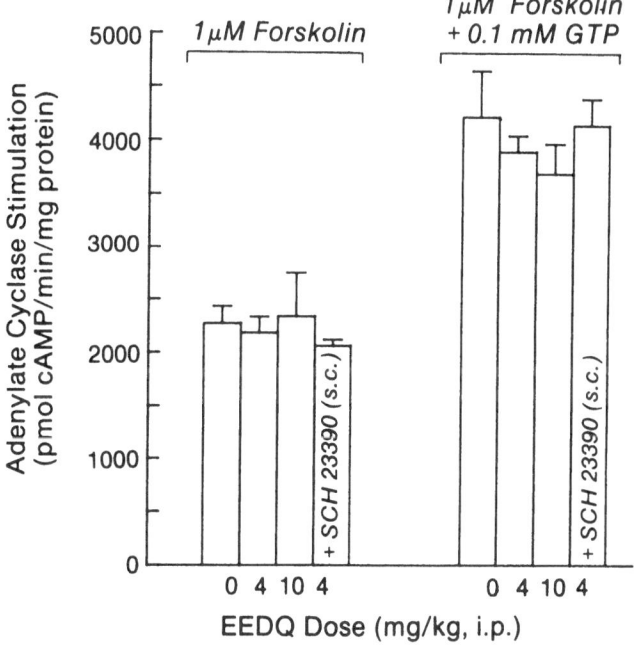

Figure 7. Effect of in vivo EEDQ administration on forskolin stimulated adenylate cyclase activity. Bars represent the mean + S.E.M. of differences between basal activity and μM forskolin (+ 0.1 mM GTP) stimulated cAMP production (n=4-6). 4 mg/kg + SCH 23390 (s.c.) bars denote treatment with 0.5 mg/kg SCH 23390 prior to 4 mg/kg EEDQ treatment. No significant differences in stimulation were observed between control and EEDQ-treated tissue.

such small changes in agonist stimulation. Additionally, Anderson et al. (1985) have suggested that not all D_1 receptors are coupled to adenylate cyclase, possibly also explaining the lack of an observed shift. Collectively, these pharmacologic and biochemical data suggest that in addition to a dopamine receptor selective upregulation, an additional upregulation also occurs at the level of either the guanine nucleotide regulatory subunit or perhaps the catalytic subunit of adenylate cyclase, leading to the small overall increase in cAMP production.

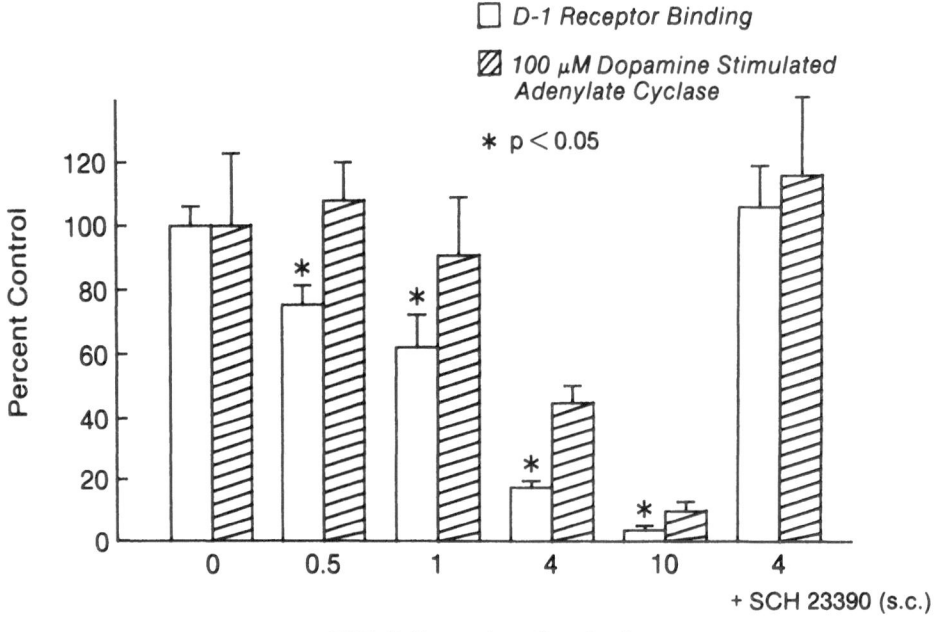

Figure 8. Dose-dependent reduction in D_1 dopamine receptor binding and receptor-mediated stimulation of adenylate cyclase after peripheral administration of EEDQ. Open bars represent the mean + S.E.M. of [³H]SCH 23390 B_{max} values as a percent of the control Bmax (47 + 7 pmoles/g tissue) and hashed bars the mean + S.E.M. of the differences between stimulation by 0.1 mM GTP alone and stimulation by 100 µM dopamine + 0.1 mM GTP as a percent of stimulation in controls (186 + 45 pmoles cAMP/min/mg protein). EEDQ-induced reductions were prevented by pretreatment with SCH 23390 (s.c. 0.5 mg/kg), denoted by bars labeled + SCH 23390 (s.c.). Asterisks denote percent Bmax significantly less than percent dopamine stimulated adenylate cyclase, p<(0.05).

Unlike chronic neuroleptic treatment, where neither an increase nor decrease in spontaneous locomotor activity was observed (Tarsy and Baldessarini, 1974), rats chronically treated with SCH 23390 (0.5mg/kg/day for 21 days) demonstrated a more than two-fold higher level of locomotor activity than control animals during habituation to the locomotor cages (p < 0.02) two days after ending the chronic drug treatment (Figure 9). Paralleling the habituation results, again in contrast to classic neuroleptics where tolerance develops to their cataleptogenic effects after chronic treatment (Ezrin-Waters and Seeman, 1977), rats receiving chronic administration of SCH 23390 for 21 days demonstrated no tolerance to its cataleptogenic action. This suggests that the neuronal network through which chronic SCH 23390 elicits its effects is different from and is not regulated in the same manner as the neuronal network through which classic neuroleptics exert their effects.

Other research supports this hypothesis. After treatment with either D_1 or D_2 selective agonists, unilaterally 6-OHDA lesioned rats demonstrate contralateral circling behavior (Arnt and Hyttel, 1984; Arnt and Hyttel, 1985; Herrera-

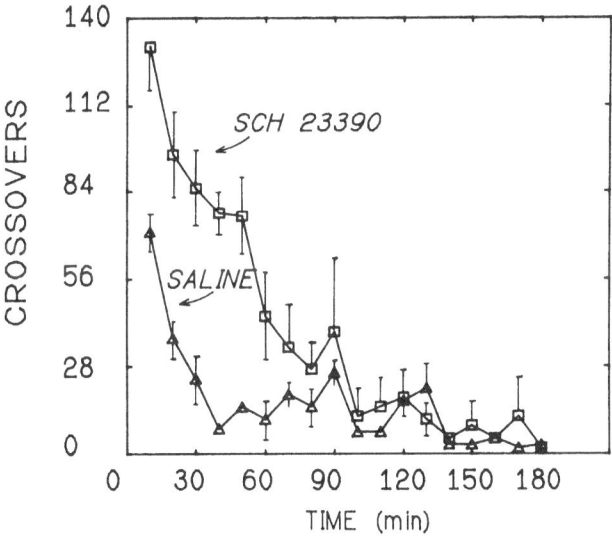

Figure 9. Photocell beam crossovers recorded during habituation to activity cages for rats chronically treated with SCH 23390 (0.5mg/kg/day s.c. for 21 days) or saline, two days after termination of the chronic drug treatment. The SCH 23390 treated rats were significantly more active (p<0.02 ANOVA).

Marschitz and Ungerstedt, 1984; Herrera-Marschitz and Ungerstedt, 1985) and reserpinized or bilaterally 6-OHDA lesioned animals demonstrate hypermotility and oral stereotypy (Arnt, 1985a, 1985b). In these cases, although similar behaviors were induced by the D_1 and D_2 receptor agonists, behaviors induced by D_2 agonists were blocked only by D_2 antagonists and similarly, D_1 antagonists only blocked D_1 agonist responses. These data suggest that although D_1 and D_2 dopamine receptor-mediated behaviors may be overtly similar or even identical, they are independently modulated and can be distinguished from each other through these various pharmacologic treatments.

In concert with these data, the chronically SCH 23390 treated rats responded to the selective D_1 dopamine receptor agonist, SKF 38393 (Setler, 1978; O'Boyle and Waddington, 1984), with potentiated locomotor behavior (Figure 10). However, the magnitude and time course of the locomotor activity as determined by beam crossovers after SKF 38393 administration was identical to the activity response seen in habituation, for both groups. Because we were unable to run the rats with a control saline injection after habituation it is unclear from these data whether the chronically SCH 23390 treated rats are indeed showing an enhanced response to SKF 38393 itself, or simply exhibiting

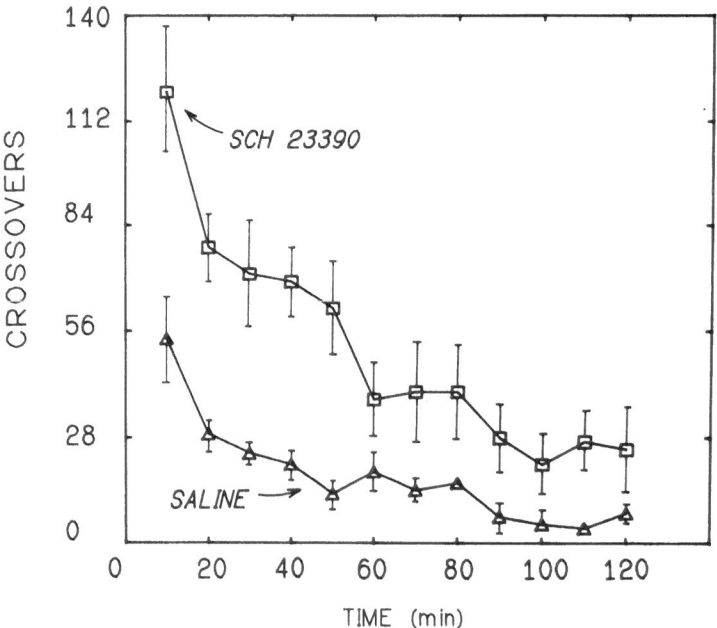

Figure 10. Photocell beam crossovers recorded in response to 3 mg/kg (s.c.) SKF 38393 after habituation in rats chronically treated with SCH 23390 or saline. The SCH 23390 treated rats were significantly more active ($p < 0.001$ ANOVA).

an enhanced spontaneous response to handling as seen in the
habituation data. However, the stereotypy observations
clearly indicate that chronic SCH 23390 does enhance the
behavioral response to SKF 38393. As seen in Figure 11,
chronic SCH 23390 treated rats showed a more intense
stereotypy response to SKF 38393 than did the chronic saline
treated rats. Unlike mixed D_1/D_2 agonists, SKF 38393 induced
stereotyped grooming in both groups of rats. This was scored
as 4 on the rating scale and accounts for the initial high
stereotypy response recorded for the chronic saline treated
rats. However, grooming quickly diminished in these rats and
they demonstrated locomotor stimulation. The chronic SCH
23390 treated rats, however, continued to groom and/or show
stereotyped sniffing and rearing in one location over the
first hour in response to SKF 38393.

Surprisingly, a similar potentiation in locomotor
activity and stereotypy was observed in chronically SCH 23390
treated rats after treatment with quinpirole (LY 171555), a
selective D_2 agonist (Tsuruta et al., 1981). Figure 12 shows
that the locomotor responses to quinpirole in both groups
was quite different from their habituation response. This
clearly indicates that the locomotor response to quinpirole
is enhanced by the chronic SCH 23390 treatment. The time
course of the response, initially low, peaking and dropping
away is explained in the stereotypy ratings (Figure 13).

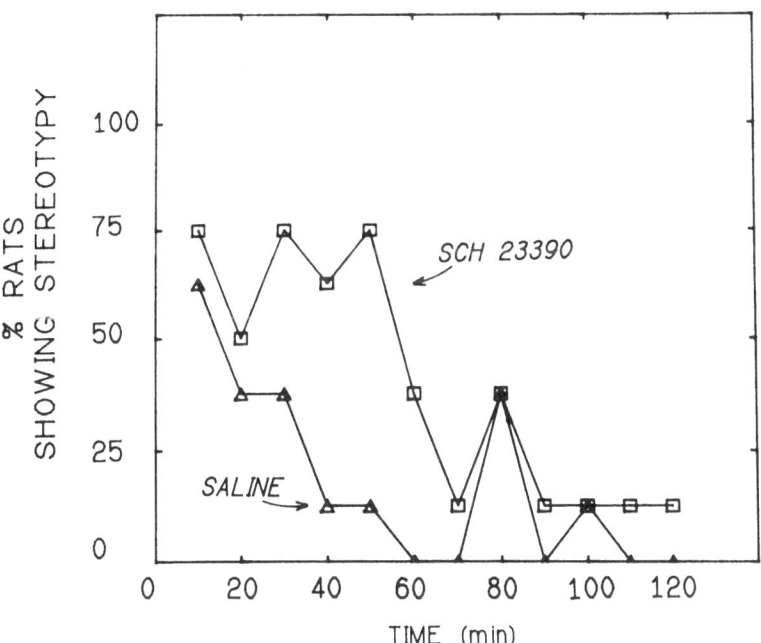

Figure 11. Mean stereotypy response to 3.0 mg/kg (s.c.) SKF
38393 of rats chronically treat with SCH 23390 or saline. The
SCH 23390 treated rats demonstrated an overall greater
stereotypy response (p < 0.005, Information Statistic).

Quinpirole initially induced intense stereotyped sniffing
and rearing in one location in both groups. Between 50 and
80 min post injection, some of the chronic SCH 23390 treated
rats were also showing stereotyped licking of the cage -
although none of the control rats showed this response. The
peak in crossovers at 140 min corresponded to the transition
from stereotyped behavior in one location to locomotor
activity. Surprisingly, locomotor activity was quickly
attenuated in the chronically SCH 23390 treated rats and each
rat "instantaneously" went from "sniff/locomotion" to
"freezing" in position. This frozen posture was maintained
for 5-10 min before the rats closed their eyes and apparently
went to sleep. Control rats did not show this freezing
behavior. This response may potentially prove to be a useful
model for the "on-off" phenomenon seen during dopamine
receptor agonist treatment of Parkinson's Disease. One might
speculate that this troublesome side effect may result from
the upregulation of D1 receptors in this disease.

In $\underline{in\ vitro}$ binding studies, quinpirole (LY 171555) has
extremely low affinity (high micromolar) for D_1 dopamine
receptors (data not shown), suggesting that it is unlikely
that this drug might elicit these behaviors through D_1

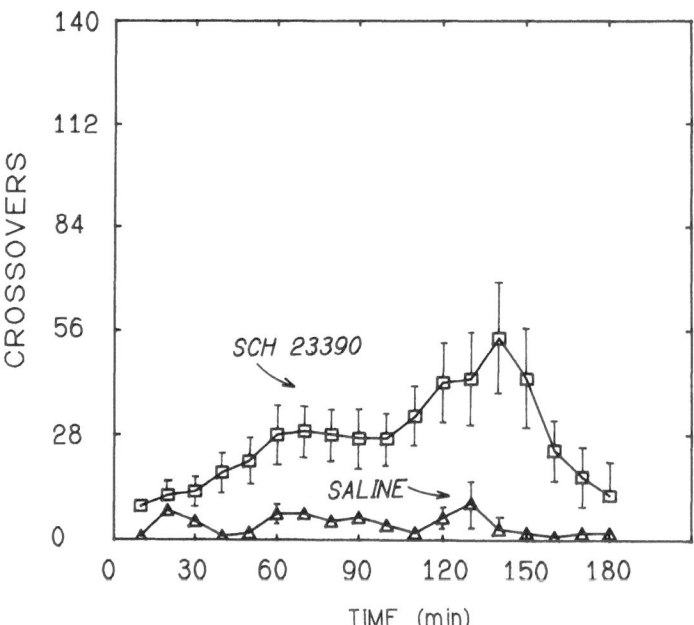

Figure 12. Photocell beam crossovers to 0.3 mg/kg (s.c.)
quinpirole after habituation in rats chronically treated with
SCH 23390 or saline. The response of the SCH 23390 treated rat
was significantly higher. ($p < 0.005$ ANOVA)

dopamine receptors <u>in vivo</u>. Thus, the behavioral effects of a D_2 dopamine agonist are potentiated after a selective D_1 receptor upregulation. Certainly this is an anomalous response given that SCH 23390 has no direct effect on D_2 dopamine receptors <u>in vivo</u>. Paralleling the results presented herein, it has been demonstrated that although SCH 23390 acts as a D_1 dopamine receptor antagonist, inducing catalepsy in rats, pretreatment with selective D_2 dopamine receptor agonists prevent this response in a dose-dependent manner (Meller et al., 1985). Likewise, the behavioral effects of the D_1 dopamine receptor agonist, SKF 38393, which include non-stereotyped sniffing, rearing and locomotor responses, could be partially reversed by the D_2 dopamine receptor antagonist metaclopramide (Molloy and Waddington, 1985). Breese and Mueller (1985) have demonstrated that SCH23390 antagonism of locomotor activity induced by quinpirole may be prevented by 6-hydroxydopamine or reserpine treatment. That is, D_1/D_2 dopamine receptor interactions are dependent on the integrity of catecholamine containing neurons. These behavioral data, then, suggest that D_1 and D_2 dopamine receptor-activated neuronal systems are not functionally isolated. Rather, the behavioral data presented herein suggest that although the networks through which D_1 and D_2 dopamine receptors mediate behavioral

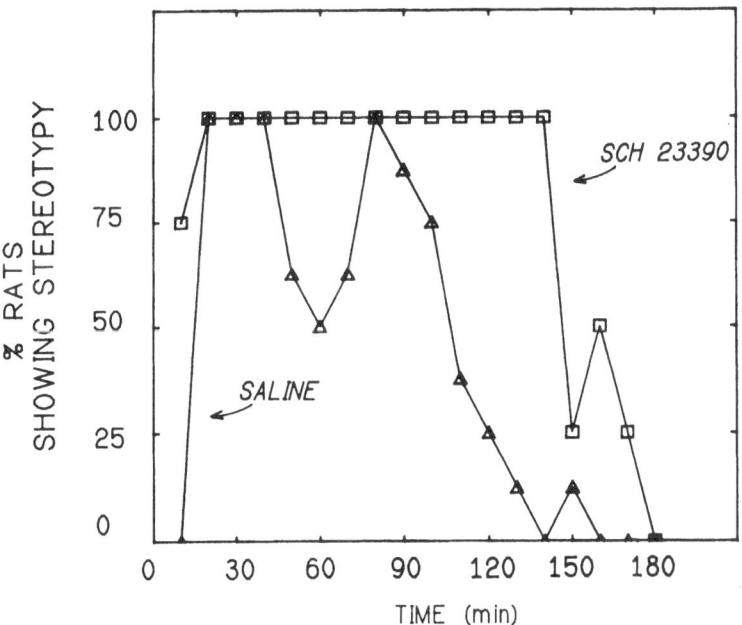

Figure 13. Mean stereotypy response to 0.3 mg/kg (s.c.) quinpirole of rats chronically treated with SCH 23390 or saline. The SCH 23390 treated rats demonstrated an overall greater stereotypy response (p < 0.005, Information Statistic).

effects appear to be functionally independent (i.e., separate, parallel systems), these systems are interactive in their modulation of motor function.

CLINICAL IMPLICATIONS

One must always be careful in drawing conclusions from animal behavioral and biochemical data that pertain to the clinical situation. With this caveat in mind, some points can be made: (1) If SCH 23390 proved to be antipsychotic, its chronic administration may still induce tardive dyskinesia, assuming the 3 week chronic treatment/enhanced behavioral agonist-sensitivity is an adequate and predictive animal model of tardive dyskinesia potential. That is, following SCH 23390 treatment the behavioral response to both D_1 and D_2 selective agonists is increased - even though there is a selective increase in only D_1 dopamine receptors. (2) Rats demonstrate tolerance to the cataleptogenic action and to the induction of acute Parkinsonian extrapyramidal side effects after chronic neuroleptic treatment. Since we did not see tolerance to the cataleptogenic action of SCH 23390, it may well continue to induce Parkinsonian side effects during clinical use. However, the validity of both of these animal models has been questioned previously for their relevance to the clinical situation and thus, the study of SCH 23390 in clinical trials may be the only tool to determine the validity of these animal models and the utility of this novel drug in the clinical situation.

ACKNOWLEDGEMENTS

This investigation was supported by NIMH Grant MH 32990, an RSDA MH 00316 to I.C., and the Scottish Rite Schizophrenia Research Program, NMJ, USA. We would like to thank Drs. George Koob and Neal Swerdlow for discussion, use of their locomotor activity cages, and statistical analyses. Drs. Andrew Norman and George Battaglia are thanked for their collaboration on many of the research papers discussed in this paper. We also thank Paula Martin for manuscript preparation.

REFERENCES

Andersen, P.H., Gronvald, F.C. and Jansen, J.A., 1985, A comparison between dopamine-stimulated adenylate cyclase and ^{3}H-SCH 23390 binding in rat striatum, Life Sci., 37:1971-1983.

Arnt, J., 1985a, Behavioural stimulation is induced by separate dopamine D_1 and D_2 receptor sites in reserpine-pretreated by not in normal rats, Eur. J. Pharmacol., 113:79-88.

Arnt, J., 1985b, Hyperactivity induced by stimulation of separate dopamine D_1 and D_2 receptors in rats with bilateral 6-OHDA lesions, Life Sci., 37:717-723.

Arnt, J. and Hyttel, J., 1984, Differential inhibition by dopamine D_1 and D_2 antagonists of circling behaviour induced by dopamine agonists in rats with unilateral 6-hydroxydopamine lesions, Eur. J. Pharmacol., 102:349-354.

Arnt, J. and Hyttel, J., 1985, Differential involvement of dopamine D_1 and D_2 receptors in the circling behaviour induced by apomorphine, SK&F 38393, pergolide and LY 171555 in 6-hydroxydopamine-lesioned rats, Psychopharmacol., 85:346-352.

Battaglia, G., Shannon, M. and Titeler, M., 1984, Guanyl nucleotide and divalent cation regulation of cortical S_2 serotonin receptors, J. Neurochem., 43:1213-1219.

Battaglia, G., Norman, A.B., Newton, P.L. and I. Creese 1985, In vitro and in vivo irreversible blockade of cortical S_2 serotonin receptors by N-ethoxycarbonyl-2-ethoxy-1,2-dihydroquinoline (EEDQ): A technique for investigating S_2 serotonin receptor recovery, J. Neurochem., (in press).

Battaglia, G., Norman, A.B., Hess, E.J. and Creese, I., 1985, D_2 dopamine receptor-mediated inhibition of forskolin-stimulated adenylate cyclase activity in rat striatum, Neurosci. Letters, 59:177-182.

Battaglia, G., Norman, A.B., Hess, E.J. and Creese, I., 1985, Functional recovery of D_1 dopamine receptor- mediated stimulation of rat striatal adenylate cyclase activity following irreversible receptor blockade, (Submitted).

Belleau, B., Ditullio, V. and Godin, D., 1969, The mechanism of irreversible adrenergic blockade by N-carbethoxy-dihydroquinolines - model studies with typical serine hydrolases, Biochem. Pharm., 18:1039-1044.

Belleau, B., Martel, R., Lacasse, G., Menard, M., Weinberg, N.L. and Perron, Y.G., 1969, N-carboxylic acid esters of 1,2 and 1,4-dihydroquinolines. A new class of irreversible inactivators of the catecholamine alpha receptors and potent central nervous system depressants, J. Am. Chem. Soc., 90:823-824.

Billard, W., Ruperto, V., Crosby, G., Iorio, L.C. and Barnett, A., 1984, Characterization of the binding of [^{3}H]SCH 23390, a selective D_1 receptor antagonist ligand, in rat striatum, Life Sci., 35:1885-1893.

Boeynaems, J.M. and Dumont, J.E., 1975, Quantitative analysis of the binding of ligands to their receptors, J. Cyclic Nucleotide Res., 1:123-142.

Breese, G.R. and Mueller, R.A., 1985, SCH 23390 antagonism of a D_2 dopamine agonist depends upon catecholaminergic neurons, Eur. J. Pharmacol., 113:109-114.

Chang, K.J., Moran, J.F. and Triggle, D.J., 1970, Mechanism of cholinergic antagonism by N-ethoxycarbonyl-2-ethoxy-1,2-dihydroquinoline (EEDQ), Pharm. Res. Comm., 2:63-66.

Christensen, A.V., Arnt, J., Hyttel, J., Larsen, J.J. and Svendsen, O., 1984, Pharmacological effects of a specific dopamine D_1 antagonist SCH 23390 in comparison with neuroleptics, Life Sci., 34:1529-1540.

Creese, I. and Chen, A., 1985, Selective D_1 dopamine receptor increase following chronic treatment with SCH 23390, Eur. J. Pharmacol., 109:127-128.

Creese, I., Burt, D.R. and Snyder, S.H., 1976, Dopamine receptor binding predicts clinical and pharmacological potencies of antischizophrenic drugs, Science, 192:481-483.

Creese, I. and Iversen, S.D., 1975, The pharmacological and anatomical substrates of the amphetamine response in the rat, Brain Res., 83:419-436.

Creese, I., Sibley, D.R., Hamblin, M.W. and Leff, S., 1983, The classification of dopamine receptors: relationship to radioligand binding, Ann. Rev. Neurosci., 6:43-71.

Cross, A.J., Crow, T.J., Ferrier, I.N., Johnstone, E.C., McCreadie, R.M, Owen, F., Owens, D.G.C. and Poulter, M., 1983, Dopamine receptor changes in schizophrenia in relation to the disease process and movement disorder, J. Neural Transmission Suppl., 18:265-272.

Ezrin-Waters, C. and Seeman, P., 1977, Tolerance to haloperidol catalepsy, Eur. J. Pharmacol., 41:321-327.

Fleminger, S., Rupniak, N.M.J., Hall, M.D., Jenner, P. and Marsden, C.D., 1983, Changes in apomorphine-induced stereotypy as a result of subacute neuroleptic treatment correlates with increased D_2 receptors, but not with increases in D_1 receptors, Biochem. Pharmacol., 32:2921-2927.

Hamblin, M.W. and Creese, I., 1983, Behavioral and radioligand binding evidence for irreversible dopamine receptor blockade by N-ethoxycarbonyl-2-ethoxy-1,2-dihydroquinoline, Life Sci., 32:2247-2255.

Heidenrich, K.A., Weiland, G.A. and Molinoff, P.B., 1980, Characterization of radiolabeled agonist binding to β-adrenergic receptors in mammalian tissues, J. Cyclic Nucleotide Res., 6:271-230.

Herrera-Marschitz, M. and Ungerstedt, U., 1984, Evidence that apomorphine and pergolide induce rotation in rats by different actions on D_1 and D_2 receptor sites, Eur. J. Pharmacol., 98:165-176.

Herrera-Marschitz, M. and Ungerstedt, U., 1985, Effect of the dopamine D_1 antagonist SCH 23390 on rotational behaviour induced by apomorphine and pergolide in 6-hydroxy-dopamine denervated rats, Eur. J. Pharmacol,. 109:349-354.

Hess, E.J., Battaglia, G., Norman, A.B. and Creese, I., 1985, In vivo EEDQ specificity for D_1 dopamine receptor blockade: Lack of effect on Ns or the catalytic subunit of adenylate cyclase, Soc. for Neurosci.Abstr., 11:313.

Hess, E.J., Battaglia, G., Norman, A.B. and Creese, I., 1985, Differential modification of striatal D1 dopamine receptors and effector moieties by N-ethoxycarbonyl-2-ethoxy-1,2-dihydroquinoline (EEDQ) in vivo and in vitro, (submitted).

Hess, E.J., Battaglia, G., Norman, A.B., Iorio, L.C. and Creese, I., 1985, Guanine nucleotide regulation of agonist interactions at [^{3}H]SCH 23390 labeled D_1 dopamine receptors in rat striatum, Eur. J. Pharmacol., in press.

Hoffman, B.B., Michel, T., Brennan, T.B. and Lefkowitz, R.J., 1982, Interactions of agonists with platelet α-2 adrenergic receptors, Endocrinology, 110:926-932.

Hoffman, D.C. and Beninger, R.J., 1985, The D_1 dopamine receptor antagonist, SCH 23390 reduces locomotor activity and rearing in rats, Pharmacol. Biochem. Beh., 22:341-342.

Hyttel, J., 1978, Effects of neuroleptics on ^{3}H-haloperidol and ^{3}H-cis(Z)-flupentixol binding and on adenylate cyclase activity in vitro, Life Sci., 23:551-556.

Hyttel, J., 1981, Flupentixol and dopamine receptor selectivity, Psychopharmacol., 75:217.

Hyttel, J., 1984, Functional evidence for selective dopamine D_1 receptor blockade by SCH 23390, Neuropharmacol., 23:1395-1401.

Iorio, L.C., Barnett, A., Leitz, F.H., Houser, V.P. and Korduba, C.A., 1983, SCH23390, a potential benzazepine antipsychotic with unique interactions of dopaminergic systems. J. Pharm. Exp. Ther., 226:462-468.

Jacobs, S. and Cuatrecasas, P., 1976, The mobile receptor hypothesis and cooperativity of hormone binding: application to insulin, Biochem. Biophys. Acta,433:482-295.

Janssen, P.A.J. and Van Brever, W.F.M., 1978, Structure-activity relationships of the butyrophenones and diphenylbutylpiperidines. In: "Handbook of Psychopharmacology", L.L. Iversen, S.D. Iversen and S.H. Snyder, eds., pp. 1-31,Plenum Press, New York.

Kebabian, J.W. and Calne, D.B., 1979, Multiple receptors for dopamine, Nature, 277:93-96.

Leff, S.E., Hamblin, M.W. and Creese, I. 1985a, Interactions of dopamine agonists with brain D_1 receptors labeled by ^{3}H-antagonists: Evidence for the presence of high and low affinity agonist-binding states, Mol. Pharmacol., 27:171-183.

Leff, S.E. and Creese, I., 1985b, Interactions of dopaminergic agonists and antagonists with dopaminergic D_3 binding sites in rat striatum: Evidence that [3H]dopamine can label a high affinity agonist-binding state of the D_1 dopamine receptor, Mol. Pharmacol., 27:184-192.

Leysen, J.E., Van Gompe, P., Verwimp, M. and Niemegeers, C.J.E., 1983, Role and localization of serotonin-2 (S_2) receptor binding sites: effects of neuronal lesions, Advance Biochem. Psychopharmacol., 37:373-383.

Limbird, L.E., 1981, Activation and attenuation of adenylate cyclase: The role of GTP-binding proteins as macromolecular messengers in receptor cyclase coupling, Biochem. J.,194:1-13.

Mailman, R.B., Schulz, D.W., Lewis, M.H., Staples, L.,Rollema, H. and Dehaven, D.L., 1984, SCH 23390: A selective D_1 dopamine antagonist with potent D_2 behavioral actions, Eur. J. Pharmacol., 101:159-160.

Meller, E., Bohmaker, K., Goldstein, M. and Friedhoff, A.J., 1985, Inactivation of D_1 and D_2 dopamine receptors by N-ethoxycarbonyl-2-ethoxy-1,2-dihydroquinoline in vivo: Selective protection by neuroleptics, J. Pharmacol. and Exp. Ther., 233:656-662.

Meller, E., Kuga, S., Friedhoff, A.J. and Goldstein, M., 1985, Selective D_2 dopamine receptor agonists prevent catalepsy induced by SCH 23390, a selective D_1 antagonist, Life Sci., 36:1857-1864.

Molloy, A.G. and Waddington, J.L., 1985, Sniffing, rearing and locomotor responses to the D_1 dopamine agonist R-SKF 38393 and to apomorphine: Differential interactions with the selective D_1 and D_2 antagonists SCH 23390 and metaclopramide, Eur. J. Pharmacol. 108:305-308.

O'Boyle, K.M. and Waddington, J.L., 1984, Selective and stereospecific interactions of R-SK&F 38393 with [3H]piflutixol but not [3H]spiperone binding to striatal D_1 and D_2 dopamine receptors: Comparisons with SCH 23390, Eur. J. Pharmacol., 98:433-436.

Onali, P., Olianas, M.C. and Gessa, G.L., 1984, Selective blockade of dopamine D_1 receptors by SCH 23390 discloses striatal dopamine D_2 receptors mediating the inhibition of adenylate cyclase in rats, Eur. J. Pharmacol., 99:127-128.

Plantje, J.F., Hanson, H.A., Davis, F.J. and Stoof, J.C., 1984, The effects of SCH 23390 (+)-YM 09151-2 and (-)-3-

PPP and some classical neuroleptics on D_1 and D_2 receptors in rat neostriatum in vitro, Eur. J. Pharmacol., 105:73-83.

Schulz, D.W., Wyrick, S.D. and Mailman, R.B., 1985, [^{3}H]SCH 23390 has the characteristics of a dopamine receptor ligand in the rat central nervous system, Eur. J. Pharmacol., 106:211-212.

Seamon, K.B., Padagett, W. and Daly, J.W., 1981, Forskolin: Unique diterpine activator of adenylate cyclase in membranes and in intact cells, Proc. Natl. Acad. Sci., 78:3363-3367.

Seeman, P., Lee, T., Chau-Wong, M. and Wong, K., 1976, Antipsychotic drug doses and neuroleptic/dopamine receptors, Nature, 261:717-719.

Seeman, P., 1981, Brain Dopamine Receptors, Pharmacol. Rev., 32:229-313.

Seeman, P., Ulpian, C., Grigoriadis, D., Pri-Bar, I. and Buchman, O., 1985, Conversion of dopamine D_1 receptors from high to low affinity for dopamine, Biochem. Pharmacol., 34:151-154.

Setler, P.E., Sarau, H.M., Zirkle, C.L. and Saunders, H.L., 1978, The central effects of a novel dopamine agonist, Eur. J. Pharmacol., 50:419.

Sibley, D.R., DeLean, A. and Creese, I., 1982, Anterior pituitary receptors: demonstration of interconvertible high and low affinity states of the D_2 dopamine receptor, J. Biol. Chem., 257:6351-6361.

Stoof, J.C. and Kebabian, J.W., 1981, Opposing roles for D_1 and D_2 dopamine receptors in efflux of cyclic AMP from rat striatum, Nature, 294:366-268.

Tarsy, D. and Baldessarini, J., 1974, Behavioural supersensitivity to apomorphine following chronic treatment with drugs which interfere with the synaptic function of catecholamines, Neuropharmacol., 13:927-940.

Tsuruta, K.,Frey, E.A., Grewe, C.W., Cote, T.E., Eskay, R.L. and Kebabian, J.W., 1981, Evidence of LY-141865 specifically stimulates the D_2 dopamine receptor, Nature, 292:463-465.

THE MULTIPLICITY OF THE D_1 DOPAMINE RECEPTOR

Richard B. Mailman[1,2,3], David W. Schulz[1,3],
Clinton D. Kilts[5], Mark H. Lewis[1], Hans
Rollema[6], and Steven Wyrick[4]

Biological Sciences Research Center[1],
Departments of Psychiatry and Pharmacology[2]
Neurobiology Curriculum[3],Department of
Medicinal Chemistry[4], University of North
Carolina School of Medicine, Chapel Hill, North
Carolina 27514

Department of Psychiatry[5], Duke University
Medical Center, Durham, N.C. 27710

Reiksuniversiteit[6], Groningen, NETHERLANDS

INTRODUCTION

Dopaminergic neurotransmission is known to modulate a
variety of behaviors, including ambulation (Ungerstedt and
Arbuthnott, 1970; Pijnenburg et al., 1976), stereotyped
behaviors (Creese and Iversen, 1973), self-stimulation
(Phillips and Fibiger, 1973), conditioned avoidance responding
(Seiden and Carlsson, 1963), stimulus control (Ho and Huang,
1975), and feeding and drinking (Ungerstedt, 1971; Fitzsimons
and Setler, 1975). It is not surprising, therefore, that drugs
which are believed to act primarily as dopamine receptor
agonists or antagonists have important clinical utility. Our
work has sought to address two questions of some
neuropharmacological importance. First, what is the nature of
mechanisms by which dopamine initiates many of these
psychopharmacological effects, and second, is it possible to
design highly specific drugs targeted only at a selected
subpopulation of dopamine receptors?

THE BIOCHEMICAL PHARMACOLOGY OF DOPAMINE RECEPTORS

The first biochemical effect linked to occupation of
dopamine receptors was the stimulation of cAMP synthesis found
in cell-free preparations derived from brain regions that
receive dense dopaminergic innervation (Kebabian et al., 1972;
Brown and Makman, 1972). This led to the proposal that
increased cAMP formation might be the essential mechanism by
which dopamine altered cellular events at its postsynaptic
target sites (Miller et al., 1974; Miller, 1975; Iversen,
1975). However, three separate types of data were inconsistent

with such changes in cAMP concentration or turnover being solely and directly responsible for the immediate psycho-pharmacological effects of drugs affecting dopamine receptors.

One line of evidence was from data using either brain slices (Palmer et al., 1973; Harris, 1976) or intact animals (Breese et al., 1979). These studies found that dopamine receptor occupation did not cause the expected effects on cAMP synthesis. Consistent with this, certain ergot alkaloids, such as lergotrile and ergotamine, were found to be potent dopamine agonists even though they failed to stimulate adenylate cyclase (Trabucchi et al., 1976; Schmidt and Hill, 1977). More recently, Vance and Blumberg (1983) reported that infusion of dopamine into the nucleus accumbens causes increases in locomotor activity without concomitant changes in cAMP formation.

However, the most convincing evidence may have come from comparing the relative potencies of many dopamine receptor antagonists in inhibiting dopamine-sensitive adenylate cyclase versus their antidopaminergic behavioral potency. While most of these compounds do inhibit dopamine-sensitive adenylate cyclase (Clement-Cormier et al., 1974; Miller, 1975; Iversen et al., 1976), the correlation between their potencies at this site versus antipsychotic potency or the blockade of dopamine-mediated behaviors is noteworthy only for some classes of antagonists (Laduron et al, 1976; Snyder et al., 1975). While it seems clear that dopamine receptor-mediated regulation of cAMP synthesis has a role in neuronal function (Greengard, 1978), this combination of data has led to the proposal that changes in cAMP concentration or turnover are probably not involved in the acute psychopharmacological effects caused by antipsychotic drugs (Seeman, 1980; Creese and Leff, 1982; Laduron, 1983).

Development of D_1-D_2 Classification

As dopaminergic radioligands became available (Burt et al., 1975; Seeman et al., 1975), the affinity of drugs for butyrophenone (e.g. haloperidol or spiroperidol) recognition sites was found to correlate well with the psychopharmacological potency of these drugs in man or laboratory animals. As noted earlier, the butyrophenones have much lower relative potency at inhibiting dopamine-mediated cAMP synthesis (Snyder, 1976; Creese et al., 1982). Thus, Kebabian and Calne (1979) formulated the widely accepted hypothesis that divides dopamine receptors into two classes on the basis of specific biochemical characteristics -- the D_1 class is linked to stimulation of cAMP synthesis by dopamine, whereas the D_2 class is not. It was the D_2 class which had high affinity for butyrophenones such as [^{3}H]-spiperone, and it was this class that was believed to mediate both antipsychotic effects in man and various antidopaminergic behavioral effects in laboratory animals or man (Kebabian and Calne, 1979; Calne, 1980; Creese and Leff, 1982; Creese et al. 1983; 1982; Costentin et al. 1983). Although there was a period during which multiplicity of dopamine receptors was actively hypothesized, the recent trend has been to accept this general scheme.

Despite the elegance of the D_1- D_2 hypothesis, it appears to have a number of shortcomings. Some investigators have questioned whether [^{3}H]-spiperone (Leysen et al. 1978) labels dopamine receptors in a competitive manner (Leysen and Gommeren, 1981; Seiler and Markstein, 1982; Bacopoulos et al., 1983), and an allosteric interaction has been suggested (Bacopoulos, 1984). It has been stated that there are approximately twice as many antagonist binding sites as agonist sites in dopamine-terminal regions, leading to the proposal that a single dopamine receptor may consist of separate subunits for high-affinity agonist and antagonist binding (Leysen et al., 1979).

Quantitatively, it has been hypothesized that there may be about four times as many D_1 dopamine receptors as there are D_2 sites in the striatum (Leff et al., 1984). Lesioning studies in the striatum have led to the idea that dopamine-stimulated adenylate cyclase resides primarily on neurons intrinsic to this region (Creese et al., 1981; Schwarcz et al., 1978; Quik et al., 1979). Moreover, these data suggest that the ratio of D_1:D_2 receptors on interneurons and projection neurons may be very high (e.g., 10:1). Even if one hypothesizes that that dopamine has a greater affinity for D_2 receptors (Seeman, 1980), it would be difficult to explain the presence of so many "non-functional" dopamine receptors that are linked with adenylate cyclase activation. These dat together probably led to the comment by Laduron (1983) that the D_1 class is "a receptor in search of a function".

Hypotheses Underlying This Work

In light of the preceding data, on solely teleological grounds, it seemed likely that D_1, as well as D_2, dopamine receptors had important psychopharmacological effects, and this became an underlying hypothesis of our studies. Moreover, similar reasoning suggested that there was likely to be profound, functionally relevant, microheterogeneity of dopamine receptors throughout the brain. Although the recognition characteristics of these receptors might fit into categories similar to those inherent in the D_1-D_2 scheme (i.e., catechols act on both sites; ergots only the latter), the functional consequences of receptor occupation also were likely to be influenced by the cellular location of the receptors.

Several experimentally testable hypotheses were derived from these general ideas, and two of these will be discussed in this chapter. One was that D_1-like dopamine receptors in brain can mediate profound antidopaminergic behavioral effects. The second was that there are D_1-like receptors which are not linked to cAMP synthesis. It is important to note our use of the term "D_1-like". This usage expresses our opinion that a more general definition of the D_1 dopamine receptor may be appropriate. One alternative would be as simple as using only ligand recognition characteristics: this class of receptors recognizing substituted benzazepines (e.g., SCH23390 or SKF38393) with much greater affinity than it recognizes various butyrophenones, benzamides, or ergots. In such a redefinition, the D_1 class of recognition sites as originally outlined by Kebabian and Calne (1979) would really be one subpopulation. However, since such an idea is not generally accepted, we shall use the term "D_1-like", with the hope that the data presented herein may cause reconsideration of this point.

INITIAL STUDIES WITH SCH23390

Biochemical Pharmacology

The strongest and most direct data supporting the functional importance of D_1 receptors came from studies with the compound synthesized by Schering Corp., SCH23390 [(+)-7-hydroxy-8-chloro-2,3,4,5-tetrahydro-3-methyl-5-phenyl-1H-3-benzazepine]. The abstract of Iorio et al. (1981) reported that SCH23390 potently inhibited dopamine-sensitive adenylate cyclase, whereas it had much less affinity for [^{3}H]-spiperone binding sites, data later expanded by others (Iorio et al. 1983; Cross et al. 1983; Hyttel et al. 1983). Our early in vitro studies with SCH23390 confirmed that it was extremely potent at inhibiting dopamine-stimulated adenylate cyclase, with a K_i value of < 1 nM (Mailman et al. 1984a; 1984b). Pifluthixol or cis-flupenthixol is frequently used to label D_1 sites because they are potent inhibitors of dopamine-stimulated adenylate cyclase (Hyttel 1978), although they also have D_2 properties. The potency of SCH23390 at antagonizing dopamine-stimulated adenylate cyclase was as great as these thioxanthenes, whereas cis-flupenthixol is about three orders of magnitude more potent than SCH23390 at displacing [^{3}H]-spiperone. We have also confirmed that while SCH23390 is a potent antagonist of dopamine-stimulated adenylate cyclase, it displays very little ability, in vitro, to compete with [^{3}H]-spiperone, [^{3}H]-dopamine, or [^{3}H]-dipropyl-5,6-ADTN for binding to recognition sites in striatal homogenates (Mailman et al. 1984a; 1984b).

Psychopharmacological Effects

On the basis of this evidence that SCH23390 is a selective D_1 dopamine receptor antagonist, it was to be expected that SCH23390 would have little effect on dopamine-mediated behaviors (Calne 1980; Creese et al. 1983). Consistent with this, Iorio et al. (1983) initially reported that SCH23390 had relatively low potency in antagonizing several apomorphine-induced behaviors, or in releasing prolactin. However, we found that SCH23390, administered to rats intraperitoneally (ip) rather than orally, is at least as potent (ID_{50} = 0.03 mg/kg) as haloperidol at antagonizing amphetamine-induced locomotor behavior (Mailman et al. 1984a; 1984b). Moreover, it has a similar potency in inhibiting all of the stereotyped behaviors induced by apomorphine (Mailman et al. 1984a; 1984b), or the locomotor stimulation and stereotyped behavior induced by dipropyl-5,6-ADTN. This unexpected potency of SCH23390 was also reported by Christensen et al. (1984), among others.

EFFECTS OF SCH23390 ON DOPAMINE SYNTHESIS AND RELEASE

Iorio et al. (1983) also reported that, consistent with its designation as a selective D_1 antagonist, SCH23390 had relatively little potency at increasing rates of dopamine

56

TABLE 1
Effects of SCH23390 and haloperidol on concentrations of dopamine, DOPAC, and HVA in various rat brain regions

TREATMENT	Dopamine	DOPAC	HVA
		(ng/mg protein $\pm$ SEM)	
STRIATUM			
Vehicle	79.6 + 5.2	15.2 + 1.0	9.6 + 0.6
SCH23390	78.9 + 2.8	*22.0 + 0.6	13.2 + 1.2
Haloperidol	83.6 + 4.3	*#47.2 + 2.5	*#30.8 + 2.1
NUCLEUS ACCUMBENS			
Vehicle	56.4 + 3.0	27.6 + 3.6	5.6 + 0.7
SCH23390	54.5 + 2.4	25.7 + 1.6	*9.1 + 0.7
Haloperidol	51.5 + 4.2	*#57.0 + 2.9	*#23.4 + 1.4
FRONTAL CORTEX			
Vehicle	3.1 + 0.6	0.9 + 0.1	1.2 + 0.1
SCH23390	2.4 + 0.1	0.7 + 0.1	1.4 + 0.2
Haloperidol	2.8 + 0.5	*#2.5 + 0.2	*#4.0 + 0.6

* Significantly different from Vehicle ($p < 0.05$).
# Significantly different from SCH23390 ($p < 0.05$).

Values are the mean $\pm$ SEM of four animals per point, using treatments of 0.3 mg/kg (i.p.) of either vehicle (0.1% tartaric acid), SCH23390, or haloperidol 60 min prior to sacrifice.

synthesis or increasing secretion of prolactin. This is in contrast to what is observed following administration of typical D_2 dopamine antagonists. Like Iorio et al. (1983), we failed to detect dramatic neurochemical changes in the same rats in which SCH23390 had profound antidopaminergic behavioral effects (Mailman et al. 1984a; 1984b). For example, one study compared SCH23390 (0.3 mg/kg) and haloperidol (0.3 mg/kg) directly. Whereas haloperidol caused increases of 150-300% in DOPAC and HVA concentrations (a measure of dopamine turnover), no dose of SCH23390 increased DOPAC or HVA in any region by more than 60% (Table 1). In microdissection of dopamine-rich areas throughout brain there was also no evidence of changes in dopamine synthesis and release as estimated by either metabolite concentrations, or rate of dopamine utilization after synthesis inhibition. Other antipsychotic drugs showed dramatic (and regionally specific) effects using both techniques.

As would be expected from these findings, SCH23390 also failed to affect release of either dopamine or acetylcholine using the electrically-stimulated, perfused rabbit striatal slice preparation (per Niedzwiecki et al. 1984). SCH23390 did not cause any reversal of the apomorphine- or nomifenisine-induced inhibition of dopamine release at concentrations of 1 uM, whereas haloperidol caused dramatic changes at concentrations 100 times lower. Interestingly, SCH23390 had some effects on the efflux of acetylcholine, but these effects required concentrations greater than 1 uM. Thus, the lack of effect of SCH23390 on transmitter overflow in this system was in contrast with other drugs that had similar behavioral potency.

We have also concluded studies on the effects of SCH23390 on the firing of dopamine neurons in the substantia nigra (Napier et al. 1986). In identified dopaminergic neurons, apomorphine caused a dose-dependent inhibition of firing that is reversed by classical neuroleptics, also in a dose-dependent fashion. Conversely, SCH23390 would not reverse the apomorphine-induced inhibition of firing even at doses of 5 mg/kg i.v.--these doses being more than 100 times the behavioral (i.p.) ID_{50}. At the very high doses (but not the lower ones), SCH23390 by itself does cause some increase in firing; the relevance of this finding is unclear at present.

EFFECTS OF SCH23390 ON IN VIVO RECEPTOR BINDING

Feenstra and coworkers (1983a; 1983b; 1983c; Rollema et al., 1986) have demonstrated that there is saturable accumulation of the dopamine agonist dipropyl-5,6-ADTN in striatal membranes, and that the ED_{50} for this accumulation is the same as the ED_{50} for the induction of stereotyped behavior (Feenstra et al. 1983a; 1983c). Moreover, various antipsychotic drugs were found to displace this specific accumulation of dipropyl-5,6-ADTN at the same doses that inhibited the behavioral effects of the agonist (Feenstra et al. 1983a; 1983c). Interestingly, the ED_{50} for neurochemical changes (i.e., decreases in DOPAC and HVA) caused by dipropyl-5,6-ADTN treatment was much lower than for the effects on specific binding or induction of stereotypy, consistent with the greater sensitivity of dopamine autoreceptors for agonists (REFERENCE). When we performed a similar series of experiments with SCH23390, this drug blocked the behavioral effects of dipropyl-5,6-ADTN, yet as shown in Figure 1, no displacement of dipropyl-5,6-ADTN whatsoever was seen (Mailman et al. 1984a). Conversely, in the same experiments cis-flupenthixol and haloperidol, but not trans-flupenthixol, did cause the expected displacement of dipropyl-5,6-ADTN.

OTHERS ASPECTS OF SCH23390 PHARMACOLOGY

Effects of Various Routes of Administration

The apparent contradiction between some of the psychopharmacological data of Iorio et al. (1983) and others (Mailman et al. 1984a; 1984b; Christensen et al. 1984) could simply be due to SCH23390 being subject to extensive first-pass metabolism. Consistent with this, we found that SCH23390 administered into the lateral ventricles was effective at reversing amphetamine-induced hyperactivity with an ID_{50} of 1 ug, thus making SCH23390 five times as potent as fluphenazine when the latter drug is given by the same route (Lewis et al., 1983; Mailman et al. 1984a; 1984b). This latter experiment also suggests that it is neither a metabolite of SCH23390 that is responsible for its behavioral effects, nor does SCH23390

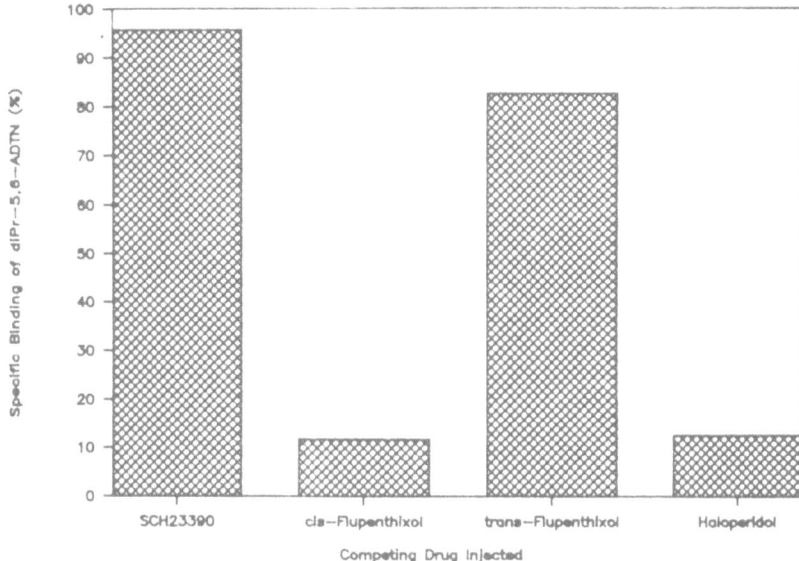

Figure 1. The effects of SCH23390 on the _in vivo_ binding
of dipropyl-5,6-ADTN. Values shown are the
specific binding of dipropyl-5,6-ADTN defined
per Feenstra et al., 1983. Doses of competing
drugs used were: SCH23390 - 1.07 mg/kg; cis-
or trans-flupenthixol - 5 mg/kg; and
haloperidol - 1 mg/kg [reprinted by permission
of _Psychopharmacol. Bull._ from Mailman et al.,
(1986)].

given parenterally act by inhibiting the entry of amphetamine
or other dopamine agonists into the brain. Consistent with the
hypothesis that pharmacokinetics are important, the ID_{50} of
SCH23390 given orally is about 100-fold higher than after
intraperitoneal administration (Iorio et al. 1983; Mailman et
al. 1984a; 1984b).

Quantification of SCH23390 in Biological Matrices

To confirm directly the points mentioned above, we
developed an HPLC method using solvent extraction, reverse
phase (RP-8) separation, and electrochemical detection to
quantify SCH23390 and electrochemically active metabolites in
extracts of brain and blood (Kilts et al. 1985). The most
significant early finding using this method relates to the
time course of SCH23390 distribution and metabolism after
intraperitoneal injection with SCH23390. There is a rapid
disappearance of SCH23390 from the blood (plasma half-life < 1
hr), and it appears that the compound has an extremely large
volume of distribution after oral administration. Of greater
interest, however, is the fact that after an intraperitoneal
dose of 0.1 mg/kg, the brain concentrations of SCH23390 are
still near maximal two hrs post-injection, whereas the plasma
concentrations are undetectable at this time (Kilts et al.,
1985; Schulz et al. 1985a). Thus, it might be predicted that
SCH23390 may cause persistent biochemical and behavioral
effects because of its prolonged presence in brain (vide
supra). Many antipsychotic drugs (e.g., chlorpromazine or
thioridazine) are often found at a ten-fold higher

concentration in brain than in blood at peak times, although the washout of these drugs from both compartments follows a similar time course (Kilts et al. 1984; Cohen et al. 1980; Jorgensen et al. 1969). As noted above, there does not appear to be bioconcentration of SCH23390 in brain compared to blood, nor do the blood and brain have the same kinetics of clearance.

Persistent Effects of SCH23390

The finding of SCH23390 in brain after clearance from the circulation suggested that there may be residual functional effects of this drug. Thus, we investigated the persistence of the effect of SCH23390 on two functional endpoints: inhibition of amphetamine-induced locomotion in vivo; and inhibition of dopamine-stimulated adenylate cyclase in vitro in membranes of rats pretreated with SCH23390. As noted, studies with many other antipsychotic drugs have shown a parallel disappearance of the parent drug and/or active metabolites from the blood concomitantly with a decrease in brain concentration. Attenuation of direct biological effects also occurs. Unlike other dopamine receptor blockers, a single injection of SCH23390 (0.1 mg/kg) caused significant inhibition of the locomotor stimulatory effects of amphetamine for at least 8 hrs after treatment. Yet, this occurred despite the fact that there is no detectable circulating concentration of SCH23390 2 hrs after treatment. Moreover, the synthesis of cAMP in striatal membranes of rats pretreated with SCH23390 was significantly less at saturating (i.e., 100 uM) concentrations of dopamine than it was in membranes from untreated rats handled otherwise identically. In vitro studies have shown that a large excess of dopamine can completely reverse the effects of SCH23390 on dopamine-stimulated adenylate cyclase, suggesting that the actions of the drug are reversible.

BIOCHEMICAL PHARMACOLOGY OF SCH23390

SCH23390 Effects on Non-Dopamine Systems

One possibility is that SCH23390 has generalized effects on cAMP systems. Since both norepinephrine (Grabowska-Anden, 1977; Mogilnicka and Braestrup, 1976) and adenosine (Snyder et al. 1981) are two likely candidates in the CNS that can also influence the actions of dopamine systems, we investigated the effects of SCH23390 on norepinephrine-stimulated adenylate cyclase and adenosine-stimulated adenylate cyclase in CNS regions which also contained dopamine-stimulated adenylate cyclase. As shown in Figure 2, in the dorsomedial frontal cortex, SCH23390 completely antagonized dopamine-stimulated adenylate cyclase, while it inhibited only that portion of norepinephrine-stimulated adenylate cyclase which could be attributed to stimulation of DA receptors (Bockaert et al. et al. 1977).

In striatal homogenates, there is also an adenylate cyclase which is stimulated by activation of A_2-adenosine receptors (Daly 1977; Daly et al. 1981). The A_2 ligand 2-chloroadenosine stimulated adenylate cyclase 60% above basal levels, and this activation was reversed by the adenosine antagonist 3-isobutyl-1-methylxanthine, but not by SCH23390.

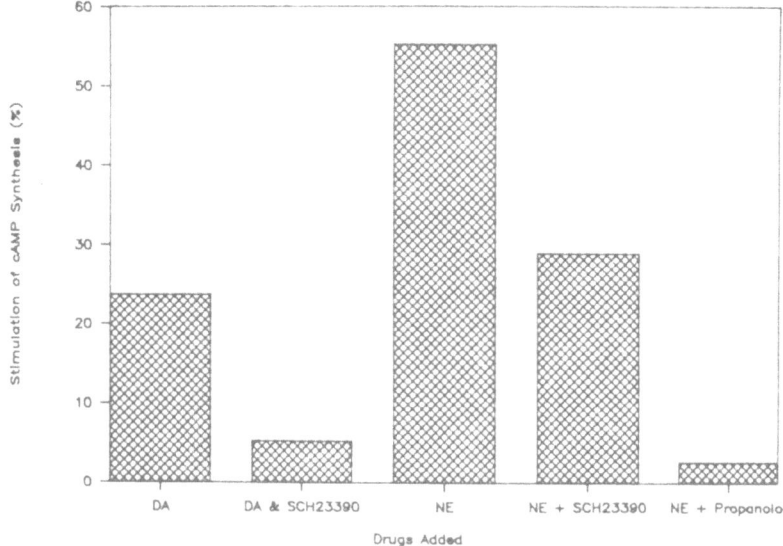

Figure 2. Effects of SCH23390 on dopamine- and norepinephrine stimulated cAMP synthesis in homogenates of prefrontal cortex. The concentrations of each drug used were: dopamine-100 uM; norepinephrine-100 uM; SCH23390-100 nM; and propanolol-10 uM. As can be noted, SCH23390 blocks essentially all of the dopamine induced synthesis of cAMP, but only a portion of the norepinephrine-induced synthesis.

In addition, in the NG108-15 cultured cell line, SCH23390 was inactive at affecting the regulation of cAMP synthesis mediated via opiate, muscarinic or a_2-adrenergic receptors (per Smith and Harden 1984). It also did not affect the binding of the B-adrenergic ligand iodocyanobenzylpindolol to brain membranes (per Doss et al. 1981). Finally, SCH23390 does not inhibit basal adenylate cyclase activity in any system we have tested, nor does it inhibit the increase in cAMP synthesis induced by forskolin. Thus, it appears that SCH23390 does not act simply by interfering nonspecifically with the catalytic unit of adenylate cyclase, the nucleotide binding protein, or the process by which non-DA stimulatory ligands couple with adenylate cyclase. Finally, we have determined that SCH23390 does not affect phosphodiesterase activity.

Binding sites for [³H]SCH23390

We have synthesized [9-³H]SCH23390 (Wyrick and Mailman 1985), and characterized the binding of this purportedly selective antagonist of D_1 dopamine receptors (Schulz et al. 1984b; 1985b). The regional distribution of high-affinity, specific [³H]SCH23390 binding sites in the rat brain correlated well with levels of endogenous dopamine. As shown in Table 2, receptor densities were greatest in corpus striatum, nucleus accumbens, and olfactory tubercle; intermediate levels were found in several limbic and cortical areas, while few sites were detectable in cerebellum, brainstem, and olfactory bulb (Schulz et al. 1984b; 1985b).

TABLE 2

Regional distribution of [³H]SCH23390 binding in rat central
nervous system.

Brain region	[³H]-SCH23390 bound* (fmol/mg protein + SEM)
caudate-putamen	113.9 ± 5.8
olfactory tubercle	109.0 ± 15.5
nucleus accumbens	97.0 ± 9.7
dorsomed. prefront. cortex	23.1 ± 2.6
lateral preoptic area	21.1 ± 2.8
globus pallidus	18.1 ± 1.5
amygdala	16.9 ± 1.1
lateral septum	14.6 ± 2.7
parietal cortex	14.5 ± 2.1
hippocampus	10.4 ± 0.3
hypothalamus	9.3 ± 3.8
olfactory bulb	7.0 ± 1.8
cerebellum	4.6 ± 0.5
brainstem	4.3 ± 1.7

* Tissue was incubated with 0.5 nM [³H]-SCH23390 for 15
minutes. Nonspecific binding was defined by addition of
1 uM SCH23390 (data from Schulz et al., 1985b).

Specific binding in caudate-putamen was found to be both
temperature- and pH-dependent, with optima at 25-30°C and pH
7.8-8.0. Scatchard or Woolf analyses of binding in caudate-
putamen suggest that the majority of sites are either of a
single class or of classes with similar characteristics (K_d =
0.7 ± 0.1 nM, B_{max} = 347 ± 35 fmol/mg protein). Both dopamine
and cis-flupenthixol altered the slope but not the intercept
of lines generated by Scatchard (1949) analysis, suggesting a
competitive mode of inhibition of [³H]-SCH23390 binding.
Competition for binding by dopamine or the D_1 agonist SKF38393
was inhibited by guanine nucleotides, whereas GTP had little
effect on the competition for binding by the antagonist cis-
flupenthixol. The competition for [³H]SCH23390 binding sites
by dopamine was much more sensitive to GTP than was
competition for [³H]spiperone binding (Schulz et al. 1985b).
These data support the hypotheses that [³H]SCH23390 binds to
recognition sites which differ from those previously described
using other radiolabeled dopamine antagonists, and that these
sites have the characteristics expected of dopamine receptors.

DIFFERENTIAL DISTRIBUTION OF A DOPAMINE SENSITIVE ADENYLATE
CYCLASE AND [³H]-SCH23390 BINDING SITES

Cellular Subfractionation of the Striatum

The accepted definition of the D_1 dopamine receptor is
the one linked to dopamine-mediated increases in cAMP
synthesis. One way to test the hypothesis that there are more
than one population of receptors with D_1-like recognition
characteristics is to perform cellular subfractionation of the
rat corpus striatum using differential centrifugation (Cotman,

1974; Laduron et al., 1983). These studies demonstrated that [^{3}H]-SCH23390 binding sites had a significantly different distribution from dopamine-sensitive adenylate cyclase among the various cellular fractions.

As shown in Figure 3, the [^{3}H]-SCH23390 binding sites tended to be concentrated in lighter cellular fractions relative to dopamine-sensitive adenylate cyclase. Moreover, when the mitochondrial or microsomal fractions were further subfractionated on a continuous sucrose gradient, the [^{3}H]-SCH23390 still resided in lighter fractions than did the dopamine-sensitive adenylate cyclase activity. These data suggest either the presence of spare receptors (and their cellular localization in structures different than dopamine-sensitive adenylate cyclase, or that the D_1 class of dopamine receptors is actually comprised of more than one population.

Absence of Dopamine-Sensitive Adenylate Cyclase in the Amygdala

Consistent with the second of these hypotheses, we have found that although basal cAMP synthesis rates are very high in tissue homogenates of rat amygdala, there is no detectable

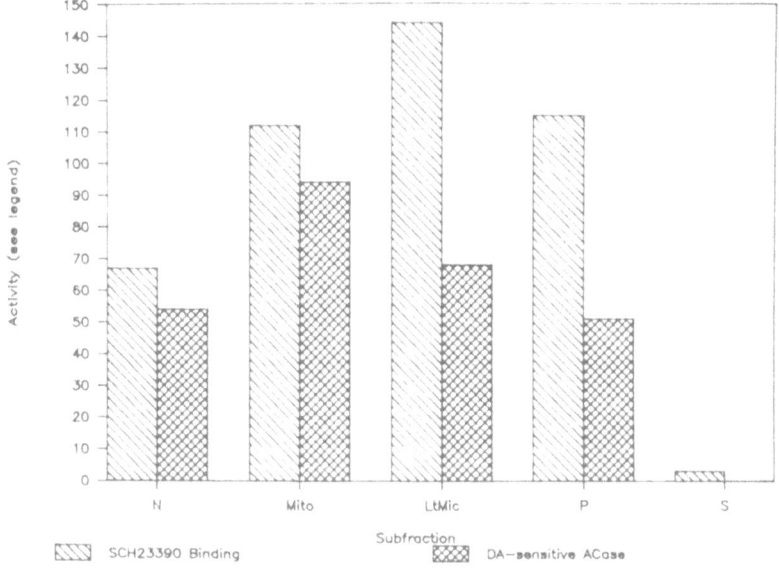

Figure 3. Distribution of [^{3}H]-SCH23390 Binding and dopamine-stimulated adenylate cyclase in subcellular fractions of striatal homogenates. Fractions prepared basically according to Laduron et al. (1983) are: N-nuclear; Mito-mitochondrial; LtMito-light mitochondrial; P-microsomal; and S-supernatant. Values are listed in fmol/mg protein for binding of 0.5 nM [^{3}H]-SCH23390 (Schulz et al., 1984b; 1985b) and pmol/mg/min for dopamine (100 uM) stimulated adenylate cyclase activity (Schulz and Mailman, 1984).

stimulation by addition of dopamine. Dopamine did cause a pronounced dose-dependent increase in cAMP synthesis in tissue from the same animals taken from adjacent areas of the caudal caudate nucleus in the same animals. SCH23390 did not increase or decrease cAMP synthesis in the amygdala. Despite the absence of DA-stimulated adenylate cyclase in the amygdala, there are significant concentrations of high affinity $[^3H]$-SCH23390 recognition sites in this brain region. These data lend further support to the hypothesis that not all D_1 receptors are linked to cAMP synthesis.

SUMMARY

SCH23390 Acts via Dopamine Recognition Sites

The utility of SCH23390 (or similar compounds) as a selective ligand for D_1-like receptors first requires that the biological actions of this compound (or its congeners) be due principally to effects at sites normally receptive to dopamine. One possibility, is that SCH23390 interacts with a receptor for another neurotransmitter or neuromodulator, thus causing its antidopaminergic effects. This seems unlikely for several reasons. First, SCH23390 has significantly lower potency (relative to inhibition of dopamine-sensitive adenylate cyclase) at every other biochemical index in which it has been tested. Second, it is well known that neuromodulators (e.g., various neuropeptides) that modulate dopaminergic function cause marked effects on dopamine turnover and release (e.g., Kalivas et al. 1983; Govoni et al. 1982; Nemeroff et al. 1983; Widerlov et al. 1982). It is clear that SCH23390 does not cause such effects at behaviorally active doses. Finally, it is also seems clear that SCH23390 does not have generalized effects on cAMP systems, as demonstrated by its inactivity in stimulating or inhibiting several non-dopamine receptors that influence cAMP synthesis (Mailman et al. 1984a; 1984b).

There are multiple lines of evidence consistent with the conclusion that SCH23390 is active at dopamine recognition sites. Structure-activity studies of the potencies of various dopamine agonists at stimulating adenylate cyclase have led to the suggestion that the actual binding site of dopamine most closely resembles the D_1 receptor (Seiler and Markstein, 1982). Clearly, the structure of SCH23390 (i.e., it contains the elements of dopamine), and the structure-activity data that is currently available on various benzazepines (e.g., O'Boyle and Waddington, 1984), is consistent with a requirement for a catecholamine-like configuration. The in vitro biochemical pharmacology of SCH23390 is remarkably consistent with actions at dopamine recognition sites. For example, $[^3H]$-SCH23390 binding sites have a distribution similar to dopamine (Schulz et al. 1984b; 1985b), and the pharmacology of these binding sites is consistent only with a dopamine-like recognition site (Schulz et al. 1984b; 1985b; Billard et al. 1984).

At the functional level, an important observation is the temporal parallel between changes in SCH23390 concentrations in brain and behavioral or biochemical functional effects. After a single intraperitoneal dose, the drug is metabolized rapidly and cleared from the periphery yet brain concentrations are detectable for many hours. There is inhibition of amphetamine-induced locomotion in vivo, and dopamine sensitive-adenylate cyclase from isolated striatal membranes for up to 12 hours after treatment (Schulz et al. 1985a). This parallel of presence of drug in brain and two functional antidopaminergic effects is also consistent with actions at dopamine receptors.

Redefinition of the D_1 Dopamine Receptor

Although Kebabian and Calne's (1979) division of dopamine receptors into two classes has been conceptually useful, are available data consistent with this categorization? As an aside, it should be noted that those authors acknowledged the possibility of subclasses with their divisions. Thus, in the absence of specific supporting data, there would seem no reason to believe that the class of dopamine receptor labeled by Kebabian and Calne (1979) as D_1 is of necessity homogeneous. Similarly, while the ability of dopamine to stimulate cAMP synthesis seems to reside with this general type of receptor, it is also possible that different biochemical mechanisms (other second messengers, ionophores, etc.) may be involved in the action of sites with similar ligand recognition characteristics, hence the term "D_1-like".

As noted earlier, a teleological approach predicted previously unrecognized functional effects of D_1 dopamine receptors (e.g., psychopharmacological effects), and also the possibility that there is a profound microheterogeneity of dopamine receptors throughout the brain. The data summarized in the previous sections provides specific evidence to support the idea of multiple D_1 receptors. Naturally, the recognition characteristics of these multiple D_1 receptors are similar (they all bind SCH23390), and consistent with the D_1-D_2 scheme (i.e., catechols act on both sites; ergots only the latter).

Since this book provides a forum for both review, and for speculation, the latter may be somewhat excusable. As noted in various points of this chapter and this volume, it seems clear that SCH23390 can indirectly modulate what has formerly been regarded as D_2 receptor function. We would like to propose a crude model (shown in Figure 4) that is built on these data. If one accepts our hypothesis that D_1 receptors are heterogeneous, a scenario may be constructed loosely based on the model of the acetylcholine receptor. Thus, while there are some D_1 sites that are linked to cAMP synthesis, there may also be a single postsynaptic complex having both D_1 and D_2 receptors. In Figure 4, this is shown as an ionophore (the tooth-like-structure in the Figure, one not found in the dentate gyrus). Both the D_1 and D_2 sites on this complex would normally recognize dopamine, their endogenous ligand, with the D_1 site modulating the D_2 site. The two sites may have significantly different affinities for this endogenously released catecholamine. Thus, under normal situations, the

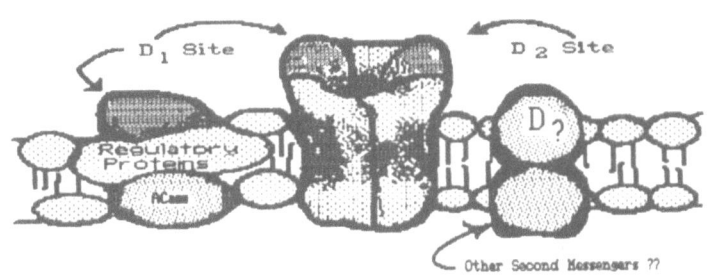

Figure 4. Model of D_1 dopamine receptors in membrane, illustrating the lack of identity of some of the [^{3}H]-SCH23390 binding sites with the dopamine receptor linked to stimulation of cAMP synthesis. This model also shows how D_1 and D_2 binding sites might interact to modulate each others function.

postsynaptic consequences of the firing of dopamine neurons may depend markedly on the rate of firing and release.

Such a model leads to several predictions, many of which can be tested empirically. Functional inactivation of the receptor complex may occur with an appropriate antagonist at either the D_1 or D_2 site. Conversely, the actions of a pure agonist for one site will be modulated by the presence of an agonist for the other site. Finally, endogenous dopamine is likely to be very important in the expression of actions of any agonist. Although psychopharmacological and physiological approaches are likely to be very useful in testing such ideas, it would seem that the most convincing evidence can come from biochemical and molecular biological approaches. However, if valid, this model raises even more important questions.
Are all D_1 receptors a product of the same gene? Are functional differences a consequence of dissimilar primary structures, or does posttranslational processing or the local cellular milieu also play a role? What is the ontogeny of the different receptors, and what factors mediate their expression? Answers to such questions have important potential for both basic and clinical neuropharmacology. It may be possible to design new, truly "atypical", antipsychotic drugs with much greater selectivity. More importantly, the same issues are relevant to developing new insights into the neurobiology of dopamine-receptive neurons and dopaminergic neurotransmission. The data we have presented provide clear evidence that the basis for classification of DA receptors into the D_1 and D_2 categories must now be redefined, or at least be made less restrictive. It may also be appropriate to introduce fresh ideas into our concepts of dopamine receptor pharmacology.

ACKNOWLEDGEMENTS

The authors would like to thank Carl Anderson, Eddie Stanford, and Dr. T. K. Harden for technical assistance. This work was supported in part by PHS grants MH40537, ES01104, MH37404, HD16834, MH39967, and Center Grant HD03110.

REFERENCES

Bacopoulos, N.G., 1984, Dopaminergic ^{3}H-agonist receptors in rat brain, New evidence on localization and pharmacology, Life Sci., 34: 307.

Bacopoulos, N.G., Brown, S.J., Ware, P.L., and Thron, C.D., 1983, On the mechanism of inhibition of dopamine receptor by fluphenazine, Biochem. Pharmac., 32: 930.

Billard W., Ruperto V., Crosby G., Iorio L.C., and Barnett A., 1984, Characterization of the binding of ^{3}H-SCH 23390, a selective D-1 receptor antagonist ligand, in rat striatum, Life Sci., 35: 1885.

Bockaert, J., Tassin, J.P., Thierry, A.M., Glowinski, J. and Premont, J., 1977, Characteristics of dopamine and beta-adrenergic sensitive adenylate cyclase in the frontal cerebral cortex of the rat. Comparative effects of neuroleptics on frontal cortex and striatal dopamine sensitive adenylate cyclases, Brain Res., 122: 71.

Breese, G.R., Mueller, R.A. and Mailman, R.B., 1979, Effect of dopaminergic agonists and antagonists on in vivo cyclic nucleotide content: Relation of guanosine 3',5'-monophosphate (cGMP) changes in cerebellum to behavior, J. Pharmacol. Exp. Ther., 209: 262.

Brown, J.H. and Makman, M.H., 1972, Stimulation by dopamine of adenylate cyclase in retinal homogenates and of adenosine 3',5'-cyclic monophosphate formation in intact retina, Proc. Nat. Acad. Sci. (U.S.), 69: 539.

Calne, D.B., 1980, Clinical relevance of dopamine receptor classification, Trends Pharmacol. Sci., 3: 412.

Christensen, A.V., Arnt, J., Hyttel, J., Larsen, J.-J. and Svendsen, O., 1984, Pharmacological effects of a specific dopamine D1 antagonist SCH23390 in comparison with neuroleptics, Life Sci., 34: 1529.

Clement-Cormier, Y.C., Kebabian, J.W., Petzold, G.L. and Greengard, P., 1974, Dopamine-sensitive adenylate cyclase in mammalian brain: A possible site of action of antipsychotic drugs, Proc. Nat. Acad. Sci. (U.S.), 71:1113.

Cohen, B.M., Herschel, M., Miller, E. Mayberg, H. and Baldessarini, R.J., 1980, Radioreceptor assay of haloperidol tissue levels in the rat, Neuropharmacol., 19: 663.

Costentin, J., Dubuc, I. and Protais, P., 1983, Behavioral data suggesting the plurality of central dopamine receptors, in: "CNS Receptors: From Molecular Pharmacology to Behavior", pp. 289-297. Mandel, P. and DeFeudis, F.V. (eds) Raven Press, New York, 1983.

Cotman, C.W., 1974, Isolation of synaptosomal and synaptic plasma membrane fractions, Meth. Enzymol., 31: 445.

Creese, I. and Leff, S.E., 1982, Dopamine receptors: A classification, J. Clin. Psychopharmacol., 2:329.

Creese, I., Morrow, A.L., Leff, S.E., Sibley, D.R. and
    Hamblin, M.W., 1982, Dopamine receptors in the central
    nervous system, Intl. Rev. Neurobiol., 23: 255.
Creese, I., Sibley, D.R., Hamblin, M.W. and Leff, S.E., 1983,
    The classification of dopamine receptors: relationship to
    radioligand binding, Annu. Rev. Neurosci., 6: 43.
Cross, A.J., Mashal, R.D., Johnson, J.A. and Owen, F., 1983,
    Preferential inhibition of ligand binding to calf
    striatal dopamine D1 receptors by SCH 23390,
    Neuropharmacol., 22: 1327.
Daly, J., 1977, "Cyclic Nucleotides in the Nervous System".
    Plenum Press, New York.
Daly, J.W., Bruns, R.F. and Snyder, S.H., 1981, Adenosine
    receptors in the central nervous system: Relationship to
    the central actions of methylxanthines, Life Sci., 28:
    2083.
Doss, R.C., Perkins, J.P. and Harden, T.K., 1981, Recovery of
    beta-adrenergic receptors following long-term exposure of
    astrocytoma cells to catecholamines. role of protein
    synthesis, J. Biol. Chem., 251: 12282.
Feenstra, M.G.P., Rollema, H., Mulder, T.B.A., DeVries, J.B.
    and Horn, A.S., 1983b, In vivo dopamine receptor agonist
    binding in rat brain: Relation with pharmacological
    effects, Eur. J. Pharmacol., 90: 433.
Feenstra, M.G.P., Rollema, H., Mulder, T.B.A., Westerink,
    B.H.C. and Horn, A.S., 1983a, In vivo dopamine receptor
    binding of a non-radioactively labelled agonist,
    dipropyl-5,6-ADTN, Acta Pharm. Sci. Suppl., 2: 203.
Feenstra, M.G.P., Rollema, H., Mulder, T.B.A., Westerink,
    B.H.C. and Horn, A.S., 1983c, In vivo dopamine receptor
    binding studies with a non-radioactively labelled
    agonist, dipropyl-5,6-ADTN, Life Sci., 32: 1313.
Govoni, S., Yang, H.Y.T., Bosio, A., Pasinetti, G. and Costa,
    E., 1982, Possible interaction between cholecystokinin
    and dopamine. in: "Regulatory Peptides: From Molecular
    Biology to Function", E. Costa and M. Trabucchi, eds.,
    Raven Press, New York, p. 437.
Grabowska-Anden, M., 1977, Modification of amphetamine-
    induced stereotypy in rats following inhibition of
    noradrenaline release by FLA-136, J. Pharm. Pharmacol.,
    29: 566.
Greengard, P., 1978, Phosphorylated proteins as physiological
    effectors, Science, 199: 146.
Haldane, J.B.S., 1957, Graphical methods in enzyme chemistry,
    Nature, 179: 832.
Harris, J.E., 1976, Beta adrenergic receptor-mediated
    adenosine cyclic 3',5'-monophosphate accumulation in rat
    corpus striatum, Mol. Pharmacol., 12: 546.
Ho, B.T. and Huang, J.T., 1975, Role of dopamine in d-
    amphetamine-induced discriminative responding, Pharmacol.
    Biochem. Behav., 3: 1085.
Hyttel, J., 1978, Effects of neuroleptics on ^{3}H-haloperidol
    and ^{3}H-cis(z)-flupenthixol binding and on adenylate
    cyclase activity in vitro, Life Sci., 23: 551.
Hyttel, J., 1983, SCH 23390 - The first selective dopamine D-
    1 antagonist, Eur. J. Pharmacol., 91: 153.
Hyttel, J., 1981, Similarities between the binding of ^{3}H-
    piflutixol and ^{3}H-flupentixol to rat striatal dopamine
    receptors in vitro, Life Sci., 28: 563.
Iorio, L.C., Barnett, A., Leitz, F.H., Houser, V.P. and
    Korduba, C.A., 1981, SCH23390, a potential benzazepine

antipsychotic with atypical effects on dopaminergic systems, <u>Pharmacologist</u>, 23: 137.

Iorio, L.C., Barnett, A., Leitz, F.H., Houser, V.P. and Korduba, C.A., 1983, SCH23390, a potential benzazepine antipsychotic with unique interactions on dopaminergic systems, <u>J. Pharmacol. Exp. Ther.</u>, 226: 462.

Iversen, L.L., 1975, Dopamine receptors in brain, <u>Science</u>, 188: 1084.

Iversen, L.L., Rogawski, M.A. and Miller, R.J., 1976, Comparison of the effects of neuroleptic drugs on pre- and postsynaptic dopaminergic mechanisms in the rat striatum, <u>Mol. Pharmacol.</u>, 12: 251.

Jorgensen, A.L., Hansen, V., Larsen, U.D. and Khan, A.R., 1969, Metabolism, distribution and excretion of flupenthixol, <u>Acta Pharmacol. et Toxicol.</u>, 27: 301.

Kalivas, P.W., Widerlov, E., Stanley, D., Breese, G. and Prange, A.J., 1983, Enkephalin action on the mesolimbic system: A dopamine-dependent and a dopamine-independent increase in locomotor activity, <u>J. Pharmacol. Exp. Ther.</u>, 227: 229.

Kebabian J.W., Petzold G.L. and Greengard P., 1972, Dopamine-sensitive adenylate cyclase in caudate nucleus of rat and its similarity to the "dopamine receptor", <u>Proc. Nat. Acad. Sci. (U.S.)</u>, 69: 2145.

Kebabian, J.W. and Calne, D.B., 1979, Multiple receptors for dopamine, <u>Nature</u>, 277: 93.

Kilts, C.D., Knight, D.L. Mailman, R.B., Widerlov, E. and Breese, G.R., 1984, <u>J. Pharmacol. Exp. Ther.</u> 231: 334.

Kilts, C.D., Dew, K.L., Ely, T.D. and Mailman, R.B., 1985, Quantification of SCH23390 [R-(+)-7-chloro-8-hydroxy-1-phenyl-2,3,4,5-tetrahydro-1<u>H</u>-3-methyl-3-benzazepine] in brain and blood by use of reverse phase HPLC with electrochemical detection, <u>J. Chromatog.</u>, 432: 452.

Laduron, P.M., Verwimp, M., Janssen, P.F.M, and Leysen, J.E., 1976, Subcellular localization of dopamine-sensitive adenylate cyclase in rat brain striatum. <u>Life Sci.</u>, 18: 433.

Laduron, P.M., 1983, Commentary: Dopamine-sensitive adenylate cyclase as a receptor site, <u>in</u>: "Dopamine Receptors", Kaiser, C. and Kebabian, J.W., eds., p. 22. American Chemical Society, Washington, D.C.

Laduron, P.M., Janssen, P.F.M. and Ilien, B., 1983, Analytical subcellular fractionation of rat cortex: Resolution of serotonergic nerve endings and receptors, <u>J. Neurochem.</u>, 41: 84.

Lewis, M.H., Widerlov, E., Knight, D.L., Kilts, C.D. and Mailman, R.B., 1983, N-oxides of phenothiazine antipsychotics: effects on in vivo and in vivo dopaminergic function, <u>J. Pharmacol. Exp. Ther.</u>, 225: 539.

Leysen J.E., Gommeren W. and Laduron P.M., 1978, Spiperone: a ligand of choice for neuroleptic receptors. 1. Kinetics and characteristics of in vitro binding, <u>Biochem. Pharmacol.</u>, 27:307.

Leysen, J.E. and Gommeren, W., 1981, Optimal conditions for ^{3}H-apomorphine binding and anomalous equilibrium binding of ^{3}H-apomorphine and ^{3}H-spiperone to rat striatal membranes: Involvement of surface phenomena versus multiple binding sites, <u>J. Neurochem.</u>, 36: 201.

Leysen J.E., Gommeren W. and Laduron P.M., 1979, Distinction between dopaminergic and serotonergic components of

neuroleptic binding sites in limbic brain areas, <u>Biochem.</u>
<u>Pharmacol.</u>, 28: 447.

Mailman, R.B., Rollema, H., Schulz, D.W., DeHaven, D.L. and
Lewis, M.H., 1984a, Dopamine receptor multiplicity: when
the D-1 antagonist is a D-2 antagonist, <u>Fed. Proc.</u>, 43:
1095.

Mailman, R.B., Schulz, D.W., Lewis, M.H., Staples, L.,
Rollema, H. and DeHaven, D.L., 1984b, SCH-23390: A
selective D-1 dopamine antagonist with potent D-2
behavioral actions, <u>Eur. J. Pharmacol.</u>, 101: 159.

Mailman, R.B. Schulz, D. W., Kilts, C.D., Lewis, M.H.,
Rollema, H., Wyrick, S., 1986, Multiple forms of the D_1
dopamine receptor: its linkage to adenylate cyclase and
psychopharmacological effects. <u>Psychopharmacol. Bull.</u>,
(in press).

Miller, R.J., 1975, Comparison of the inhibitory effects of
neuroleptic drugs on adenylate cyclase in rat tissues
stimulated by dopamine, noradrenaline, and glucagon,
<u>Biochem. Pharmacol.</u>, 25: 537.

Miller, R.J., Horn, A.S. and Iversen, L.L., 1974, Effects of
dopamine-like drugs on rat striatal adenyl cyclase have
implications for CNS dopamine receptor topography.
<u>Nature</u>, 250: 238.

Mogilnicka, E. and Braestrup, C., 1976, Noradrenergic
influence on the stereotyped behavior induced by
amphetamine, phenylethylamine and apomorphine, <u>J. Pharm.</u>
<u>Pharmacol.</u>, 28: 253.

Napier, T,C., Givens, B.S., Schulz, D.W., Bunney, B.S.,
Breese, G.R. and Mailman, R.B., 1986, SCH23390 effects on
apomorphine-induced responses of nigral dopaminergic
neurons, <u>J. Pharmacol. Exp. Ther.</u>, (in press)

Nemeroff, C.B., Luttinger, D., Hernandez, D.E., Mailman, R.B.,
Mason, G.A., Davis, S.D., Frye, G.D., Beaumont, K.,
Breese, G.R. and Prange, A.J., 1983, Interactions of
neurotensin with brain dopamine systems: biochemical and
behavioral studies, <u>J. Pharmacol. Exp. Ther.</u>, 225: 337.

Niedzwiecki, D.N., Mailman, R.B. and Cubeddu, L.X., 1984,
Greater potency for mesoridazine and sulforidazine than
thioridazine on striatal dopamine autoreceptors, <u>J.</u>
<u>Pharmacol. Exp. Ther.</u>, 228: 686.

O'Boyle, K.M., Molloy, A.G., and Waddington, J.L., 1984,
Benzazepine derivatives: Nature of the selective and
stereospecific interactions of SK&F 38393 and SCH 23390
with brain D-1 receptors, <u>in</u>: "Dopamine Systems and their
Regulation", G.N. Woodruff, ed., McMillan Press, London.

Palkovits, M., 1973, Isolated removal of hypothalamic or other
brain nuclei of the rat, <u>Brain Res.</u>, 59: 449.

Palmer G.C., Sulser F., and Robison G.A., 1973, Effects of
neurohumoral and adrenergic agents on cyclic AMP levels
in various areas of the rat brain in vitro,
<u>Neuropharmacol.</u>, 12: 327.

Phillips, A.G. and Fibiger, H.C., 1973, Dopaminergic and
noradrenergic substrates of positive reinforcement:
Differential effects of d- and l-amphetamine, <u>Science</u>,
179: 575.

Pijnenburg, A.J.J., Honig, W.M.M., Van der Heyden, J.A.M., and
Van Rossum, J.M., 1976, Effects of chemical stimulation
of the mesolimbic dopamine system upon locomotor
activity, <u>Eur. J. Pharmacol.</u>, 35: 45.

Rollema, H., Feenstra, M.G.P., Grol, C.J., Lewis, M.H.,
Staples, L. and Mailman, R.B., 1986, (-)-Dipropyl-

5,6-ADTN as an in vivo dopamine receptor ligand: relation between displacement by dopamine agonists and their pharmacological effects. Naunyn-Schmiedeberg's Arch. Pharmacol., (in press).

Quik M., Emson P.C. and Joyce E., 1979, Dissociation between the presynaptic dopamine-sensitive adenylate cyclase and [^{3}H]-spiperone binding sites in rat substantia nigra, Brain Res., 167: 355.

Scatchard, G., 1949, The attraction of proteins for small molecules, Ann. N.Y. Acad. Sci., 51: 660.

Schmidt, M.J. and Hill, L.E., 1977, fects of ergots on adenylate cyclase activity in the corpus striatum and pituitary. Life Sci.,20: 789.

Schulz, D.W. and Mailman, R.B., 1984, An improved, automated adenylate cyclase assay utilizing preparative HPLC: Effects of phosphodiesterase inhibitors, J. Neurochem., 42: 764.

Schulz, D.W., Lewis, M.H., Petitto, J. and Mailman, R.B., 1984a, Ascorbic acid decreases [3H]-dopamine binding in striatum without inhibiting dopamine-sensitive adenylate cyclase, Neurochem. Int., 6: 117.

Schulz, D.W., Wyrick, S.D., and Mailman, R.B. 1984b. [^{3}H]-SCH23390 has the characteristics of a dopamine receptor ligand in the rat central nervous system, Eur. J. Pharmacol., 106: 211.

Schulz, D.W., Staples, L.J. and Mailman, R.B., 1985a, SCH23390 causes persistent antidopaminergic effects in vivo: evidence in longterm occupation of receptors. Life Sci. 36: 1941.

Schulz, D.W., Stanford, E.J., Wyrick, S.B. and Mailman, R.B. 1985b. Binding of [^{3}H]SCH23390 in rat brain: regional distribution, inhibition by competing ligands, and effects of assay conditions suggest interactions at D_1-like dopamine receptors. J. Neurochem., 45: 1601.

Schwarcz, R., Creese, I. and Coyle, J.T., 1978, Dopamine receptors localized on cerebral cortical afferents to rat corpus striatum, Nature 271: 766.

Seeman, P., Chau-Wong, M., Tedesco, J., and Wong, K., 1975, Brain receptors for antipsychotic drugs and dopamine: Direct binding assays. Proc. Nat. Acad. Sci. (U.S.A.), 72: 4376.

Seiler, M.P. and Markstein, R., 1984, Further characterization of structural requirements for agonists at the striatal dopamine D2 receptor and a comparison with those at the striatal dopamine D1 receptor. Studies with a series of monohydroxyaminotetralins on acetylcholine release from rat striatum, Mol. Pharmacol., 26: 452.

Smith, M.M. and Harden, T.K., 1984, Modification of receptor-mediated inhibition of adenylate cyclase in NG108-15 neuroblastoma x glioma cells by N-ethylmaleimide, J. Pharmacol. Exp. Ther., 228: 425.

Snyder, S.H., 1976, The dopamine hypothesis of schizophrenia: focus on the dopamine receptor, Amer. J. Psychiatry , 133: 197.

Snyder, S.H., Creese, I. and Burt, D.R., 1975, The brain's dopamine receptor: Labeling with [^{3}H]-dopamine and [^{3}H]-haloperidol, Psychopharmacol. Commun., 1:663.

Snyder, S.H., Katims, J.J., Annau, Z., Bruns, R.F. and Daly, J.W., 1981, Adenosine receptors and behavioral action of methylxanthines, Proc. Natl. Acad. Sci. (U.S.), 78: 3260.

Trabucchi, M., Spano, P.F., Tonon, G.C., and Frattola, L.,
    1976, Effects of bromocriptine on central dopaminergic
    receptors, Life Sci., 19: 225.
Ungerstedt, U. and Arbuthnott, G.W., 1970, Quantitative
    recording of rotational behavior of rats after 6-hydroxy-
    dopamine lesions of the nigrostriatal dopamine system,
    Brain Res., 24: 485.
Vance, M.A. and Blumberg, J.B., 1983, Effect of catecholamines
    on locomotor activity and cyclic AMP in nucleus accumbens
    in rats, J. Pharm. Pharmacol., 35: 402.
Widerlov, E., Kilts, C.D., Mailman, R.B., Nemeroff, C.B.,
    Prange, A.J. and Breese, G.R., 1982, Increase in dopamine
    metabolites in rat brain by neurotensin, J. Pharmacol.
    Exp. Ther., 223: 1.

THE DOPAMINE D_1 RECEPTOR: BIOCHEMICAL AND BEHAVIORAL ASPECTS

Peter H. Andersen and Erik B. Nielsen

NOVO INDUSTRI A/S
Department of Pharmacology
Novo Allé
DK-2880 Bagsvaerd
Denmark

INTRODUCTION

Research on the role of dopamine (DA) in the control of behavior was initiated with the studies by Randrup and colleagues in the early 60'es (e.g., Randrup et al., 1965). However, the direct study of DA receptors began with the discovery in 1972 of DA sensitive adenylate cyclase in rat striatum (Kebabian et al., 1972). In 1975, tritiated haloperidol was introduced as a compound for direct labelling of DA receptors (Creese et al., 1975; Burt et al., 1975; Seeman et al., 1975). Comparing the pharmacological characteristics of DA stimulated adenylate cyclase and ^{3}H-haloperidol binding, it was readily apparent that ^{3}H-haloperidol does not label the same site as the one through which DA exerts its effects on adenylate cyclase. These discrepancies between binding data and functional data, resulted a few years later in the postulated existence by Kebabian and Calne (1979) of two types of DA receptors designated D_1 and D_2. The D_1 receptor was defined by means of its coupling in a stimulatory fashion to the adenylate cyclase while the D_2 receptor was associated in an inhibitory fashion to or uncoupled from the same effector system. However, due to the lack of specific D_1 compounds, research on D_1 receptor biochemistry and D_1 receptor mediated behavior has been limited. Until recently, the only available ligands for D_1 receptor binding were the tritiated thioxanthenes, i.e. ^{3}H-flupentixol and ^{3}H-piflutixol. Since these ligands exhibit similar affinities for both D_1 and D_2 receptors, and have high non-specific binding (30-70% of total binding; Hyttel 1978, 1981; Leff et al., 1985) they were not ideal tools for investigating D_1 receptors.

In 1983, a novel benzazepine, SCH 23390, was described as a new type of neuroleptic compound (Iorio et al., 1983), however, with unusual characteristics. SCH 23390 was later discovered by Hyttel (1983) to be a specific D_1 antagonist. This finding initiated intensive biochemical and behavioral research on the D_1 receptor.

^{3}H-SCH 23390 RECEPTOR BINDING IN VITRO

Saturation Studies

^{3}H-SCH 23390 is now widely used as D_1 receptor ligand. It is superior to the tritiated thioxanthenes due to its low level of nonspecific binding and high specific activity (Billard etal., 1984; Schulz et al., 1984, 1985; Andersen et al., 1985). Most publications describing the use of ^{3}H-SCH-23390 (or the iodinated analog) utilize assay conditions with high ionic strength (Billard et al., 1984; Schulz et al., 1984, 1985; Pinoule et al., 1985; Porceddu et al., 1985; Seeman et al., 1985; Sidhu and Kebabian, 1985). However, high ionic strength of the assay medium diminishes the stimulation of adenylate cyclase by DA. Therefore, assays measuring D_1 receptor function always require low ionic strength and hypotonic assay medium (Kebabian et al., 1972; Clement-Cormier et al., 1974; Miller et al., 1974; Palmer and Manian 1976). The use of different assay conditions makes a comparison between D_1 binding data and D_1 function difficult.

In order to overcome these problems, we have used ^{3}H-SCH 23390 for D_1 receptor binding in a previously described adenylate cyclase assay preparation of rat striatal membranes (Kebabian et al., 1979). In this preparation (Andersen et al., 1985), ^{3}H-SCH 23390 binding at 30°C is stable and reversible. Further, the binding is saturable and the maximal number of binding sites is about 90 fmol/mg tissue (Fig 1).

However, the B_{max} is highly dependent upon the presence of heavy metal ions and detergents. Thus, only slight changes in the quality of the water used for buffer preparation, or remaining cleaning detergent on the glass, negatively affect

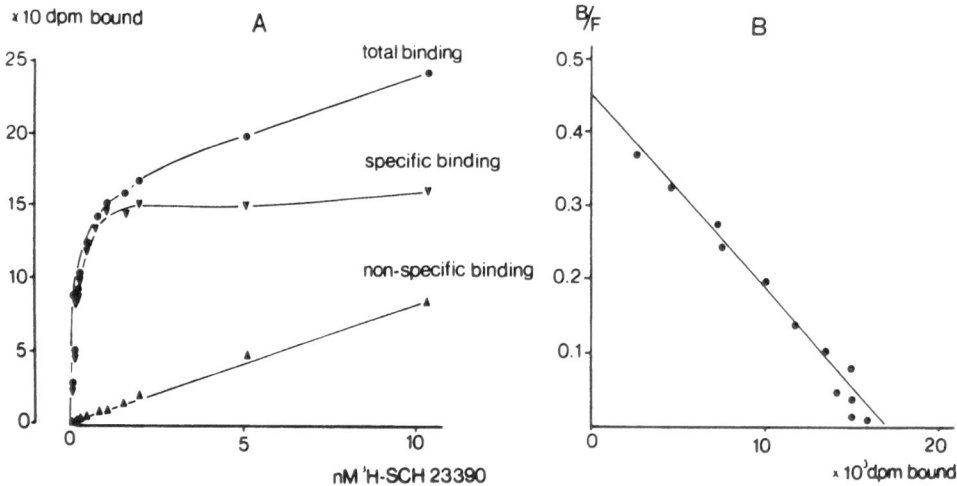

Fig 1.A. Saturation of ^{3}H-SCH 23390 binding in rat striatum as a function of increasing concentration of ^{3}H-SCH 23390 (0.01-10 nM), nonspecific binding was defined as the amount of binding in the presence of 1 μM cis-flupentixol.

B. Scatchard analysis of specifically bound ^{3}H-SCH 23390. Data from Andersen et al. (1985)

74

Table 1. Dopamine D_1 Receptor Number in Rat Striatum

Ligand	B_{max} (fmol/mg tissue)	Reference
^{3}H-flupentixol	78	Hyttel 1978
^{3}H-flupentixol	61	Cross & Waddington 1981
^{3}H-flupentixol	200	Murrin 1983
^{3}H-piflutixol	76	Hyttel 1981
^{3}H-piflutixol	70	Fleminger et al., 1982
^{3}H-piflutixol	88	Fleminger et al., 1984
^{3}H-piflutixol	122	Jenner et al., 1984
^{3}H-piflutixol	157	Nielsen et al., 1984
^{3}H-piflutixol	145*	unpublished
^{3}H-SCH 23390	69	Billard et al., 1984
^{3}H-SCH 23390	49	Schulz et al., 1984,1985
^{3}H-SCH 23390	86	Andersen et al., 1985
^{3}H-SCH 23390	98	Hyttel and Arnt, in press
^{125}I-SKF 83692	91	Sidhu & Kebabian, 1985

* Assay performed as described for ^{3}H-SCH 23390 (Andersen et al., 1985) with addition of 3 nM spiperone to the assay. Non-specific binding was defined with 1 μM SCH 23390.

in a powerful way the level of B_{max}. Table 1 shows a review of B_{max} levels reported in the literature (and some unpublished values) for the D_1 receptor using both tritiated thioxanthenes and ^{3}H-SCH 23390.

The B_{max} for the D_1 receptor labelled by either ^{3}H-flupentixol, ^{3}H-piflutixol or ^{3}H-SCH 23390, appears to converge to a B_{max} at 90-100 fmol/mg tissue. Interestingly, ^{3}H-piflutixol seems to label a substantially higher number of sites in highly diluted tissue preparations (Nielsen et al., 1984) or in hypotonic assay medias with low ionic strength (unpublished and personal communication, M. Nielsen).

In similar experiments performed on prefrontal cortex tissue, ^{3}H-SCH 23390 also labels a single site with the same K_d but the level of B_{max} is somewhat lower (9-13 fmol/mg tissue; Schulz et al., 1984; Andersen et al., 1985).

Pharmacological Characterization

The pharmacological characterization of the ^{3}H-SCH 23390 binding are shown in table 2 and fig 2. It is readily apparent that the characteristics of ^{3}H-SCH 23390 binding, performed in the presently used hypotonic medium, is very similar to those previously described for ^{3}H-piflutixol (Hyttel, 1985). Thus, D_2-compounds (e.g. pimozide, domperidone and 1-sulpiride) were inactive as inhibitors while compounds previously known to exhibit D_1 or mixed D_1-D_2 activity, were potent inhibitors.

An opposite rank order of potencies was obtained with ^{3}H-spiperone binding. Inhibition of ^{3}H-SCH 23390 binding by all tested compounds, occurred in a strictly competitive fashion and further, no antagonist inhibited specifically bound ^{3}H-SCH 23390 from more than a single site.

Table 2. Pharmacological Characteristics of ^{3}H-SCH 23390,
[3]H-Piflutixol and ^{3}H-Spiperone Binding (K_i-nM)

Compound	^{3}H-SCH 23390	^{3}H-piflutixol	^{3}H-spiperone
Benzazepines			
SCH 23390	0.14	3.0	895
SKF 38393	18	170	9,300
SKF 75670	1.9	-	840
SKF 82526	3.1	-	170
Thioxanthenes			
cis-flupentixol	0.32	3.2	0.34
trans-flupentixol	474	670	100
cis-piflutixol	0.16	0.66	0.12
trans-piflutixol	30	40	31
Phenothiazines			
chlorpromazine	25	380	4.6
fluphenazine	4.5	32	0.84
perphenazine	44	72	0.95
thioridazine	21	100	9.5
Butyrophenones			
haloperidol	76	1,000	2.6
spiperone	360	5,400	0.11
Diphenylbutylpiperidines			
pimozide	1,420	610	0.38
domperidone	10,500	11,000	0,72
Benzamides			
l-sulpiride	>15,000	>100,000	34
d-sulpiride	10,900	>100,000	1,300
metoclopramide	>10,000	>100,000	10.2
clebopride	820	18,000	1.3
Dibenzepines			
clozapine	55	680	90
fluperlapine	85	680	245
clothiapine	8	56	7.6
dibenzepine	>1,000	-	>1,000
dibenzadiazepine	>1,000	-	>1,000
Serotonergic compounds			
serotonin	>5,000	-	12,500
ketanserin	204	-	395
ritanserin	175	-	14.8
8-OH-PAT	>1,000	-	395
methysergide	980	-	95
buspirone	>1,000	>100,000	310
Dopamine agonists			
DA	380	>10,000	660
apomorphine	87	850	98
ADTN	5,120	2,500	1,370r
pergolide	400	103,700	7.8
(+)-3P	>1,000	>100,000	1,300
(-)-3P	>1,000	50,000	190
NPA	480	-	4.1
lisuride	29	-	1.2
terguride	35	-	0.6
Miscellaneous			
(+)-butaclamol	0.95	25	0.9
(-)-butaclamol	>9,000	>100,000	6,700
bulbocapnine	270	-	4,500

(Table legend: see following page)

In conclusion, ^{3}H-SCH 23390 seems to label selectively the D_1 receptor. Further, the characteristics of the binding are almost identical to those of the site labeled by ^{3}H-piflutixol, but very different from those of the ^{3}H-spiperone labeled site. Despite of the fact that SCH 23390 exhibits relatively high affinity for 5-HT$_2$ receptors (K_i = 30 nM, unpublished), ^{3}H-SCH 23390 does not under the present conditions label this receptor site.

Agonist Displacement

Agonist effects on the D_1 receptor have previously been evaluated using ^{3}H-agonists such as dopamine or apomorphine (Creese et al., 1984, Leff and Creese, 1985) or, as mentioned above, the triated thioxanthenes (Huff and Molinoff, 1984, Leff et al., 1985) and recently ^{3}H-SCH 23390 (Seeman et al., 1985). All of these studies, using hyper- or isotonic assay media with high ionic strength, demonstrated an effect of guanyl nucleotides on agonist displacement. In the presently used preparation, inhibition of ^{3}H-SCH 23390 binding by DA indicated the existence of multiple binding sites for DA (n_H = 0.6-0.7) (see fig 3). Addition of GTP steepen the DA

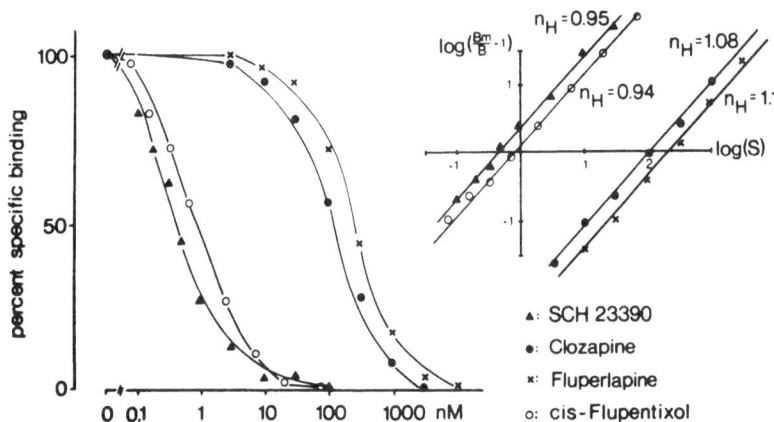

Fig. 2. Inhibition ^{3}H-SCH 23390 binding by SCH 23390, cis-flupentixol, clozapine and fluperlapine. Results are means of 2-6 independent experiments. Insert shows Hill-plot of the data.

Table 2. Legend

K_i-values were measured using the relationship
K_i = IC$_{50}$/(1+(L/K$_d$)) where IC$_{50}$ is the drug concentration able to inhibit 50% of specifically bound ^{3}H-SCH 23390/^{3}H-spiperone, respectively. L is the radioligand concentration (0.19 and 0.05 nM, respectively) used, while K$_d$ is the dissociation constant of ^{3}H-SCH 23390 (0.14 nM) or ^{3}H-spiperone (0.08 nM). Displacement studies with agonists were performed in the absence of GTP. Data from ^{3}H-piflutixol binding are from Hyttel (1985), while other data are from Andersen et al., (1985).

displacement curve and, at a concentration of 300 μM GTP, inhibition of ^{3}H-SCH 23390 occurred from just a single site with an IC_{50} = 4 μM (Andersen et al., 1985). However, the sensitivity of this preparation to GTP was somewhat higher than reported when using different assay conditions (Seeman et al., 1985, Leff and Creese 1985, Leff et al., 1985).

[3]H-SCH 23390 BINDING IN VIVO

The previously available ligands for D_1 binding, e.g. ^{3}H-flu-pentixol, are not well-suited for in vivo studies. This is largely due to the fact that these ligands have similar affinities for both D_1 and D_2 receptors and, further, that the ligands bind with high affinity to a variety of non-dopaminergic receptors, i.e. alpha-adrenergic and serotonergic.

As mentioned above (see Table 2), ^{3}H-SCH 23390 is highly specific for DA D_1 receptors, and is, thus, expected also to be ideal for labeling D_1 receptors in vivo.

Several methods have been published for determining receptors in vivo (Chang and Snyder, 1978; Laduron et al., 1978; Braestrup et al., 1982; Owen et al., 1983; Kohler et al., 1985). In principle, these methods are all very similar. A labelled ligand is administered, usually via the tail vein. After a predetermined time interval, in which the radioligand reaches the brain, the animals are decapitated, the brain rapidly removed (eventually dissected) and, homogenized and filtered under vacuum through Whatman glass filters. These manipulations are performed very quickly (usually within 30-40 sec) in order to minimize redistribution of the radioligand after decapitation.

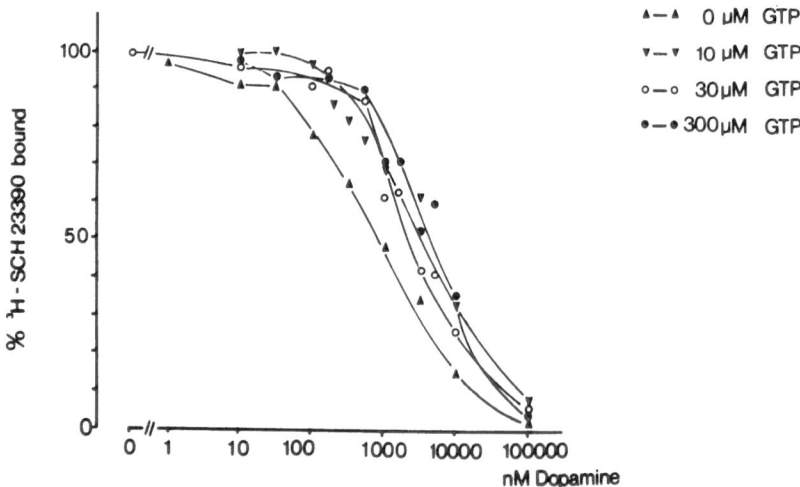

Fig. 3. Influence of GTP on DA displacement of specifically bound ^{3}H-SCH 23390. Increasing concentrations of DA (1-100,000 nM) were allowed to compete with 0.2 nM ^{3}H-SCH 23390 in the absence (▲----▲) or presence of different concentrations of GTP (▼----▼) 10 μM, o----o 30 μM ●----● 300 μM, respectively).

Kinetics and Saturation Studies In Vivo

After injection of 4 µCi of ^{3}H-SCH 23390 into the tail vein, a rapid increase in the amount of brain radioactivity is observed (Fig. 4). After 15 min, the level of radioactivity in the brain reaches a plateau, and thereafter declines. The approximate half-life of the binding is 33 min. The level of nonspecific binding (5-15% of total binding) increases rapidly, reaches a plateau after 10-15 min (Fig. 4), and is then stable for more than 40 min.

The very short half-life of specifically bound ^{3}H-SCH 23390 is in agreement with the short duration of action of the compound (Christensen et al., 1984). When in vivo binding was evaluated as a function of increasing ligand concentration (Fig. 5A) saturation is achieved. Scatchard analysis indicated the presence of only a single binding site (Fig. 5B). Assuming that the brain tissue density is 1 (1g = ml), a K_d of 12.3 nM and a B_{max} of 14.1 fmol/mg tissue is determined. The obtained K_d in vivo is approximately a hundred times higher than the K_d obtained in vitro (0.15 nM in mouse brain, unpublished). The calculated B_{max} is in close agreement with in vitro results from mouse brain, where the combined number of binding-sites in striatum and prefrontal cortex accounts for 10.2 fmol/mg tissue relative to the whole brain (Andersen and Groenvald, in press).

Pharmacological Characterization

The pharmacological characteristics of the ^{3}H-SCH 23390 binding in vivo is shown in table 3. It is apparent that the pharmacological characteristics of ^{3}H-SCH 23390 binding in vivo and in vitro, are very similar (Table 3).

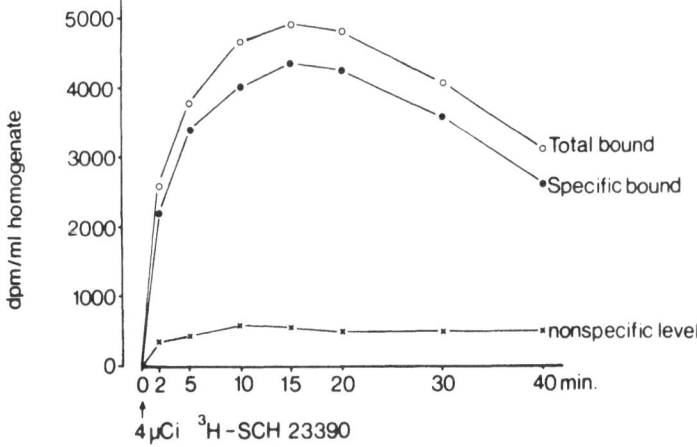

Fig. 4. Time-dependency of bound ^{3}H-SCH 23390 in whole mouse brain (minus cerebellum) following i.v. injection of 4 µCi of the ligand. Each point represents the average of data from 4-6 mice. Labels are: ●——● specific bound, o——o total bound and x——x nonspecific bound. Data from Andersen and Groenvald (in press).

Thus, D_2-specific antagonists (e.g. pimozide, metoclopramide and spiperone) were almost inactive as inhibitors of the binding, while antagonists previously known to exhibit D_1-specific or mixed D_1-D_2 activity were potent displacers. The column, "ratio", in table 3 indicates the ratio between in vivo/in vitro potency. It is evident that most "typical" neuroleptics exhibit ratios >200. However, atypical neuroleptics of the dibenzepine class (e.g. clozapine, fluperlapine and perlapine) and sulpiride and molindone have ratios below 200. This indicates, that the compounds are more potent in vivo than in vitro. As pointed out previously (Andersen et al., 1986), some agreement between ED_{50}'s on ^{3}H-SCH 23390 binding in vivo and average clinical dose exists. On the basis of these results, it is tempting to speculate that the antipsychotic efficacy of the presently-studied neuroleptics, with low in vivo/in vitro ratio, is due to a blockade of brain D_1 receptors.

When using agonists as inhibitors of the ^{3}H-SCH 23390 binding, the D_1 specificity is less pronounced. Thus, the selective D_1-agonist, SKF 75670 potently inhibits ^{3}H-SCH 23390 binding whereas another D_1 selective agonist, SKF 38393, inhibits ^{3}H-SCH 23390 binding only at high doses. D_2-selective agonists, such as pergolide and NPA displaced bound ^{3}H-SCH 23390 in doses which were lower than those observed with SKF 75670. Another D_2-selective agonist, LY 171555, inhibited the ^{3}H-SCH 23300 binding only in extreme doses.

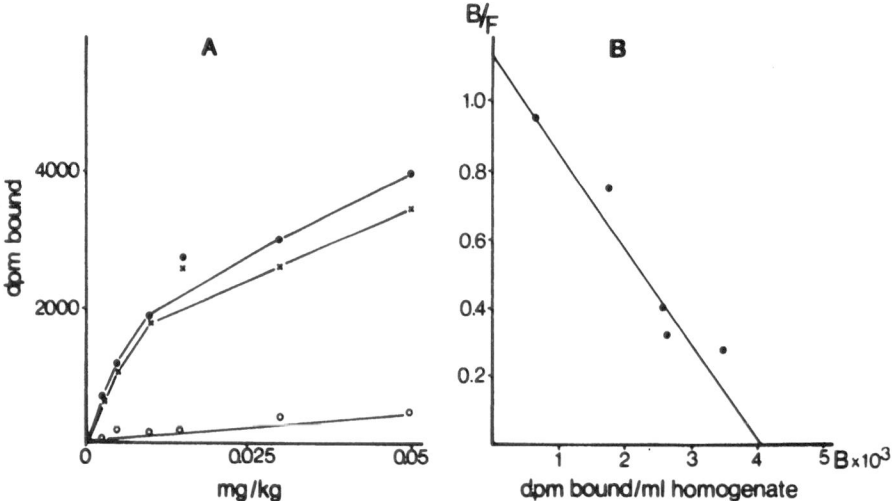

Fig 5 A. Saturation of ^{3}H-SCH 23390 in vivo binding as a function of increasing ^{3}H-SCH 23390 (7.225 Ci/mmol) concentration (0.005-0.05 mg/kg). Nonspecific binding was defined as the amount of bound ^{3}H-SCH 23390 after pretreatment of the animals with 20 mg/kg (i.p., 2 h) cis-flupentixol. Labels are ●——● total binding, o——o nonspecific binding and x——x specific binding. Data from Andersen and Groenvald (in press).

B. Scatchard analysis of specifically bound ^{3}H-SCH 23390.

Table 3. Pharmacological Characterization of ^{3}H-SCH 23390 Binding In Vivo and In Vitro

Compound	^{3}H-SCH 23390 binding		
	in vivo[b] ED$_{50}$ (μg/kg)	in vitro[c] K$_i$ (nM)	in vivo / in vitro ratio x 10^3
Benzazepines			
SCH 23390 (s.c. 1/2)	17	0.14	120
[d]SKF 38292 (s.c. 1 h)	52,500	18	2.900
[d]SKF 75670 (s.c. 1 h)	400	1.9	210
Thioxanthenes			
cis-flupentixol	400	0.32	1.250
trans-flupentixol[a]	192,000	474	400
thioridazine	9,000	21	430
Phenothiazines			
chlorpromazine	7,300	25	290
fluphenazine	2,800	4.5	620
Butyrophenones			
haloperidol	72,500	76	950
spiperone	168,000	360	470
Diphenylbutylpiperidines			
pimozide	190,000	1,420	135
Benzamides			
(+)-sulpiride	90,600	>15,000	<6
clebopride	126,000	820	154
remoxipride	>150,000	>10,000	>15
metoclopramide	185,000	>10,000	>18.5
Dibenzepines			
clozapine (s.c. 1 h)	10,200	55	185
fluperlapine	800	85	9.4
clothiapine	1,300	8	163
perlapine	1,600	97	17
loxapine	300	16	19
dibenzepine	>100,000	>100,000	>100
dibenzadiazepine	>100,000	>100,000	>100
DA agonists			
pergolide (s.c. 1 h)	11,500	400	29
LY 171555 (s.c. 1 h)	250,000	>5,000	<50
NPA (s.c. 1/2 h)	35,000	450	78
Miscellaneous			
(+)-butaclamol	300	0.95	316
(-)-butaclamol[a]	194,000	>9,000	>22
ketanserin	21,000	205	102
molindone	51,000	>10,000	<5

Compounds were administered i.p. 2 h before decapitation except when otherwise indicated.
a) Inactive isomer.
b) The ED$_{50}$ value is the dose which reduces the specific binding of ^{3}H-SCH 23390 in vivo by 50%. Each value is the mean of 2-8 values, determined in separate experiments. In each experiment, 1-6 doses of test substance were administered to groups of at least two mice. Data are from Andersen et al., 1986, and Andersen and Groenvald (in press).
c) K$_i$-values calculated as described in Table 2.
d) DA D$_1$ specific agonists.

In conclusion, ^{3}H-SCH 23390 labels the D_1 receptor both in vivo and in vitro. Relative to D_1 selective agonists (e.g. SKF 38393 and SKF 75670), some D_2 agonists possess high potencies in inhibiting ^{3}H-SCH 23390 binding in vivo. This may indicate the selectivity of D_2 receptor agonists for a possible antagonist state of the D_1 receptor.

DA-STIMULATED ADENYLATE CYCLASE

GTP-Dependency

Homogenates of rat striatum are able to accumulate cAMP when exposed to DA (Kebabian et al., 1972). However, when such membranes are purified intensively using several homogenization/centrifugation steps, DA no longer stimulates cAMP production (Kebabian et al., 1979). By adding supernatant from one of the centrifugation steps, or by adding GTP, DA stimulation is restored (Kebabian et al., 1979). Thus, GTP (or its analogs) is essential for DA stimulation. These effects of GTP have also been observed for other hormone sensitive adenylate cyclases. The GTP-dependency of the presently used preparation is shown in Fig. 6.

DA-Stimulation

DA dose-dependently increased cAMP formation in the present preparation. From dose-response relationships, an EC_{50} for DA is calculated to be 43 ± 22 μM (mean $\pm$ SD, N=10; Fig. 7). This value is somewhat higher than that reported for assays using raw homogenate (2-5 μM; Kebabian et al., 1972a; Clement-Comier et al., 1974; Miller et al., 1974).

Both unstimulated and DA stimulated activity was very stable. Thus, both activities were observed to increase linearly for at least 2 hours (Fig. 8) when using 15 μM GTP as standard and 1.5 mM ATP in the assay (Andersen et al., 1985).

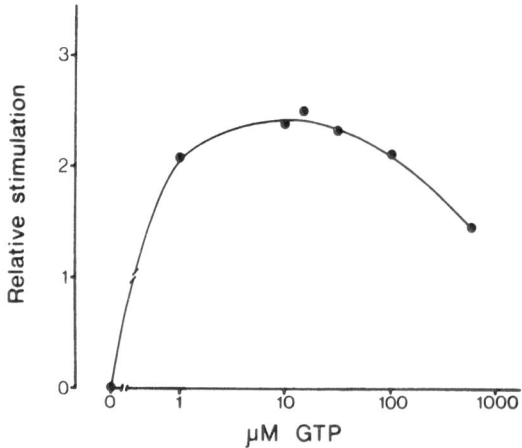

Fig. 6.   GTP-dependency of DA stimulated adenylate cyclase activity in rat striatal membranes. Data from Andersen et al. (1985).

Pharmacological Characterization

DA stimulated adenylate cyclase in raw homogenate has been characterized intensively. The characteristics of the presently used preparation are shown in Table 4.

It is readily apparent that the characteristics of DA sensitive adenylate cyclase are similar to those of ^{3}H-SCH-23390 binding. It is interesting, however, that most K_i values obtained in the adenylate cyclase assay are very different

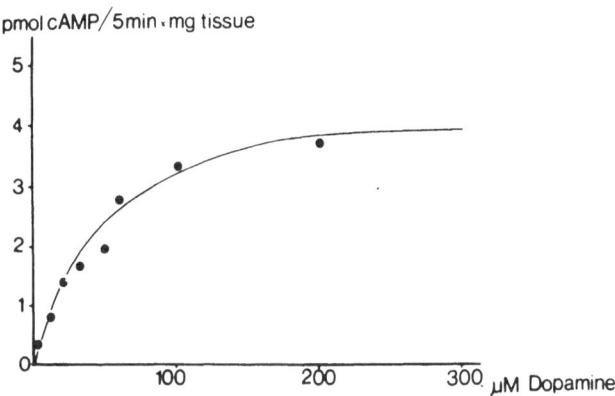

Fig. 7. Dose-response relationship for DA stimulated adenylate cyclase in rat striatum. Shown as an increase in activity. The concentration of DA ranged from 1 to 300 μM. Unstimulated activity was 3.45 ± 0.75 pmol cAMP/5 min x mg tissue. The results represent means of 10 separate experiments. Data from Andersen et al. (1985).

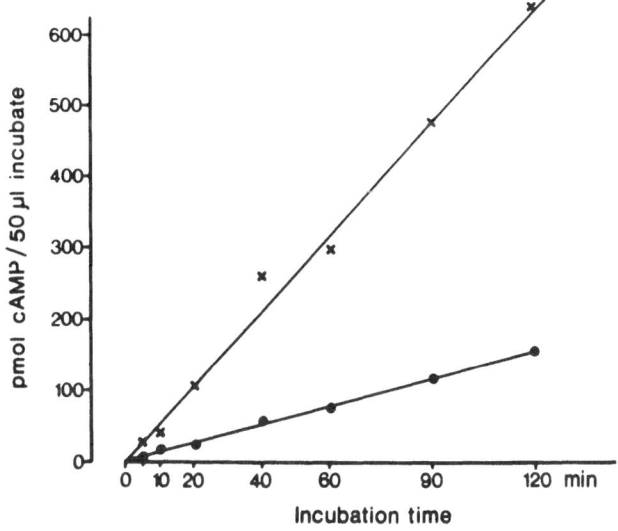

Fig. 8. Time-dependency of unstimulated (●————●) and DA stimulated (x————x) cAMP synthesis in rat striatal membranes.

Table 4. Pharmacological Characteristics of DA
Stimulated Adenylate Cyclase and ^{3}H-SCH
23390 Binding

Compound		K_i (nM) DA-stimulation	^{3}H-SCH 23390 binding
Benzazepines			
SCH 23390		39.9	0.14
SKF 38393	(0.45)	190*#	18
SKF 75670	(0.25)	30*#	1.9
Thioxanthenes			
cis-flupentixol		40.0	0.32
trans-flupentixol		1,200	474
Phenothiazines			
chlorpromazine		463	25
fluphenazine		212	4.5
Butyrophenones			
spiperone		1,720	360
Diphenylbutylpiperidines			
pimozide		>5,000	1,420
domperidone		>5,000	10,520
Benzamides			
l-sulpiride		>5,000	>15,000
Dibenzepines			
clozapine		32.5	55
fluperlapine		26.6	85
clothiapine		34.5	8
dibenzepine		>5,000	>1,000
dibenzadiazepine		>5,000	>1,000
DA agonists			
DA	(1)	43,000*	380
apomorphine	(0.7)	2,700*	87
3,4-DNH	(0.3)	57,000*	>1,140
Miscellaneous			
(+)-butaclamol		81.8	0.95
(-)-butaclamol		>5,000	>5,000
bulbocapnine		865	270
serotonin		>5,000	>5,000

K_i values for inhibiting DA stimulated adenylate cyclase were
calculated from Schild analysis using three different
inhibitor concentrations and 5 different DA concentrations.
The K_i values are mean of data from 2-9 separate experiments.
K_i values from ^{3}H-SCH 23390 binding were obtained using the
relationship $K_i = IC_{50}/(1+(L/K_d))$ where IC_{50} is the drug
concentration which inhibits 50% of the specifically bound ^{3}H-
SCH23390. "L" is the radio-ligand concentration (0.2 nM) and
K_d the dissociation constant (0.14 nM).
* Km values for stimulating adenylate cyclase; relative effi-
cacies are shown in brackets.
estimated values; dose-response relationship does not
conform to Michaelis-Menten kinetics.
3,4-DHN: 3,4-dihydroxynomifensine.

from the K_i values obtained in inhibiting ^{3}H-SCH 23390 binding. Most drugs exhibit a several-fold selectivity towards inhibiting ^{3}H-SCH 23390 binding, with two interesting exceptions, the atypical dibenzepine neuroleptics clozapine and fluperlapine. These compounds had the highest affinity for inhibiting DA-stimulation. Schild analysis of the effect of these two compounds, SCH 23390 and cis-flupentixol, is shown in Fig 9.

These results suggest that ^{3}H-SCH 23390 and DA label two separate binding sites. However, the almost identical pharmacological characteristics (Table 4) indicate that the binding sites are very closely related. This raises two possibilities: 1)that ^{3}H-SCH 23390 and DA label different states of the D_1 receptor or 2)that ^{3}H-SCH 23390 and DA binds to different, but closely, allosterically coupled, sites on the D_1 receptor moiety.

D_1 RECEPTOR: BEHAVIORAL ASPECTS

The pharmacologic characterization of SCH 23390 revealed, for the first time, a compound which has very little D_2 receptor blocking property in vitro, but yet has several of the properties of classical D_2 antagonists (e.g., the drug induces catalepsy, antagonizes DA-dependent stereotyped behavior and blocks conditioned avoidance behavior; Arnt, 1985). SCH 23390 differs, however, from classical DA-antagonists with respect to the relative inability (following systemic administration) to influence DA turnover or firing rate of DA neurons (Morelli and Chiara, 1985). SCH 23390 also does not readily elevate prolactin levels in the blood, a classical D_2 receptor mediated effect. (Apud et al., 1985).

The existence of a DA-receptor subtype, which is dissimilar pharmacologically from the D_2 receptor, was, however,

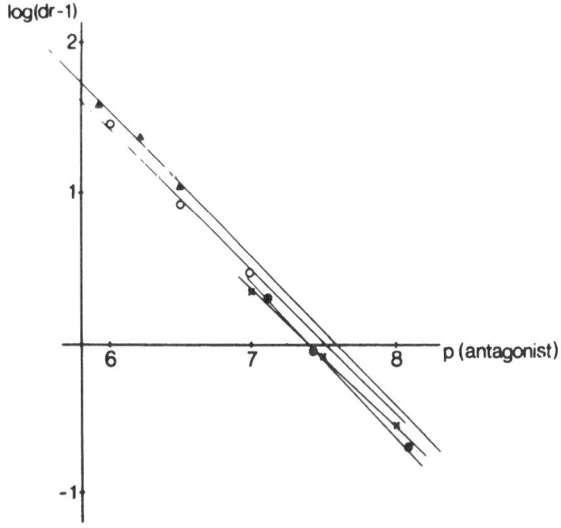

Fig. 9.   Schild analysis of inhibition of DA stimulated adenylate cyclase by SCH 23390 (x———x), cis-flupentixol (●———●), clozapine (o———o) and fluperlapine (▲———▲).

already indicated by the early work on SKF 38393 by Setler et al. (1978). Here, SKF 38393 was found to produce rotational behavior in rats with unilateral 6-hydroxydopamine (6-OHDA) lesions of the substantia nigra, although the drug failed to produce stereotyped behavior, a prototypic behavioral response mediated by DA receptors.

Several lines of evidence indicate that D_1 and D_2 receptors, under normal conditions, are closely coupled (below). Furthermore, the study of D_1 receptor function has been complicated by the fact that a _full_ agonist for D1 receptors has not yet been described. Thus, SKF 38393, the prototypic D_1 agonist, is a partial agonist (45% efficacy; table 4) as determined by its ability to stimulate adenylate cyclase activity. The ability of SKF 38393 to cause rotational behavior in 6-OHDA-lesioned animals, or hyperactivity and stereotyped behavior in animals given chronic reserpine (Arnt, 1985), may be explained by the possibility that supersensitive DA-receptors develop under such conditions. Consonant with this hypothesis is the observation that partial D_2 agonists (e.g. 3-PPP) behave in a similar fashion.

Nevertheless, the lesion models have been important with respect to providing functional evidence for pharmacologically specific DA-receptor subtypes. Thus, in these models, SKF 38393-mediated activity is blocked only by a D_1 antagonist while D_2 antagonists are ineffective, and _vice versa_ for D_2 agonist-mediated activity. This situation suggests that endogenous DA or some (other) presynaptic factor, is necessary for the D_1/D_2 coupling which is otherwise present under normal physiological conditions.

The data obtained with SCH 23390 indicates that its ability to influence D_2 function is not mediated by a direct effect on the D_2 receptor; thus, SCH 23390 does not affect _in vivo_ binding of ^{3}H-spiperone to D_2 receptors in striatum (unpublished observations), nor does SCH 23390 block DA effects in tissues which lack D_1 receptors (e.g. changes in the firing rate of DA neurons or elevation of prolactin-levels). Since D_1 receptors appear to be closely linked to D_2 receptors, it is expected that a D_1 agonist could simply mimic the effect of a D_2 agonist. Consistent with this notion is the observation that SKF 38393 mimics the effects of D_2 agonists in DA receptor hypersensitive animals (above). However, in normosensitive animals, SKF 38393 produces only partially the effect of a full agonist (e.g., increased grooming and slight hyperactivity) consistent with the partial agonist efficacy in biochemical models. SKF 38393 does appear to produce some effects which may be related to non-D_2 receptor-linked D_1 receptors. Thus, SKF 38393 produces EEG desynchronization in rabbits and rats (Ongini et al., 1985), an effect which was blocked by SCH 23390 but not by sulpiride. Furthermore, SKF 38393 has also been found to produce discriminative stimulus effects which are blocked by SCH 23390 but not by haloperidol suggesting, again, non-D_2 linked D_1 receptor effects (Cunningham et al., 1985). In this respect, it should also be noted that the motor effects produced by SKF 38393 are not blocked by metoclopramide (a specific D_2 antagonist; Mollpy and Waddington, 1984). Further characterization is, however, necessary for validation of the involvement of the D_1 receptor in the above findings.

So far, relatively little success has been obtained with respect to elucidating the role of D_1 receptors in behavior. Thus, a specific D_1 "behavior" has not been demonstrated, i.e. a behavior which is not also produced by D_2 compounds.

GENERAL CONCLUSION

^{3}H-SCH 23390 labels the DA D_1 receptor both in vitro and in vivo (Billard et al. 1984; Schulz et al., 1984, 1985; Andersen et al., 1985; Andersen and Groenvald, in press). The characteristics of the ^{3}H-SCH 23390 labelled site (Tables 2,3,4) are very similar to those of the ^{3}H-piflutixol labelled site and the site by which DA stimulates adenylate cyclase. The pharmacological characteristics of D_1 binding and function suggest that ^{3}H-SCH 23390 binding in vitro and DA stimulated adenylate cyclase label two closely related but different sites. On basis of the present data, it is not possible to clarify if these two sites are allosterically coupled with both located on the D_1 receptor or, if they represent different states of the same receptor. Irradiation experiments show that ^{3}H-piflutixol (Nielsen et al., 1984) and ^{3}H SCH 23390 (Nielsen and Hyttel, personal communication, and our own unpublished observations) label a target size protein of 75,000 daltons while the DA stimulated adenylate cyclase target size is 205,000 daltons. This indicates that the DA D_1 receptor may exist both coupled to or uncoupled from adenylate cyclase.

The K_d obtained in vivo for ^{3}H-SCH 23390 binding (12.3 nM) is close to the 39.9 nM calculated for SCH 23390 in inhibiting DA-stimulated adenylate cyclase in vitro. These results suggest that ^{3}H-SCH 23390 in vivo labels a D_1 receptor coupled to adenylate cyclase. On the other hand, ^{3}H-SCH 23390 seem to label in vitro a D_1 receptor which is uncoupled from adenylate cyclase.

Interestingly, some atypical neuroleptics exhibit selectivity for adenylate cyclase-coupled D_1 receptor while mixed D_1/D_2, but otherwise typical neuroleptics, selectively bind to the uncoupled D_1 moiety. It is tempting to speculate that the antipsychotic efficacy of atypical neuroleptic drugs are due to a blockade of the DA D_1 receptors which are coupled to the adenylate cyclase.

Since agonist displacement of ^{3}H-SCH 23390 in vitro is sensitive to GTP, a G-protein must somehow be involved. Two possibilities can be ruled out: 1)that the coupled or un-coupled DA D_1 receptor exists in an equilibrium with each other; 2) or that the uncoupled D_1 receptor is associated with a G-protein. No data exist which supports the existence of an equilibrium between the adenylate cyclase coupled or uncoupled D_1 receptor. This means that the ^{3}H-SCH 23390 labelled D_1 receptor is associated with a G-protein. It is tempting to speculate that the D_1 receptor, besides the adenylate cyclase, is associated with an additional effector system, as has been observed with the muscarinic receptor and beta-receptor (Haga et al., 1985; Brown and Brown, 1984; Maguire, 1984, and Hirata et al., 1979). The results from functional studies of the D_1 receptor have indicated that there may exist both D_2 coupled and non-coupled D_1 receptors in the brain. Since a demonstration of D_1/D_2 receptor coupling has been lacking in biochemical experiments, it can be speculated that the "coupling" may be of an anatomical nature; i.e. neurons with only D_1 receptors may be interneurons. The possibility that DA receptors themselves subserve a role for specific pharmacologic responses await further characterization.

REFERENCES

Andersen P.H., Groenvald F.C., and Jansen J. A., 1985, A comparison between dopamine-stimulated adenylate cyclase and ^{3}H-SCH 23390 binding in rat striatum, Life Sci., 37:1971-1983.

Andersen, P.H. and Groenvald F.C., Specific binding of ^{3}H-SCH 23390 to dopamine D_1 receptors in vivo. Life Sci., in press.

Andersen P.H., Nielsen, E.B., Groenvald F.C. and Braestrup C., Some atypical neuroleptics inhibit ^{3}H-SCH 23390 binding in vivo, Eur. J. Pharmacol., 120:143-144.

Apud J.A., Masotto C., Ongini E. and Racagni G., 1985, Interaction of SCH 23390, a D_1 selective antagonist with the anterior pituitary D_2 receptors and prolactin secretion in the rat, Eur. J. Pharmacol., 112:187-193.

Arnt J., 1984, Differential inhibition by dopamine D_1 and D_2 antagonists of circling behaviour induced by dopamine agonists in rats with unilateral 6-OHDA lesions, Eur. J. Pharmacol., 102:349-354.

Arnt J., 1985, Hyperactivity induced by stimulations of separate D_1 and D_2 receptors in rats with bilateral 6-OHDA lesions, Life Sci., 37:717-723.

Braestrup C., Schmiechen R., Nielsen M. and Petersen E.N., 1982, Benzodiazepine receptor ligands, receptor occupancy,pharmacological effect and GABA receptor coupling. In: The Pharmacology of Benzodiazepine, Usdin E., Skolnick P., Tallman J.F., Greenblatt D. and Paul S.M. (eds) pp 71-85, MacMillan Press, London, UK.

Billard W., Ruperto G., Grosby L.C., Iorio L.C., and Barnett A., 1984, Characterization of the binding of ^{3}H-SCH 23390, a selective D_1 receptor antagonist ligand, in rat striatum, Life Sci., 35:1885-1893.

Brown J.H. and Brown S.L., 1984, Agonists differentiate muscarinic receptors that inhibit cyclic AMP formation from those that stimulate phosphoionsitide metabolism, J. Biol. Chem., 259:3777-3781.

Burt D.R., Enna S.J., Creese I. and Snyder S.M., 1975, Dopamine receptor binding in the corpus striatum of mammalian brain, Proc. Natl. Acad. Sci., USA, 72:4655-4659.

Chang R.S.L. and Snyder S.H.,1978, Benzodiazepine receptors:Labeling in intact animals with ^{3}H-flunitrazepam, Eur. J. Pharmacol., 48:213-218.

Christensen A.V., Arnt J., Hyttel J., Larsen J.-J. and Svendsen O., 1984, Pharmacological effects of a specific dopamine D_1 antagonist SCH 23290 in comparison with neuroleptics, Life Sci., 34:1529-1540.

Clement-Cormier Y.C., Kebabian J.W., Petzold G.L., and Greengard P., 1974, Dopamine-sensitive adenylate cyclase in Mammalian brain: A possible site of action of antipsychotic drugs, Proc. Natl. Acad. Sci., USA, 71: 1113-1117.

Creese I., Burt D.R. and Snyder S.H., 1975, Dopamine receptor
    binding: differentiation of agonist and antagonist states
    with ^{3}H-dopamine and ^{3}H-haloperidol, Life Sci., 17:993-
    1002.
Creese I., Sibley D.R. and Leff S.E., 1984, Agonist
    interactions with dopamine receptors: focus on radiolig
    and-binding studies, Fed. Proc., 43:2779-2784.
Cross A.J. and Waddington J.L., 1981, Kainic acid lesions
    dissociate ^{3}H-spiperone and ^{3}H-flupentixol binding sites
    in rat striatum, Eur. J. Pharmacol., 71:327-332.
Cunningham K.A., Callahan P.M. and Appel J.B., 1985, Dopamine
    D_1 receptor mediation of discriminative stimulus
    properties of SKF 38393, Eur. J. Pharmacol., 119:121-125.
Fleminger S., Jenner P., Marsden C.D. and Rupniak N.M., 1982,
    Dopamine receptor supersensitivity produced by repeated
    neuroleptic administration correlates with D_2 receptors.
    Br. J. Pharmacol., 77:456P.
Fleminger S., Hall M.D., Jenner P., Kilpatrick G., Mann S.,
    Marsden C.D. and Rupniak N.M., 1984, Differential effects
    of administration of haloperidol, sulpiride or clozapine
    for 12 months on rat striatal function, Br. J.
    Pharmacol., 82:288P.
Haga K., Haga T., Ichiyama A., Katada T., Kurose H., and Ui
    M., 1985, Functional reconstitution of purified
    muscarinic receptors and inhibitory quanine nucleotide
    regulatory protein, Nature, 316:731-733.
Hirata F., Strittmatter W.J. and Axelrod J., 1979, Beta-
    adrenergic receptor agonists increase phospholipid
    methylation, membrane fluidity and beta-adrenergic
    receptor adenylate cyclase coupling, Proc. Natl. Acad.
    Sci., USA 76:368-372.
Huff R.M., Molinoff P.B., 1985, Assay of dopamine receptors
    with ^{3}H-flupentixol, J. Pharm. Exp. Ther., 232:57-61.
Hyttel J., 1978, Effects of neuroleptics on ^{3}H-haloperidol
    binding and ^{3}H-flupentixol binding and on adenylate
    cyclase in vitro, Life Sci., 23:551-556.
Hyttel J., 1981, Similarities between the binding of ^{3}H-
    piflutixol and ^{3}H-flupentixol to rat striatal dopamine
    receptors in vitro, Life Sci., 28:563-569.
Hyttel J., 1983, SCH 23390 - The first selective D_1
    antagonist, Eur. J. Pharmacol., 91:153-154.
Hyttel J., 1984, Dopamine D_1 and D_2 receptors.
    Characterization and differential effects of
    neuroleptics, VIIIth Int. Symposium on Med. Chem., (eds.)
    Dahlbom R. and Nilsson J.L.G. ,Swedish Pharmaceutical
    Press. Stockholm, pp 426-439.
Hyttel J. and Arnt. J., Characterization of binding of ^{3}H-SCH
    23390 to D_1 receptors. Correlation to other D_1 and D_2
    measures and effects of selective lesions. J.
    Neurotransm., in press.
Iorio L.C., Barnett A., Leitz F.H., Houser V.P. and Korduba
    C.A., 1983, SCH 23390, a potential benzazepine
    antipsychotic with unique interactions on dopaminergic
    systems. J. Pharmacol. Exp. Ther., 226:462-468.
Jenner P., Kilpatrick G.J. and Marsden C.D., 1984, CHAPS
    solubilizes D_2 but not D_1 binding sites from rat striatal
    preparations, Br. J. Pharmacol., 81:52P.
Kebabian J.W. and Greengard P., 1972, Dopamine-sensitive
    adenyl cyclase: Possible Role in Synaptic Transmission,
    Science, 174:1346-1349.

Kebabian J.W., Chen T.C. and Cote T.E., 1979, Endogenous
    Guanyl nucleotides: components of the striatum which
    comfort Dopamine-sensitivity to adenylate cyclase, Comm.
    in Psychopharmacol., 3:421-428.
Kebabian J. W. and Calne D.B., 1979, Multiple receptors for
    dopamine, Nature, 277:93-96.
Kohler C., Hall H., Oegren S.-O. and Gawell L., 1985, Specific
    in vitro and in vivo binding of ^{3}H-Raclopride, Biochem.
    Pharmacol., 34:2251-2259.
Laduron P., Janssen P.F.M. and Leysen J.E., 1978, Spiperone: A
    ligand of choice for neuroleptic receptors, Biochem.
    Pharmacol, 27:317-321.
Leff S.E. and Creese I., 1985, Interactions of dopaminergic
    agonists and antagonists with dopaminergic D3 binding
    sites in rat striatum, Mol. Pharmacol., 27:184-192.
Leff S.E., Hamblin M.W., and Creese I., 1985, Interactions of
    dopamine agonists with brain D_1 receptors labelled by ^{3}H-
    antagonists, Mol. Pharmacol., 27:171-183.
Maguire M.E., 1984, Hormone sensitive magnesium transport and
    magnesium regulation of adenylate cyclase, TIPS, 5:73-77.
Miller R.J., Horn A.S. and Iversen L.L., 1974, The action of
    neuroleptic drugs on dopamine-stimulated adenosine cyclic
    3',3'-monophosphate production in rat neostriatum and
    limbic forebrain, Mol. Pharmacol., 10:759-766.
Molloy A.G. and Waddington J.L., 1984, Dopaminergic behaviour
    stereospecifically promoted by the D_1 agonist R-SKF 38393
    and selectively blocked by the D_1 antagonist SCH 23390,
    Psychopharmacol., 82:409-410.
Morelli M. and Di Chiara G., 1985, Catalepsy induced by SCH
    23390 in rats, Eur. J. Pharmacol., 37:717-723.
Murrin L.C., 1983, Characteristics of ^{3}H-flupentixol bindingin
    rat striatum, Life Sci., 33:2179-2186.
Nielsen M., Klimek V. and Hyttel J., 1984, Distinct target
    size of dopamine Da and D_2 receptors in rat striatum,
    Life Sci., 35:325-332.
Ongini E., Caporali M.G. and Massotti M., 1985, Stimulation of
    dopamine D_1 receptors by SKF 38393 induces EEG
    desynchronization and behavioral arousal, Life Sci., 37:
    2377-2333.
Owen F., Poulter M., Mashal R.D., Crow T.J., Veall N. and
    Zanelli G.D., 1978, ^{77}Br-p-Bromospiperone; A ligand for
    in vivo labelling of dopamine receptors, Life Sci., 33:
    765-768.
Palmer G.C. and Manian A.A., 1976, Actions of Phenothiazine
    analogues on dopamine-sensitive adenylate cyclase in
    neuronal and glial-enriched fractions from rat brain,
    Biochem. Pharmacol., 25:63-71.
Pinoule C., Schoemaker H., Reynolds G.P., and Langer S.Z.
    1985, ^{3}H-SCH 23390 labeled D_1 dopamine receptors are
    unchanged in schizophrenia and parkinson's disease, Eur.
    J. Pharmacol., 114:235-237.
Proceddu M.L., Ongini E. and Biggio G., 1985, ^{3}H-SCH 23390
    binding sites increase after chronic blockade of D_1
    dopamine receptors, Eur. J. Pharmacol., 118:367-370.
Randrup A., Munkvad I., 1965, Special antagonism of
    amphetamine induced abnormal behaviour,
    Psychopharmacologia, 7:416-422.
Schulz D.W., Wyrick S.D., and Mailman R.B., 1984, ^{3}H-SCH 23390
    has the characteristics of a dopamine receptor ligand in
    the rat central nervous system, Eur. J. Pharmacol.,
    106:211-212.

Schulz D.W., Stanford E.J., Wyrick S.W., and Mailman R.B., 1985, Binding of ^{3}H-SCH 23390 in rat brain: Regional distribution and effects of assay conditions and GTP suggest interactions at a D_1-like dopamine D_1 receptor, J. Neurochem., 45:1601-1611.

Seeman P., Chau-Wong M., Tedesco J. and Wong K., 1975, Brain receptors for antipsychotic drugs and dopamine: direct binding assays, Proc. Natl. Acad. Sci., USA, 72: 4376-4380.

Seeman P., Ulpian C., Grigoriadis D., Pri-Bar I. and Buchman O., 1985, Conversion of Dopamine D_1 receptors from high to low affinity for dopamine, Biochem. Pharmacol., 34: 151-154.

Setler P.E., Sarau H.M., Zirkle C.L. and Saunders H.L., 1978, The central effects of a novel dopamine agonist, Eur. J. Pharmacol., 50:419-430.

Sidhu A. and Kebabian J.W, 1985, An Iodinated ligand identifying the D_1 dopamine receptor, Eur. J. Pharmacol., 113:437-440.

White F.J. and Wang R.Y., Electrophysiological evidence for the existence of both D_1 and D_2 dopamine receptors in the rat nucleus accumbens, Mol. Neurosci., in press.

QUANTITATIVE AUTORADIOGRAPHIC LOCALIZATION OF CENTRAL DOPAMINE D-1 AND

D-2 RECEPTORS

Ted M. Dawson, Donald R. Gehlert* and James K. Wamsley

Departments of Psychiatry and Pharmacology
University of Utah School of Medicine
Salt Lake City, Utah 84132

*Present address:
National Institutes of Health
National Heart, Lung and Blood Institute
Bethesda, MD 20205

INTRODUCTION

Interest in the role of dopamine (DA) as a neurotransmitter within the central nervous system has been increasing markedly over the last several years (Kaiser and Jain, 1985); in fact, it has become the "most extensively investigated neurotransmitter in the nervous system" (Kaiser and Jain, 1985). One area that has been the subject of intensive research is the study of DA receptors. Controversies exist on the actual number of different types of DA receptors, but based on dopamine stimulated adenylate cyclase activity (Kebabian and Calne, 1979; Stoof and Kebabian, 1984) there are primarily two subtypes of DA receptors. The dopamine type-1 (D-1) receptor which is positively associated with adenylate cyclase, and the dopamine type-2 (D-2) receptor which is not associated with this enzyme or, more appropriately, negatively linked.

The recent development of selective agents for these receptor subtypes (for review see Kaiser and Jain, 1985) has greatly facilitated investigations in this area. As a direct result of the availability of these selective compounds, there is now a better understanding of the individual role, function, biochemistry and localization of DA receptors. This chapter will review the application of in vitro receptor autoradiography (Young and Kuhar, 1979), using selective agents for the localization of D-1 and D-2 receptors in the central nervous system (CNS).

LABELING OF DOPAMINE RECEPTORS

Radioligand binding techniques (see Yamamura, Enna and Kuhar, 1985, for review) have been used to identify and characterize dopamine receptors. Initial studies of the DA receptors involved the use of radiolabeled neuroleptics (Baudry et al., 1977; Laduron and Leysen, 1977; Hollt et al., 1977). One of these neuroleptics, [^{3}H]-spiperone, was found to label the D-2 receptor with high affinity (Creese et al., 1977; Fields et al., 1977) and it has subsequently been used extensively as a D-2 receptor ligand. The microscopic localization of DA receptors was made possible by applying radioligand binding techniques to in vivo binding studies (Kuhar et al., 1978; Hollt and Schubert, 1978), as had originally been accomplished for cholinergic receptors (Yamamura et al., 1974; Kuhar and Yamamura, 1975, 1976). These studies and others (Klemm et al., 1979; Murrin and Kuhar, 1979) showed that by using in vivo binding conditions spiperone distributed in high concentrations in areas of the brain known to contain dopaminergic projections. Palacios et al. (1981) used in vitro receptor labeling techniques (Young and Kuhar, 1979) to localize [^{3}H]-spiperone binding sites at the light microscopic level. Use of this technique allowed a more precise anatomical delineation of these binding sites. Furthermore, Palacios et al. (1981) were able to confirm that [^{3}H]-spiperone not only labels D-2 receptors but also labels serotonin type-2, alpha-1-adrenergic and the "spirodecanone site" with high affinity (Howlett et al., 1979; Leysen et al., 1981; Morgan et al., 1984). Despite [^{3}H]-spiperone deficiencies as a D-2 receptor ligand, it was possible to localize D-2 receptors to several cell bodies and terminal fields associated with the dopaminergic systems in the rat CNS (Palacios et al., 1981; Palacios and Wamsley, 1984).

Several agents are now available which are relatively selective and specific for D-1 and D-2 receptors. DA receptor agonists that are selective for the D-1 receptor include SKF 38393 (Setler et al., 1978) and SKF 82526 (fenoldopam) (Hahn et al., 1982), tetrahydro-3-benzazepine derivatives (Frey et al., 1982), and 3',4'-dihydroxynomifensine (Dandridge et al., 1984). Selective and potent D-1 antagonists are tetrahydro-3-benzazepine derivatives such as SCH 23390 (Iorio et al., 1983; Hyttel, 1983; Christensen et al., 1984) and SKF 83566 (Berkowitz et al., 1984). There are also a number of compounds which are potent D-2 receptor agonists and antagonists. LY 171555, an octahydropyrazolo [3,4-g] quinoline derivative (Titus et al., 1983); RU 24213 and RU 24926, meta-tyramine derivates (Euvard et al., 1980; Summers et al., 1981); and N-0434 and N-0437, n,n-disubstituted 2-aminotetralin derivates (Horn et al., 1984; Beaulieu et al., 1984) are several selective D-2 receptor agonists that are now available. Many D-2 receptor antagonists exist, but selectivity and specificity are limited to a few compounds. The benzamide derivatives such as S(-)sulpiride (Jenner and Marsden, 1981; Jenner et al., 1982), iodosulpride (Martres et al., 1985a,b), YM-09151-2 (Grewe et al., 1982; Terai et al., 1983), and (-)-DO710 (Jenner and Marsden, 1981; Jenner et al., 1982; Sokoloff et al., 1985), the benzimidazolone, domperidone (Denef and Follebouckt, 1978; Baudry et al., 1979) and the pyrroloisoquinolone RO 22-1319 (Nakajima et al., 1983) are selective D-2 antagonists. Extensive radioligand binding studies have been performed using some of the agents mentioned above. [^{3}H](-)-sulpiride (Theodorou et al., 1979; Freedman et al., 1981a,b; Woodruff and Freedman, 1981; O'Connor and Brown, 1982; Memo et al., 1983), [^{3}H]-domperidone (Baudry et al., 1979; Lazareno and Nahorski, 1982; Sokoloff et al., 1980), [^{3}H](-)-DO 710 (Sokoloff et al., 1985) and [^{125}I]-iodosulpride (Martres et al., 1985a,b) have been shown, and subsequently have been confirmed by classical competition experiments for the respective radioligands, to be selective and potent D-2 receptor antagonists. A few selective D-1 agents have been radiolabeled, such as [^{3}H]-SCH 23390 (Billard et al., 1984; Schulz et al., 1985b,c), [^{3}H]-SKF 82526 (Flaim et al., 1985), [^{3}H]-SKF 38393 (Scatton and Dubois, 1985) and [^{125}I]-SKF 83692 (Sidhu and Kebabian, 1985). By performing appropriate displacement experiments, it was possible to confirm the results of previous investigations which demonstrated the selectivity of these compounds as D-1 agents.

Table I. Incubation Conditions for Autoradiographic Localization of DA Receptors

A. Conditions used for the labeling of D-1 receptors

Ligand	Concentration (nM)	Buffer	Incubation Procedure	Rinse Procedure	Exposure Time	References
[3H]-SCH 23390	1	50mM Tris-HCl, 120mM NaCl, 5mM KCl, 2mM CaCl$_2$, 1mM MgCl$_2$, (pH 7.4)	30 min (room temp)	2x5 min (4°C)	21 days	Dawson et al., 1985, in press
[3H]-SKF 38393	1	50mM Tris-HCl (pH 7.4)	60 min (room temp)	2x5 min (4°C)	21 days	Scatton and Dubois, 1985

B. Conditions used for the labeling of D-2 receptors

Ligand	Concentration (nM)	Buffer	Incubation Procedure	Rinse Procedure	Exposure Time	References
[3H](-)-Sulpiride	15	0.17M Tris-HCl, 120mM NaCl, 5mM KCl, 2mM CaCl$_2$, 1mM MgCl$_2$, 0.01% ascorbic acid (pH 7.4)	20 min (room temp)	4x1 min (4°C)	60 days	Gehlert and Wamsley, 1984, 1985; Jastrow et al., 1985
[3H](-)-DO 710	5	50mM Tris-HCl, 120mM NaCl, 5mM KCl, 1mM CaCl$_2$, 1mM MgCl$_2$, 5.7mM ascorbic acid and 5x10^{-5}M hydroxyquinoline (pH 7.4)	30 min (room temp)	2x2 min (4°C)	14 days	Sokoloff et al., 1985
[125I]-Iodosulpride	0.3	50mM Tris-HCl, 120mM NaCl, 5mM KCl, 1mM CaCl$_2$, 1mM MgCl$_2$, 5.7mM ascorbic acid, 10uM hydroxyquinoline (pH 7.4)	30 min (25°C)	2x2 min (4°C)	5 days	Martres et al., 1985a,b

Although radioligand homogenate binding studies may be used to determine anatomical distribution and density of receptors (Yamamura, Enna and Kuhar, 1985), in vitro receptor autoradiography (Young and Kuhar, 1979) provides the means to localize receptors at the light microscopic level. Furthermore, one is able to quantitate the actual density of receptors (Unnerstall et al., 1982) by using radiolabeled standards. A detailed discussion of quantitative in vitro receptor autoradiography is beyond the scope of this chapter, but several excellent reviews on this technique exist (please see Wamsley and Palacios, 1983; and Kuhar, 1985b).

[^{3}H](-)-sulpiride was the first selective D-2 compound used to localize D-2 receptors (Gehlert and Wamsley, 1984, 1985; Jastrow et al., 1984). However, under appropriate conditions, Palacios et al. (1981) had previously been able to use [^{3}H]-spiperone to identify D-2 receptors. Since these studies, [^{3}H](-)-DO 710 (Sokoloff et al., 1985) and [^{125}I]-iodosulpride (Martres et al., 1985a,b) have also been used to microscopically localize the D-2 receptor to areas of the rat CNS. The first definitive localization of D-1 receptors was performed by Dawson et al. (1985a, in press) using the selective D-1 antagonist [^{3}H]-SCH 23390. Scatton and Dubois (1985) subsequently confirmed these results using the D-1 agonist [^{3}H]-SKF 38393. The conditions used to label the D-1 and D-2 receptors are summarized in Table I.

CHARACTERIZATION OF DOPAMINE RECEPTOR LIGANDS

[^{3}H]-SCH 23390 (Dawson et al., 1985a, in press) and [^{3}H](-)-sulpiride (Gehlert and Wamsley, 1984,1985; Jastrow et al., 1984) were the selective ligands chosen to localize D-1 and D-2 receptors, respectively. To ensure that the binding sites observed autoradiographically were DA receptors, classic competition experiments needed to be performed. Detailed studies have shown that [^{3}H](-)-sulpiride is very selective for the D-2 receptor (Freedman et al., 1981a,b; Memo et al., 1983; Zahniser and Dubocovich, 1983). Saturation studies yielded a K_d of 17.9nM and a B_{max} of 191 fmol/mg protein (Memo et al., 1983). The same pharmacologic profile was observed for binding to slide mounted tissue sections (Gehlert and Wamsley, 1985). The pharmacologic profile of both [^{3}H](-)-sulpiride and [^{3}H]-SCH 23390 to striatal membrane preparations are summarized in Table II. Of interest is the observation that the isomer of (-)sulpiride, (+)sulpiride, exhibits reversed stereospecificity for D-1 and D-2 receptors in the CNS (Leff et al., 1984) and in the periphery (Shepperson et al., 1982; Goldberg and Kohli, 1982) suggesting the possibility of putative DA_1 and DA_2 receptors (Shepperson et al., 1982; Goldberg and Kohli, 1982).

Displacement studies were performed for the binding of [^{3}H]-SCH 23390 to striatal membrane preparations (Billard et al., 1984) (see Table II) and allowed the demonstration of the relative selectivity of [^{3}H]-SCH 23390 for D-1 receptors. Dawson et al. (in press) confirmed these findings for several areas of the brain by combining classic competition studies with quantitative autoradiography. The pharmacological profile for [^{3}H]-SCH 23390 is shown for the frontal cortex, substantia nigra pars reticulata, caudate-putamen and nucleus accumbens in Figure 1. Stereospecificity of the binding to slide mounted tissue sections was assured, in that cis-(Z)-piflutixol inhibited specific binding about 1000 times more potently than trans-(E)-piflutixol (Dawson et al., in press). Furthermore, (-)-sulpiride had a K_i value of greater than 10,000 in all areas examined and [^{3}H]-SCH 23390 interacted minimally with the serotonergic system (Dawson et al., in press). Saturation studies

Table II. Pharmacologic Profile of [³H]-SCH 23390 and [³H](-)-Sulpiride to Rat CNS

A. Inhibition Constants

Drug	[³H]-SCH 23390 K_i (nM)	[³H](-)-Sulpiride K_i (nM)
SCH 23390(R)	0.3	*
SCH 23388(S)	192	
cis-(Z)-Flupentixol	4.3	1.8
trans-(E)-Flupentixol	907	220
(+)Butaclamol	14.6	3.1
Spiperone	8.400	0.08
Haloperidol	835	1100
Sulpiride(R)	30,000	7.9
Sulpiride(S)	>100,000	180
Chlorpromazine	74	950
Dopamine	1450	300
Methysergide	217	
Ketanserin	1005	**
Serotonin	44,000	

B. Saturation Data

Method	K_d (nM)	B_{max} (fmol/mg tissue)	K_d (nM)	B_{max} (fmol/mg protein)
Striatal			17.9	191
Membranes	0.59	69.0	5.9	590
Tissue				
Sections	1.86	72.91	11.2	52 (fmol/mg tissue)
Quantitative				
Autoradio-				
graphy	2.9	220.7	--	--

Comparison of the pharmacologic profiles of [³H]-SCH 23390 and [³H](-)-sulpiride. These data are taken from Billard et al., 1984; Memo et al., 1983; Zahniser and Dubocovich, 1983; Dawson et al., in press; Gehlert and Wamsley, 1985. *A 10^{-6}M concentration of SCH 23390 failed to displace [³H](-)-sulpiride binding. **A 10^{-6}M concentration of ketanserin failed to displace [³H](-)-sulpiride binding.

performed on striatal membrane preparations yielded a K_d of 0.59nM and a B_{max} of 69 fmol/mg tissue (Billard et al., 1984); similar results were obtained for slide mounted tissue sections (see Table IIB). Hill coefficients approached unity in all cases, suggesting binding to a single population of receptors.

Combining computer-modeling techniques coupled with classic competition experiments to investigate the interaction of dopaminergic agonists and antagonists with [³H]-antagonist labeled D-1 or D-2 receptors, several investigators have shown that antagonist/ [³H]-antagonist competition curves model to a single D-1 or D-2 receptor whereas agonist/[³H]-antagonist competition curves model best to high and low affinity agonist binding of the D-1 or D-2 receptor (Creese et al.,

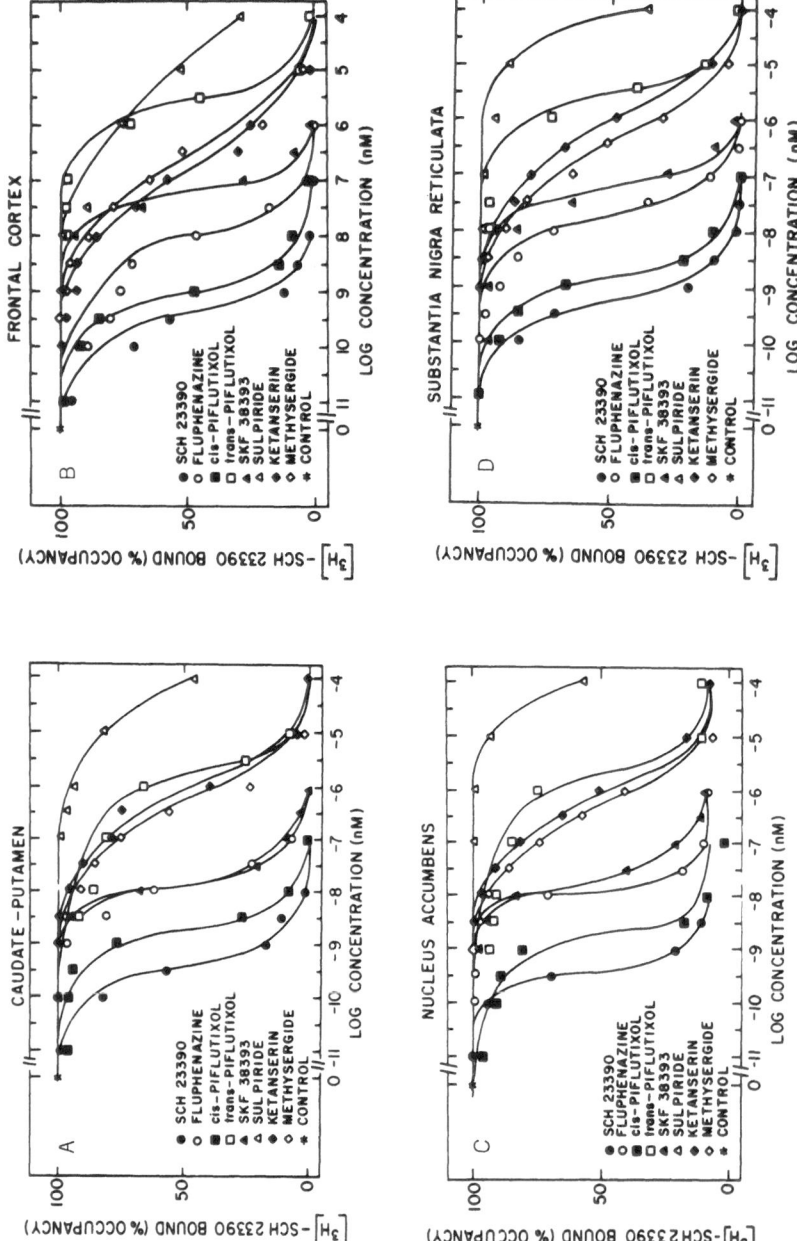

Figure 1. Competition curves for [^{3}H]-SCH 23390 binding. A. Caudate-Putamen. B. Frontal Cortex-Lamina VI. C. Nucleus Accumbens. D. Substantia Nigra Pars Reticulata. Competition curves were produced by combining classic displacement studies with quantitative autoradiography. K_i values for these respective curves appear in Dawson et al. (in press).

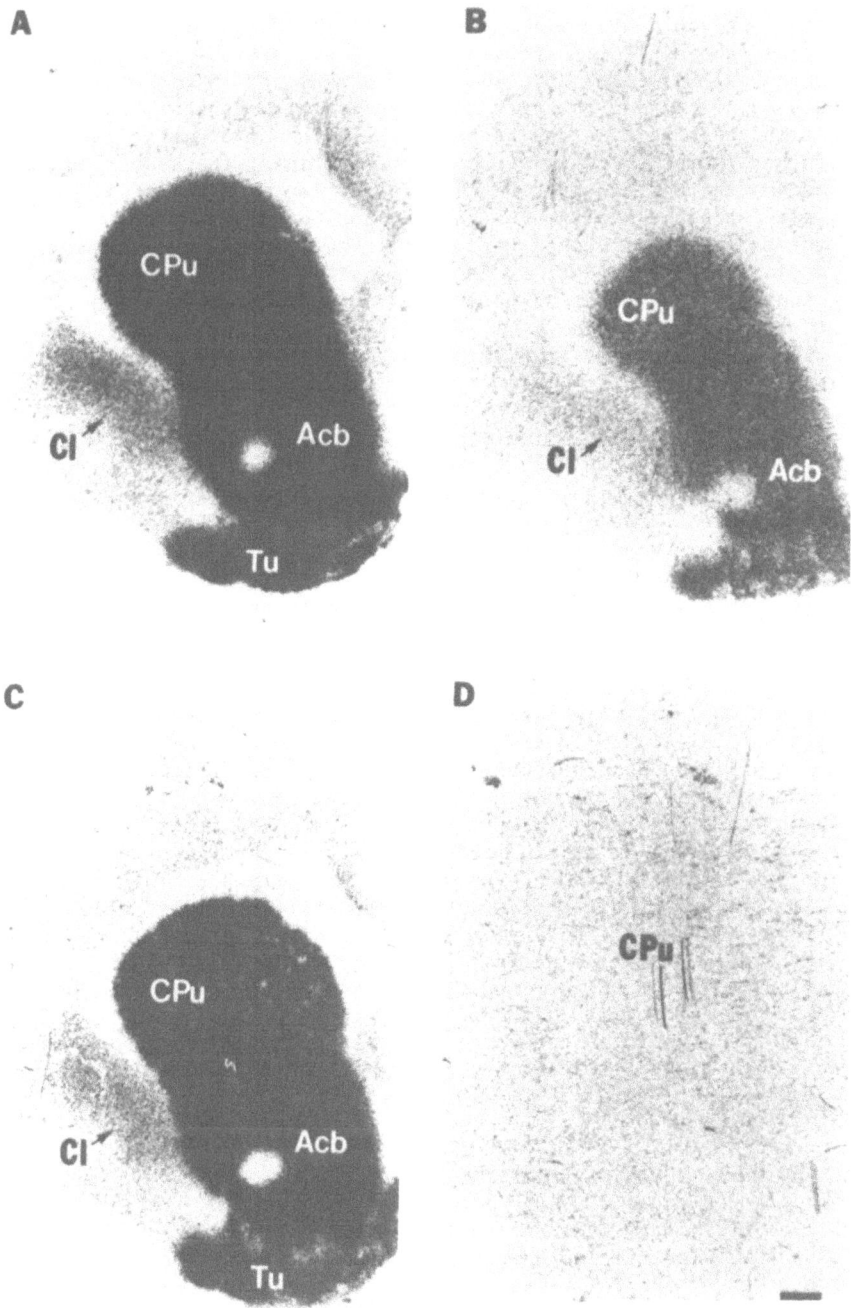

Figure 2. Guanine nucleotide effects on agonist (SKF 38393)
displacement of [^{3}H]-SCH 23390.   A. Photomicrograph of an
autoradiogram which was produced by incubating with 1nM
[^{3}H]-SCH 23390 (see Table I).   Note the high concentrations
of autoradiographic grains (D-1 receptors) in the caudate-
putamen (CPu), nucleus accumbens (Acb), and olfactory tubercle
(Tu).   In addition, note the moderate concentration of D-1
receptors in the claustrum (Cl).   B. Shown here is an
autoradiogram incubated under identical conditions with the
addition of 10^{-7}M SKF 38393 in order to displace the high
affinity agonist state of [^{3}H]-SCH 23390 binding to D-1

(Continued overleaf)

receptors. Note the significant decrease in D-1 receptor density; thus, predominantly all the high affinity receptors are not being labeled. C. Photomicrograph of an autoradiogram incubated with 1nM [^{3}H]-SCH 23390, 10^{-7}M SKF 38393, and 10 micromolar Gpp(NH)p in order to shift the high affinity state to the low affinity state. As can be seen, there is now dramatic increase in D-1 receptor density from that shown in B; thereby, visually demonstrating, the shift from a high to low agonist affinity state with the addition of guanine nucleotides. D. This autoradiogram is from a section which was incubated in the additional presence of 10^{-6}M fluphenazine to define nonspecific binding. The relative paucity of autoradiographic grains indicates that the binding seen in A, B and C is due to specific [^{3}H]-SCH 23390 binding. Bar = 500 microns.

1984; Leff et al., 1985; Grigoriadis and Seeman, 1985; Creese and Leff, 1982; Freedman et al., 1981b; George et al., 1985; Leff and Creese, 1985; Seeman et al., 1985; Schulz et al., 1985b). Saturating concentrations of 5'-guanylylimidodiphosphate (Gpp(NH)p), a non-metabolizable analog of GTP, is able to steepen and shift the agonist/[^{3}H]-antagonist competition curves to the right (Creese et al., 1984; Leff et al., 1985; Seeman et al., 1985; Schulz et al., 1985b). This data is best explained by a ternary complex, similar to that proposed for other cyclase linked receptors (Limbird, 1981).

By performing detailed displacement experiments with dopamine agonists on [^{3}H]-SCH 23390 and [^{3}H](-)-sulpiride binding (Dawson et al., 1985b, unpublished observations), and by using quantitative autoradiography it was shown that the displacement curves were shallow and exhibited GTP effects in several areas of the brain. Thereby, suggesting distinct or possibly predominant populations of either the high or low agonist affinity state of the D-1 or D-2 receptor as has been shown for the muscarinic cholinergic receptors (Wamsley et al., 1980,1984). Figures 2 and 3 illustrate the dramatic shift of the high affinity state to the low affinity state by adding Gpp(NH)p to the incubation media for the D-1 and D-2 receptor, respectively. The capability to distinguish high and low agonist states of the dopamine receptors will enable investigators to more precisely determine and characterize receptor alterations due to either a pathologic process or an experimental paradigm.

LOCALIZATION OF DOPAMINE RECEPTORS

Based on several biochemical and anatomical studies, dopamine cell bodies and terminal fields have been localized within the CNS to eight major systems by the Falck-Hillarp formaldehyde histofluorescence (Haggendal and Malmfors, 1963; Anden et al., 1964, 1965, 1966a,b; Bertler et al., 1964; Dahlstrom and Fuxe, 1964) and the glyoxylic acid histofluorescence (Lindvall et al., 1973; Lindvall and Bjorklund, 1974a,b) techniques (for review see Moore and Bloom, 1978; Bjorklund and Lindvall, 1984). These eight systems, according to Bjorklund and Lindvall (1984), are: (1) the mesostriatal, (2) mesolimbocortical, (3) diencephalospinal, (4) periventricular, (5) incertohypothalamic, (6) tuberohypophyseal, (7) periglomerular, and (8) the retinal dopamine systems. Other systems undoubtedly exist, such as the hippocampal DA system (Bischoff et al., 1979; Scatton et al., 1980; Ishikawa et al., 1982), but the aforementioned systems are firmly established. The DA containing systems in the CNS with their respective cells of origin and projections, and the relative density of the D-1 and D-2 receptors in

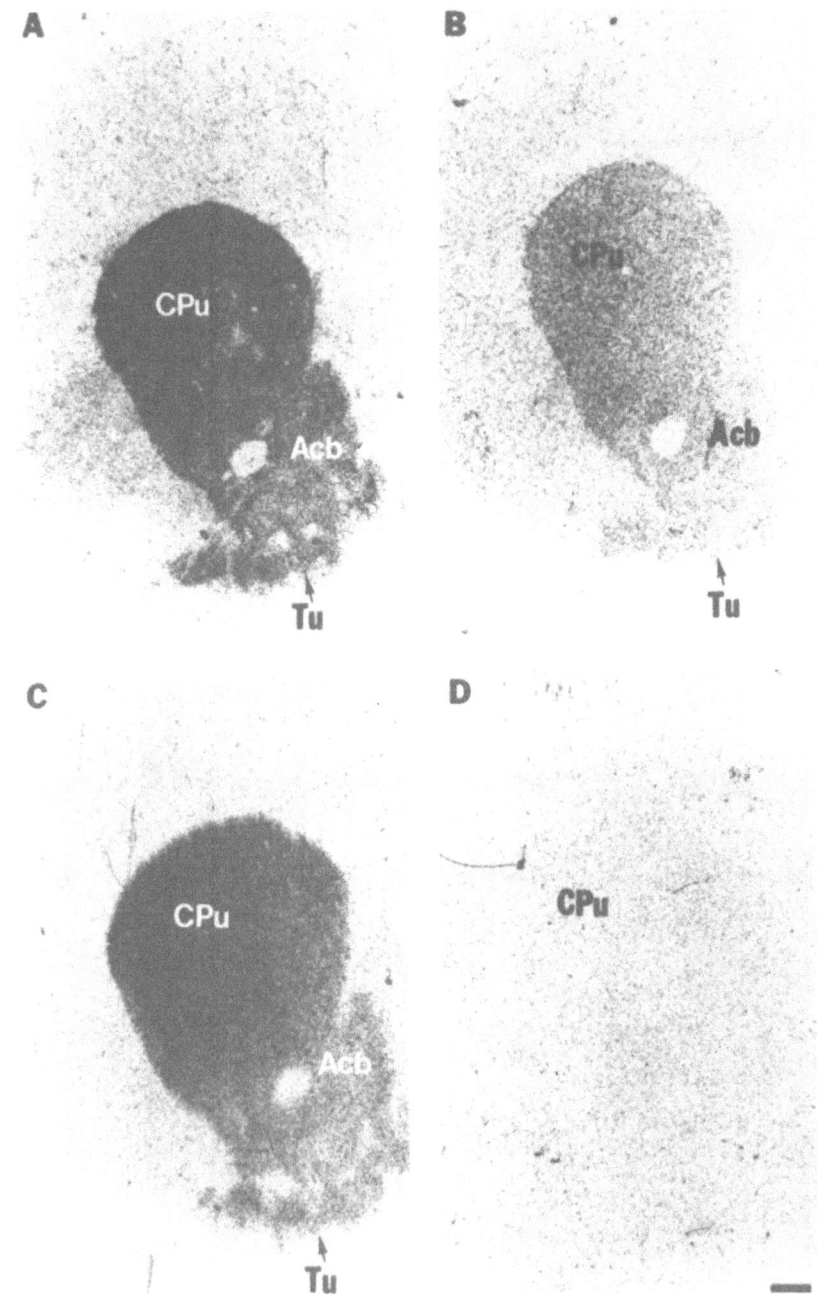

Figure 3. Guanine nucleotide effect on agonist (ADTN) displacement of [^{3}H](−)-sulpiride. A. Total binding (15nM [^{3}H](−)-sulpiride − see Table I). B. 15nM [^{3}H](−) sulpiride + 10^{-7}M ADTN. C. 15nM [^{3}H](−)-sulpiride + 10^{-7}M ADTN + 10^{-6}M Gpp(NH)p. D. 15nM [^{3}H](−)-sulpiride + 10^{-6}M haldol. Please see Figure 2, in which similar experiments were performed for the D−1 receptor, for explanation of figures and discussion of guanine nucleotide effect. Abbreviations are caudate-putamen (CPu), nucleus accumbens (Acb), olfactory tubercle (Tu). Bar = 500 microns.

Table III. Dopamine Containing Systems in the CNS and Dopamine D-1 and D-2 Receptor Densities

System	Cells of Origin[1]	Projections[1]	D-1 Receptor Density[2]	D-2 Receptor Density[3]
1. Mesostriatal	Substantia Nigra Pars Compacta (A9)		++	++
		Caudate-Putamen	++++	++++
		Globus Pallidus	++	+
		Islands of Calleja	+++	++++
		Subthalamic Nucleus	++	+
	Ventral Tegmental Area (A10)		+	+
		Accumbens Nucleus	++++	+++
		Interstitial Nucleus of the Stria Terminalis	-	
		Olfactory Tubercle	++++	++++
2. Mesolimbocortical	A9		++	++
		Supragenual Anteromedial Cortex	+,++	-
	A10		+	+
		Lateral Habenular Nucleus	-	+
		Lateral Septal Nucleus	+,++	+
		Pregenual Anteromedial Cortex	+,++	-
		Suprarhinal Cortex	+	-
		Ventral Entorhinal Cortex	++	+,++
	A9 and A10		+,++	+,++
		Amygdala	+,++,+++	-

System	Cells of Origin[1]	Projections[1]	D-1 Receptor Density[2]	D-2 Receptor Density[3]
2. Mesolimbocortical	A9	Anterior Olfactory Nuclei	++	++
		Locus Coeruleus	++	-
		Olfactory Bulb	-	-
		Perirhinal Cortex	-	+++
		Piriform Cortex	+	-
		Temporal Cortex	+	-
3. Diencephalospinal	Dorsal Hypothalamus		-	+
	Posterior Hypothalamus		+	+
	Zona Incerta		+,++	-,+
	Caudal Thalamus (All)		+	-
		Spinal Cord	-	+
4. Periventricular	Mesencephalic			
	Periaqueductal Gray	Periaqueductal Gray	-	+
	Caudal Thalamus (All)	Medial Thalamus	+	-
		Hypothalamus	-,+	+
5. Incertohypothalamic	Zona Incerta	Zona Incerta	+,++	+
	Periventricular Hypo-thalamus (A11,A13,A14)	Preoptic Hypothalamus	-	-
		Periventricular Hypothalamus	-	-
		Septum	+,++	+

(continued)

Table III. (continued)

System	Cells of Origin[1]	Projections[1]	D-1 Receptor Density[2]	D-2 Receptor Density[3]
6. Tuberohypophyseal	Arcuate and Peri-ventricular Hypothalamic Nuclei (A12,A14)		-	+
		Median Eminence	-	-
		Pars Nervosa of the Pituitary	-	-
		Pars Intermedia of the Pituitary	-	+++
7. Periglomerular Dopamine Neurons	Olfactory Bulb (A16)		-	+++
		Dendritic Processes into Olfactory Glomeruli	?	+++
8. Retinal Dopamine	Inner Nuclear Layer of the Retina		?	?
		Local Dendritic Projections	?	?

[1] From Bjorklund and Lindvall, 1984. Receptor densities are as follows: [2]D-1 receptor (Dawson et al., in press) and unpublished observations) ++++ = 15 to 25; +++ = 5 to 15; ++ = 1.5 to 5.0; + = 0.1 to 1.5. [3]D-2 receptor (Gehlert and Wamsley, 1985 ++++ = 50 to 100 fmoles/mg tissue; +++ = 20 to 50; ++ = 5 to 20; + = 1 to 5;

these areas, based on quantitative autoradiography, are summarized in Table III.

In general, areas containing DA cell bodies, terminals and/or markers show the presence of either D-1 or D-2 receptors or both. The cells of origin, interestingly, contain low concentrations of D-1 and D-2 receptors, with the noted exception of the substantia nigra pars compacta which has moderate concentrations of both D-1 and D-2 receptors. In contrast are the projection areas which show the presence of receptors ranging from very high to low or nonexistent in number. The close correlation of DA fibers or other markers with DA receptors could not be observed in a few areas. The substantia nigra pars reticulata and the central amygdaloid nucleus are good illustrative cases. The substantia nigra pars reticulata (Figure 4) has been shown to contain very low amounts of dopamine fibers and the central amygdaloid nucleus (Figure 5) has only moderate concentrations of dopamine fibers (Bjorklund and Lindvall, 1984). When one compares the density of DA receptors in these areas marked discrepancies occur, in that the substantia nigra pars reticulata has very high concentrations of D-1 receptors and the central amygdaloid nucleus shows only a low number of both D-1 and D-2 receptors. The existence of differences between the distribution of fibers and neurotransmitters and the location of receptors has been called the "mismatch" problem (Kuhar, 1985a). Several reasons for these discrepancies exist and the reader is referred to Kuhar (1985a) for further discussion.

The meso-limbocortical system illustrated in the schematics shown in Figure 4 is a fairly well characterized dopaminergic system. The cell bodies of origin are located in the ventral tegmental area and the medial substantia nigra pars compacta (Bjorklund and Lindvall, 1984). These areas have relatively low numbers of both D-1 and D-2 receptors associated with them, but are known to contain a dense population of dopamine cell bodies. The projection areas are numerous and include the anterior olfactory nuclei and piriform cortex; regions in which we were able to show low to moderate concentrations of D-1 receptors. Another projection area, the amygdaloid nuclear complex is only labeled by [^{3}H]-SCH 23390 and Figure 5 shows the location and density of D-1 receptors in several amygdaloid nuclei (Dawson et al., in press). In this projection, the DA fibers are concentrated in the intercalated, basolateral and central nuclei and moderate to sparse DA terminals are located in the cortical and medial nuclei (Lindvall and Bjorklund, 1984). Some evidence exists for a minor DA innervation of the hippocampus (Bischoff et al., 1979; Scatton et al., 1980; Ishikawa et al., 1982) and as shown in Figure 4, there is a low density of D-2 receptors in the lacunosum molecular layer of the hippocampus and a low density of D-1 receptors in the molecular layer of the dentate gyrus.

The mesocortical projections of the mesencephalic DA cell bodies are distributed into terminal fields with the deeper laminae containing a denser dopaminergic innervation. This same pattern is observed for D-1 receptors (Dawson et al., in press) with a low density of receptors existing in the superficial laminae, but with lamina VI containing approximately twice as many receptors as the superficial laminae (Figure 4). Furthermore, the distribution of D-1 receptors closely parallels DA innervation of the prefrontal cortex, in that the D-1 receptors are concentrated in the anteromedial and suprarhinal systems (shown in Figure 4). No significant amounts of D-2 receptors could be observed in the neocortex, except for a low population in laminae II and III of the anterior cingulate cortex (unpublished observations). However, when using an iodinated ligand, [^{125}I]-iodosulpride, to localize D-2 receptors, it was shown that these receptors are widely distributed in

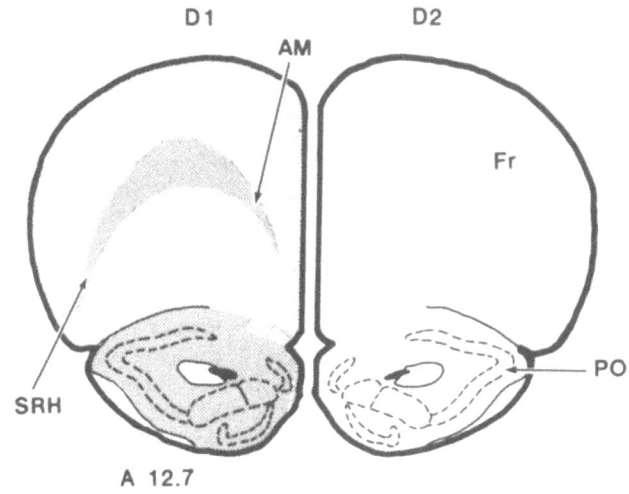

D1   D2

AM

Fr

SRH

PO

A 12.7

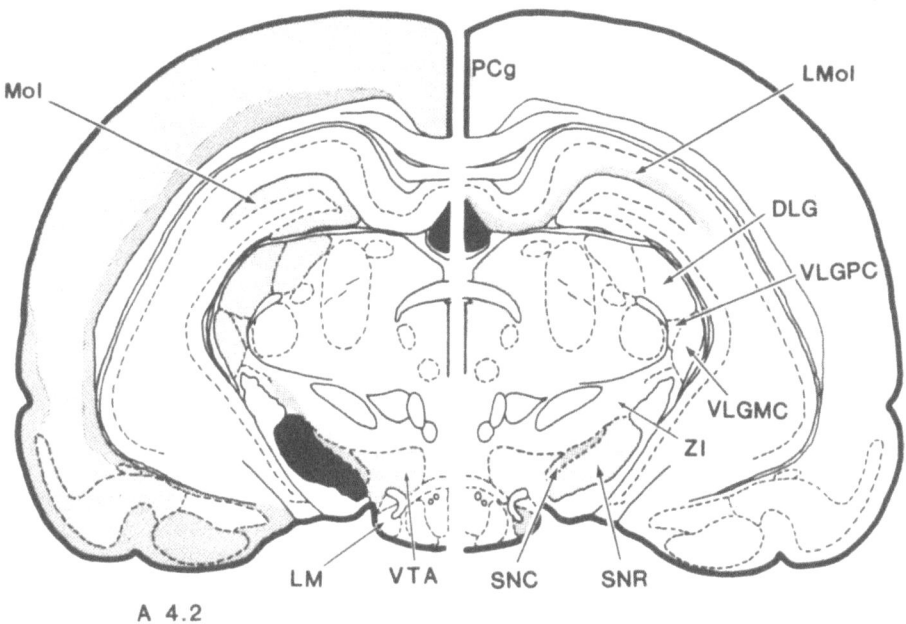

Mol

PCg

LMol

DLG

VLGPC

VLGMC

ZI

LM   VTA   SNC   SNR

A 4.2

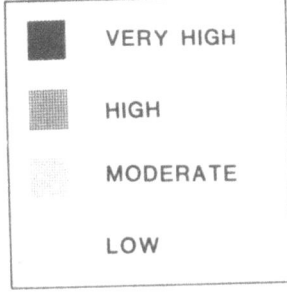

VERY HIGH

HIGH

MODERATE

LOW

Figure 4. Schematic comparison of D-1 and D-2 receptors in the rat forebrain. Receptor densities are as follows: D-1 receptors (Dawson et al., in press) Very High - 50 to 100 fmol/mg tissue; High - 20 to 50; Moderate - 5 to 20; Low - 1 to 5; D-2 receptors (Gehlert and Wamsley, 1985 and unpublished observations) Very High - 15 to 25; High - 5 to 15; Moderate - 1.5 to 5.0; Low - 0.1 to 1.5. Abbreviations are: AM - anteromedial system of the prefrontal cortex; SRH - suprarhinal system of the prefrontal cortex; Fr - prefrontal cortex; PO - primary olfactory cortex; Mol - molecular layer of the dentate gyrus; PCg - posterior cingulate cortex; LMol - lacunosum moleculare layer of the hippocampus; DLG - dorsal lateral geniculate nucleus; VLGPC - ventral lateral geniculate nucleus, parvocellular part; VLGMC - ventral lateral geniculate nucleus, magnocellular part; ZI - zona incerta; SNR - substantia nigra pars reticulata; SNC - substantia nigra pars compacta; VTA - ventral tegmental area; LM - lateral mammillary nucleus. Areas were identified according to Paxinos and Watson, 1982.

the cortices (Martres et al., 1985a). These D-2 receptors have a very unique and distinct laminar distribution when comparing them with DA nerve terminals and the distribution of D-1 receptors, in that the D-2 receptors are concentrated in lamina V and have a sparse density in laminae I to III and VI (Martres et al., 1985b).

$[^3H]$-SCH 23390 and $[^3H]$-sulpiride were also used to localize D-1 and D-2 receptors, respectively, to human brain. High concentrations of both receptor subtypes could be found in the caudate and putamen (Figure 6). The substantia nigra pars reticulata contains a moderate concentration of D-1 receptors, whereas the substantia nigra pars compacta has low to moderate concentrations of both the D-1 and D-2 receptor. The globus pallidus (Figure 6) also has low to moderate concentrations of D-1 and D-2 receptors associated with it. The cortices contain low concentrations of only the D-1 receptor and these appear with a distinct laminar distribution. The D-1 receptors are mainly concentrated in the deeper laminae, especially lamina V (unpublished observations). No D-2 receptors could be observed in the cortices when using $[^3H]$-sulpiride.

DISCUSSION

Use of the various selective agents for the D-1 and D-2 receptor has led to increasing knowledge and insight into the role that DA plays in central nervous system transmission. Autoradiographic studies employing either $[^3H]$-SCH 23390 (Dawson et al., 1985, in press) or $[^{125}I]$-iodosulpride (Martres et al., 1985a,b) have allowed the localization of DA receptors to several areas of the brain where the existence of DA nerve terminals was known, but the demonstration of DA receptors was not possible until these agents became available. Dawson et al. (in press) were able to show that there are significant areas of overlap between the D-1 and D-2 receptor distributions, with either approximately equal numbers of these receptors or a predominance of one receptor subtype existing in discrete areas of the brain. Furthermore, there are areas of the brain that appear to exhibit exclusively one DA receptor subtype, such as the amygdaloid nuclear complex which contains only D-1 receptors and the pituitary which contains only D-2 receptors. These observations will hopefully guide future investigations in selecting anatomical sites to probe when studying the dopaminergic systems.

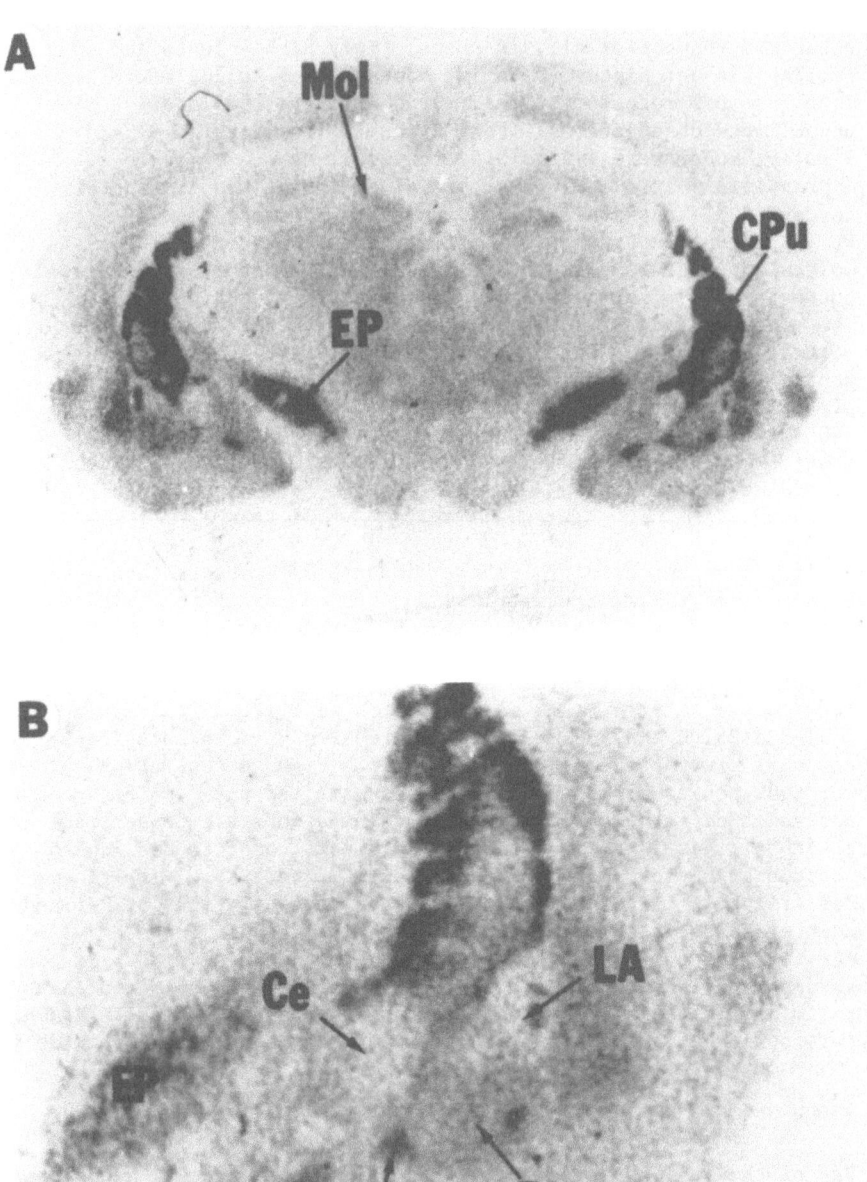

Figure 5.   A. Photomicrograph of [³H]-SCH 23390 (1nM) to
a slide mounted tissue section through an area of the
forebrain of the rat. Note the high density of D-1
receptors in the caudate-putamen (CPu), moderate density
in the entopeduncular nucleus (EP), and the low density
in the molecular layer of the dentate gyrus (Mol).
B. High power view of amygdaloid nuclear complex. Note
the low concentration of D-1 receptors in lateral nucleus
(LA) and the central amygdaloid nucleus (Ce), the moderate
density in the basolateral nucleus (BL), and the high density
in the intercalated nucleus (I).

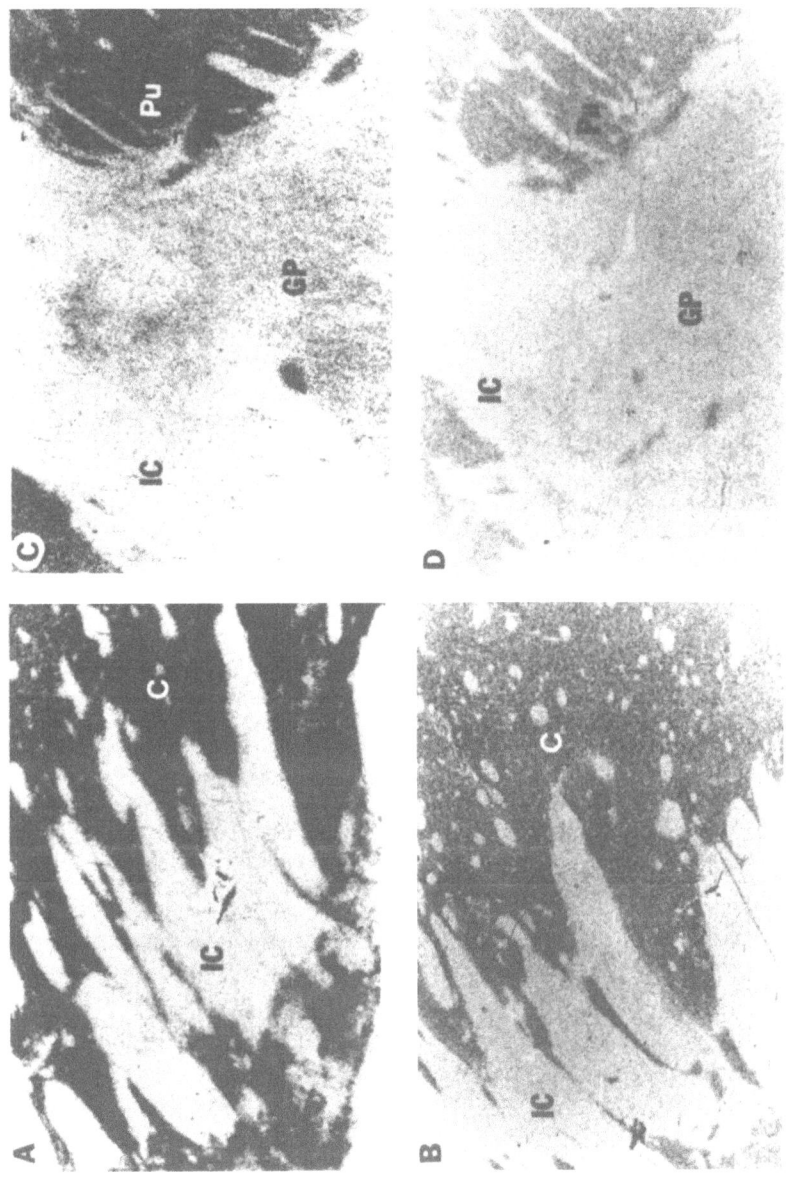

Figure 6. Dopamine receptors in human brain. A. Photomicrograph of an autoradiogram produced by incubating a section of human striatum with 15nM [^{3}H]-sulpiride. Note the high density of D-2 receptors in the caudate (C) and the relative lack of receptors in the internal capsule (IC). B. Shown in the photomicrograph is an autoradiogram produced by incubating a section of human striatum with 1nM [^{3}H]-SCH 23390. Note the high density of D-1 receptors in the caudate. C. Depicted here are D-2 receptors in the putamen (Pu) and globus pallidus (GP). D. Illustrated here are D-1 receptors in the putamen and globus pallidus.

The development and use of compounds which interact with the dopamine system, especially the more selective agents, has led to a better understanding of how stimulation of the dopamine receptor leads to a cellular response. As originally proposed by Kebabian and Calne (1979), D-1 receptors when stimulated by a dopamine agonist increase cAMP production via adenylate cyclase and D-2 receptors were unassociated with this enzyme. There is now a substantial amount of evidence indicating that agonist stimulation of the D-2 receptor decreases cAMP production via a decrease in adenylate cyclase activity (Onali et al., 1981, 1984; Enjalbert and Bockaert, 1983; Weiss et al., 1985). Furthermore, in an area which has been shown to contain moderate to high concentrations of D-1 receptors, the amygdaloid nuclear complex (Dawson et al., 1985, in press), there is no dopamine stimulated adenylate cyclase activity (Schulz et al., 1985a; Mailman et al., 1985). If this observation is substantiated, it will have far reaching implications, in that there appears to be a subpopulation of D-1 receptors which has a receptor coupling system unique from adenylate cyclase, thereby indicating the need for a further subdivision of dopamine receptor subtypes.

Another area currently being actively investigated is to determine and possibly correlate the cellular localization (i.e., presynaptic vs. postsynaptic) of the D-1 and D-2 receptor with anatomical, biochemical and physiological data. As with the controversy of the number of dopamine receptor subtypes, there is no consensus on the cellular localization of these receptors. A number of anatomical sites have been shown to contain dopamine receptors. Postsynaptic dopamine receptors are located, at least in part, on the cell bodies or dendrites of cholinergic interneurons where dopamine acts to inhibit acetylcholine release (Stoof et al., 1979). Evidence exists that a single type of DA receptor (probably D-2) mediates the dopaminergic influence on striatal cholinergic neuron activity (Scatton, 1982). DA receptors are found on the terminals of corticostriate fibers where dopamine exerts an inhibition of glutamate release (Roberts and Anderson, 1979). These receptors on the presynaptic terminals of corticostriate fibers are thought to be of the D-2 type since decortication to remove the corticostriate glutamate-containing pathway results only in the loss of $[^3H]$-spiperone binding but not adenylate cyclase activity (Schwarcz et al., 1978; Theodorou et al., 1981). Dopamine receptors are located on the terminals of strionigral and striopallidal gamma-aminobutyric acid (GABA) terminals which control GABA release (Reubi et al., 1977; Bergstrom and Walters, 1984), and striatal D-1 receptors may be influencing these striatonigral GABA neurons (Thierry et al., 1984). Cortical dopamine receptors are thought to be postsynaptic and of the D-1 subtype since lesions of the ascending DA neurons lead to enhanced DA-adenylate cyclase activity, suggesting that a denervation supersensitivity of the adenylate cyclase associated D-1 receptor occurs (Tassin et al., 1982). Our laboratory has been able to confirm the existence of postsynaptic D-1 receptors in the prefrontal cortex of the rat by showing approximately a 40% increase in the amount of $[^3H]$-SCH 23390 bound in 6-hydroxydopamine treated animals (intracerebro-ventricularly) versus control animals (unpublished observations).

There are a number of different putative anatomical locations for postsynaptic dopamine receptors as well as different hypothesized interactions and functions on various neurotransmitter systems. Other dopamine receptors (autoreceptors) are thought to exist on presynaptic dopamine terminals where dopamine acts to control its own synthesis and release (Cheramy et al., 1977). DA containing cell bodies and dendrites in the substantia nigra zona compacta and the ventral tegmental area contain these somatodendritic DA autoreceptors, such that receptor activation diminishes DA neurotransmission (Aghajanian and Bunney, 1977; Wang, 1981; White and Wang, 1984a). These dopamine autoreceptors exhibit the pharmacological characteristics of D-2 receptors (White and Wang, 1984b), but evidence exists that D-1 receptors may be presynaptic in these areas (Fujita et al., 1980). There are striatal dopamine receptors which modulate DA synthesis and release and studies provide support for both D-1 receptors (Cross and Wassington, 1981; Leff et al., 1981) and D-2 receptors (Helmreich et al., 1982; Lehmann et al., 1983; Hall et al., 1983; Stoof and Kebabian, 1981) being presynaptic in these areas. By combining the technique of autoradiography with selective lesions of various structures in the nigrostriatal pathway our laboratory has preliminary evidence that not only are there subpopulations of postsynaptic D-1 and D-2 receptors, but there are subpopulations of presynaptic D-1 and D-2 receptors (unpublished observations).

Dopamine receptor biochemistry and function appears to be amazingly more complex than originally hypothesized. Investigations, such as ours, will hopefully guide and possibly direct investigators on areas to probe for elucidating and ultimately garnishing a better understanding of DA physiology.

ACKNOWLEDGEMENTS

The authors wish to thank Linda Miller for her excellent secretarial skills and Allen Barnett for the generous donation of [^{3}H]-SCH 23390. The project was supported in part by grants from the Scottish Rite Foundation and from the Public Health Service (NS-22033). T.M. Dawson was a recipient of a PMA Medical Student Fellowship during the period when these investigations were performed. D.R. Gehlert is a recipient of a Pharmacological Research Award (PRAT) from the NIGMS.

REFERENCES

Aghajanian, G.K., and Bunney, B.S., 1977, Dopamine autoreceptors: Pharmacological characterization by microiontophoretic single-cell recording studies, Naunyn-Schmiedeberg's Arch. Pharmacol., 297:1-7.

Anden, N.E., Carlsson, A., Dahlstrom, A., Fuxe, K., Hillarp, N.A., and Larsson, K., 1964, Demonstration and mapping out of nigro-neostriatal dopamine neurons, Life Sci., 3:523-530.

Anden, N.E., Dahlstrom, A., Fuxe, K., and Larsson, K., 1965, Mapping out of catecholamine and 5-hydroxytrytamine neurons innervating the telencephalon and diencephalon, Life Sci., 4:1275-1279.

Anden, N.E., Dahlstrom, A., Fuxe, K., Larsson, K., Olson, L., and Ungerstedt, U., 1966a, Ascending monoamine neurons to the telencephalon and diencephalon, Acta. Physiol. Scand., 67:313-326.

Anden, N.E., Fuxe, K., Hamberger, B., and Hokfelt, T., 1966b, A quantitative study on the nigrostriatal dopamine neuron system in the rat, Acta. Physiol. Scand., 67:306-312.

Baudry, M., Martres, M.P., and Schwartz, J.C., 1977, In vivo binding [^{3}H]-pimozide in mouse striatum: Effects of agonists and antagonists, Life Sci., 21:1163-1170.

Baudry, M., Martres, M.P., and Schwartz, J.C., 1979, ^{3}H-Domperidone: A selective ligand for dopamine receptors, Naunyn-Schmiedeberg's Arch. Pharmacol., 308:231-237.

Beaulieu, M., Itoh, Y., Tepper, P., Horn, A.S., and Kebabian, J.W., 1984, N,N-disubstituted 2-aminotetralins are potent D-2 dopamine receptor agonists, Eur. J. Pharmacol., 105:15-21.

Bergstrom, D.A., and Walters, J.R., 1984, Dopamine attenuates the effects of GABA on single unit activity in the globus pallidus, Brain Res., 310:23-33.

Berkowitz, B.A., Zabko-Potapovich, B., Sherman, S., Hieble, J.P., Weinstock, J., and Ohlstein, E.H., 1984, Vascular effects of SK&F 83566: A selective dopamine (DA-1) receptor antagonist, Federation Proc., 43:743.

Bertler, A., Falck, B., Gottfries, C.G., Ljunggren, L., Rosengren, E., 1964, Some observations on adrenergic connections between mesencephalon and cerebral hemispheres, Acta. Pharmacol. Toxicol., 21:283-289.

Billard, W., Ruperto, V., Crosby, G., Iorio, L.C., and Barnett, A., 1984, Characterization of the binding of ^{3}H-SCH 23390, a selective D-1 receptor antagonist ligand, in rat striatum, Life Sci., 35:1885-1893.

Bischoff, S., Scatton, B., and Korf, J., 1979, Biochemical evidence for a transmitter role of dopamine in the rat hippocampus, Brain Res., 165:161-165.

Bjorklund, A., and Lindvall, O., 1984, Dopamine-containing systems in the CNS, in: "Handbook of Chemical Neuroanatomy, Vol. 2: Classical Transmitters in the CNS, Part I," A. Bjorklund and T. Hokfelt, eds., pp. 55-122, Elsevier Science Publishers, BC, Amsterdam.

Cheramy, A., Nieoullon, A., Michelot, R., and Glowinski, J., 1977, Effects of intranigral application of dopamine and substance P on the in vivo release of newly synthesized [^{3}H]-dopamine in the ipsilateral caudate nucleus of the cat, Neurosci. Lett., 4:105-109.

Christensen, A.V., Arnt, J., Hyttel, J., Larsen, J.J., and Svendsen, O., 1984, Pharmacological effects of a specific dopamine D-1 antagonist SCH 23390 in comparison with neuroleptics, Life Sci., 34:1529-1540.

Creese, I., and Leff, S.E., 1982, Dopamine receptors: A classification, J. Clin. Psychopharmacol., 2:329-335.

Creese, I., Schneider, R., and Snyder, S.H., 1977, ^{3}H-Spiroperidol labels dopamine receptors in pituitary and brain, Eur. J. Pharmacol., 46:377-381.

Creese, I., Sibley, D.R., and Leff, S.E., 1984, Agonist interactions with dopamine receptors: Focus on radioligand-binding studies, Federation Proc., 43:2779-2784.

Cross, A.H., and Waddington, J.L., 1981, Kainic acid lesions dissociate [^{3}H]-cis-flupentixol binding sites in rat striatum, Eur. J. Pharmacol., 71:327-332.

Dahlstrom, A., and Fuxe, K., 1964, Evidence for the existence of monoamine-containing neurons in the central nervous system. I. Demonstration of monoamines in the cell bodies of brain stem neurones, Acta. Physiol. Scand., 62(Suppl. 232):1-55.

Dandridge, P.A., Kaiser, C., Brenner, M., Gaitanopoulos, D., Davis, L.D., Webb, R.L., Foley, J.J., and Sarau, H.M., 1984, Synthesis, resolution, absolute stereochemistry, and enantioselectivity of 3',4'-dihydroxynomifensine, J. Med. Chem., 27:28-35.

Dawson, T.M., Gehlert, D.R., Yamamura, H.I., Barnett, A., and Wamsley, J.K., 1985a, D-1 dopamine receptors in the rat brain: Autoradiographic localization using [^{3}H]-SCH 23390, Eur. J. Pharmacol., 108:323-325.

Dawson, T.M., Gehlert, D.R., and Wamsley, J.K., 1985b, Quantitative autoradiographic demonstration of high and low affinity agonist binding of D-2 dopamine receptors, Clinical Res., 33:69A.

Dawson, T.M., Gehlert, D.R., McCabe, R.T., Barnett, A., and Wamsley, J.K., in press, D-1 dopamine receptors in the rat brain: A quantitative autoradiographic analysis, J. Neurosci.

Denef, C., and Follebouckt, J.J., 1978, Differential effects of dopamine antagonists on prolactin secretion from cultured rat pituitary cells, Life Sci., 23:431-436.

Enjalbert, A., and Bockaert, J., 1983, Pharmacological characterization of the D2 dopamine receptor negatively coupled with adenylate cyclase in rat anterior pituitary, Mol. Pharmacol., 23:576-584.

Euvard, C., Ferland, L., DiPaolo, T., Beaulieu, M., Labrie, F., Oberlander, C., Raynaud, J.P., and Boissier, J.R., 1980, Activity of two new potent dopaminergic agonists at the striatal and anterior pituitary levels, Neuropharmacol., 19:379-386.

Fields, J.Z., Reisine, T.D., and Yamamura, H.I., 1977, Biochemical demonstration of dopaminergic receptors in rat and human brain using [^{3}H]-spiroperidol, Brain Res., 136:578-584.

Flaim, K.E., Gessner, G.W., Crooke, S.T., Sarau, H.M., and Weinstock, J., 1985, Binding of a novel dopaminergic agonist radioligand [^{3}H]-Fenoldopam (SKF 82526) to D-1 receptors in rat striatum, Life Sci., 36:1427-1436.

Freedman, S.B., Mustafa, A.A., Poat, J.A., Senior, K.A., Wait, C.P., and Woodruff, G.N., 1981a, A study on the localization of [^{3}H]-Sulpiride binding sites on rat striatal membranes, Neuropharmacol., 20:1151-1155.

Freedman, S.B., Poat, J.A., and Woodruff, G.N., 1981b, Effect of guanine nucleotides on dopaminergic agonist and antagonist affinity for [^{3}H]-Sulpiride binding sites in rat striatal membrane preparations, J. Neurochem., 37:608-612.

Frey, E.A., Cote, T.E., Grewe, C.W., and Kebabian, J.W., 1982, [^{3}H]-Spiroperidol identifies a D-2 dopamine receptor inhibiting adenylate cyclase activity in the intermediate lobe of the rat pituitary gland, Endocrinol., 110:1897-1904.

Fujita, N., Saito, K., Iwatsubo, K., Hirata, A., Noguchi, Y., and Yoshida, H., 1980, Binding of [^{3}H]-apomorphine to striatal membranes prepared from rat brain after 6-hydroxydopamine and kainic acid lesions, Brain Res., 190:593-596.

Gehlert, D.R., and Wamsley, J.K., 1984, Autoradiographic localization of [^{3}H]-sulpiride binding sites in the rat brain, Eur. J. Pharmacol., 98:311-312.

Gehlert, D.R., and Wamsley, J.K., 1985, Dopamine receptors in the rat brain: Quantitative autoradiographic localization using [^{3}H]-sulpiride, Neurochem. Int., 4:717-723.

George, S.R., Watanabe, M., and Seeman, P., 1985, Dopamine D2 receptors in the anterior pituitary: A single population without reciprocal antagonist/agonist states, J. Neurochem., 4:1168-1177.

Goldberg, L.I., and Kohli, J.D., 1982, Peripheral post-synaptic dopamine (DA$_1$) receptors, in: "Advances in Dopamine Research," M. Kohsaka, T. Shohmori, Y. Tsukada and G.N. Woodruff, eds., pp. 41-49, Pergamon Press.

Grewe, C.W., Frey, E.A., Cote, T.E., and Kebabian, J.W., 1982, YM-09151-2: A potent antagonist for a peripheral D2-dopamine receptor, Eur. J. Pharmacol., 81:149-152.

Grigoriadis, D., and Seeman, P., 1985, Complete conversion of brain D2 dopamine receptors from high- to the low-affinity state for dopamine agonists, using sodium ions and guanine nucleotide, J. Neurochem., 6:1925-1935.

Haggendal, J., and Malmfors, T., 1963, Evidence of dopamine-containing neurons in the retina of rabbits, Acta. Physiol. Scand., 59:295-296.

Hahn, R.A., Wardell, J.R., Jr., Sarau, H.M., and Ridley, P.T., 1982, Characterization of the peripheral and central effects of SK&F 82526, a novel dopamine receptor agonist, J. Pharmacol. Exp. Ther., 223:305-313.

Hall, M.D., Jenner, P., Kelley, E., and Marsden, C.D., 1983, Differential anatomical location of [^{3}H]-N,n-propylnorapomorphine and [^{3}H]-spiperone binding sites in the striatum and substantia nigra of the rat, Br. J. Pharmacol., 79:599-610.

Helmreich, I., Reimann, W., Hertting, G., and Starke, K., 1982, Are presynaptic dopamine autoreceptors and postsynaptic dopamine receptors in the rabbit caudate nucleus pharmacologically different?, Neurosci., 7:1557-1566.

Hollt, V., Cztonkowiski, A., and Herz, A., 1977, The demonstration in vivo of specific binding sites for neuroleptic drugs in mouse brain, Brain Res., 130:176-183.

Hollt, V., and Schubert, P., 1978, Demonstration of neuroleptic sites in mouse brain by autoradiography, Brain Res., 151:149-153.

Horn, A.S., Tepper, P., Kebabian, J.W., and Beart, P.M., 1984, N-0434, a very potent and specific new D-2 dopamine receptor agonist, Eur. J. Pharmacol., 99:125-126.

Howlett, D.R., Morris, H., and Nahorski, S.R., 1979, Anomalous properties of [^{3}H]-spiperone binding sites in various areas of the rat limbic system, Mol. Pharmacol., 15:506-514.

Hyttel, J., 1983, SCH 23390 - the first selective dopamine D-1 antagonist, Eur. J. Pharmacol., 91:153-154.

Iorio, L.C., Barnett, A., Leitz, F.H., Houser, V.P., and Korduba, C.A., 1983, SCH 23390, a potential benzazepine antipsychotic with unique interactions on dopaminergic systems, J. Pharmacol. Exp. Ther., 226:462-468.

Ishikawa, K., Ott, T., and McGaugh, J.L., 1982, Evidence for dopamine as a transmitter in dorsal hippocampus, Brain Res., 232:222-226.

Jastrow, T.R., Richfield, E., and Gnegy, M.E., 1984, Quantitative autoradiography of [^{3}H]-sulpiride binding sites in rat brain, Neurosci. Lett., 51:47-53.

Jenner, P., and Marsden, C.D., 1981, Substituted benzamide drugs as selective neuroleptics, Neuropharmacology, 20:1285-1293.

Jenner, P., Theodorou, A., and Marsden, C.D., 1982, Specific receptors for substituted benzamide drugs in brain, in: "The Benzamides. Pharmacology, Neurobiology and Clinical Aspects," M. Stanly and J. Rostrosen, eds., Vol. 35, pp. 109-141, Raven Press, New York.

Kaiser, C., and Jain, T., 1985, Dopamine receptors: Functions, subtypes and emerging concepts, Medicinal Res. Rev., 5:145-229.

Kebabian, J.W., and Calne, D.B., 1979, Multiple receptors for dopamine, Nature, 277:93-96.

Klemm, N., Murrin, L.C., and Kuhar, M.J., 1979, Neuroleptic and dopamine receptors: Autoradiographic localization of [^{3}H]-spiperone in rat brain, Brain Res., 169:1-9.

Kuhar, M.J., 1985a, The mismatch problem in receptor mapping studies, Trends Neurosci., 8:190-191.

Kuhar, M.J., 1985b, Receptor localization with the microscope, in: "Neurotransmitter Receptor Binding," H.I. Yamamura, S.J. Enna and M.J. Kuhar, eds., pp. 153-177, Raven Press, New York.

Kuhar, M.J., Murrin, L.C., Malouf, A.T., and Klemm, N., 1978, Dopamine receptor binding in vivo: The feasibility of autoradiographic studies, Life Sci., 22:203-210.

Kuhar, M.J., and Yamamura, H.I., 1975, Light autoradiographic localization of cholinergic muscarinic receptors in rat brain by specific binding of a potent antagonist, Nature (London), 253:560-561.

Kuhar, M.J., and Yamamura, H.I., 1976, Localization of cholinergic muscarinic receptors in rat brain by light microscopic radioautography, Brain Res., 110:229-243.

Laduron, P., and Leysen, J., 1977, Specific in vivo binding of neuroleptic drugs in rat brain, Biochem. Pharmacol., 26:1003-1007.

Lazareno, S., and Nahorski, S.R., 1982, Selective labeling of dopamine (D_2) receptors in rat striatum by [^{3}H]-domperidone but not by [^{3}H]-spiperone, Eur. J. Pharmacol., 81:273-285.

Leff, S., Adams, L., Hyttel, J., and Creese, I., 1981, Kainic lesion
dissociates striatal dopamine receptor radioligand binding sites,
Eur. J. Pharmacol., 70:71-75.

Leff, S.E., Chen, A., and Creese, I., 1984, Sulpiride isomers exhibit
reversed stereospecificity for D-1 and D-2 dopamine receptors in the
CNS, Neuropharmacol., 23:589-590.

Leff, S.E., Hamblin, M.W., and Creese, I., 1985, Interactions of dopamine
agonists with brain D_1 receptors by ^{3}H-antagonists. Evidence for the
presence of high and low affinity agonist-binding states, Mol.
Pharmacol., 27:171-183.

Leff, S.E., and Creese, I., 1985, Interactions of dopaminergic agonists
and antagonists with dopaminergic D_3 binding sites in rat striatum,
Mol. Pharmacol., 27:184-192.

Lehmann, J., Briley, M., and Langer, S.Z., 1983, Characterization of
dopamine autoreceptor and ^{3}H-spiperone binding sites in vitro with
classical and novel dopamine receptor agonists, Eur. J. Pharmacol.,
88:11-26.

Leysen, J.E., Awouters, F., Kennis, L., Laduron, P.M., Vandenberk, J.,
and Janssen, P.A.J., 1981, Receptor binding profile of R 41 468, a
novel antagonist at 5-HT$_2$ receptors, Life Sci., 28:1015-1022.

Limbird, L.E., 1981, Activation and attenuation of adenylate cyclase. The
role of GTP-binding proteins as macromolecular messengers in
receptor-cyclase coupling, Biochem. J., 195:1-13.

Lindvall, O., and Bjorklund, A., 1974a, The organization of the ascending
catecholamine neuron systems in the rat brain as revealed by the
glyoxylic acid fluorescence method, Acta. Physiol. Scand., Suppl.,
412:1-48.

Lindvall, O., and Bjorklund, A., 1974b, The glyoxylic acid fluorescence
histochemical method: A detailed account of the methodology for the
visualization of central catecholamine neurons, Histochem.,
39:97-127.

Lindvall, O., Bjorklund, A., Hokfelt, T., and Ljungdahl, A., 1973,
Application of the glyoxylic acid method to vibratome sections for
improved visualization of central catecholamine neurons, Histochem.,
35:31-38.

Mailman, R.B., Schulz, D.W., and Kilts, C.D., 1985, "D$_1$-like" dopamine
receptors: Recognition sites with selectivity for SCH 23390 that are
not linked to adenylate cyclase, Soc. Neurosci. Abstr., 11:313.

Martres, M.P., Bouthenet, M.L., Sales, N., Sokoloff, P., and Schwartz,
J.C., 1985a, Widespread distribution of brain dopamine receptors
evidenced with [^{125}I]Iodosulpride, a highly selective ligand,
Science, 228:752-755.

Martres, M.P., Sales, N., Bouthenet, M.L., and Schwartz, J.C., 1985b,
Localisation and pharmacological characterization of D-2 dopamine
receptors in rat cerebral neocortex and cerebellum using
[^{125}I]Iodosulpride, Eur. J. Pharmacol., 118:211-219.

Memo, M., Govoni, S., Carboni, E., Travucchi, M., and Spano, P.F., 1983,
Characterization of stereospecific binding of [^{3}H](-)Sulpiride, a
selective antagonist at dopamine-D$_2$ receptors, in rat CNS,
Pharmacol. Res. Comm., 15:191-199.

Moore, R.Y., and Bloom, F.E., 1978, Central catecholamine neuron systems:
Anatomy and physiology of the dopamine systems, Ann. Rev. Neurosci.,
1:129-169.

Morgan, D.G., Marcusson, J.O., and Finch, C.E., 1984, Contamination
serotonin-2 binding sites by an alpha-1 adrenergic component in
assays with [^{3}H]-spiperone, Life Sci., 34:2507-2514.

Murrin, L.C., and Kuhar, M.J., 1979, Dopamine receptors in the rat
frontal cortex: An autoradiographic study, Brain Res., 177:279-285.

Nakajima, T., Iwata, K., Kuruma, I., and Nakamura, K., 1983, Binding
study of ^{3}H-RO 22-1319, a new potent antipsychotic drug - evidence
for a D$_2$ antagonist, Jpn. J. Pharmacol., 33(Suppl.):197P.

O'Connor, S.E., and Brown, R.A., 1982, The pharmacology of sulpiride - a dopamine receptor antagonist, Gen. Pharmacol., 13:185-193.

Onali, P., Schwartz, J.P., and Costa, E., 1981, Dopaminergic modulation of adenylate cyclase stimulation of vasoactive intestinal peptide (VIP) in anterior pituitary, Proc. Natl. Acad. Sci., 78:6531-6534.

Onali, P., Olianas, M.C., and Gessa, G.L., 1984, Selective blockade of dopamine D-1 receptors by SCH 23390 discloses striatal dopamine D-2 receptors mediating the inhibition of adenylate cyclase in rats, Eur. J. Pharmacol., 99:127-128.

Palacios, J.M., Niehoff, D.L., and Kuhar, M.J., 1981, [^{3}H]-Spiperone binding sites in the brain: Autoradiographic localization of multiple receptors, Brain Res., 213:277-289.

Palacios, J.M., and Wamsley, J.K., 1984, Catecholamine receptors, in: "Handbook of Chemical Neuroanatomy, Volume 3: Classical Transmitters and Transmitter receptors in the CNS, Part II," A. Bjorklund and T. Hokfelt, eds., pp. 325-351, Elsevier Science Publishers, BC Amsterdam.

Paxinos, G., and Watson, C., 1982, "The Rat Brain in Stereotaxic Coordinates", Academic Press, Inc., New York.

Reubi, J.C., Iversen, L.L., and Jessell, T.M., 1977, Dopamine selectively increases [^{3}H]-GABA release from slices of rat substantia nigra in vitro, Nature, 268:653-654.

Roberts, P.J., and Anderson, S.D., 1979, Stimulatory effect L-glutamate and related amino acids on [^{3}H]-dopamine release from rat striatum: An in vitro model for glutamate actions, J. Neurochem., 32:1539-1545.

Scatton, B., 1982, Further evidence for the involvement of D$_2$, but not D$_1$ dopamine receptors in dopaminergic control of striatal cholinergic transmission, Life Sci., 31:2883-2890.

Scatton, B., and Dubois, A., 1985, Autoradiographic localization of D$_1$ dopamine receptors in the rat brain with [^{3}H]-SKF 38393, Eur. J. Pharmacol., 111:145-146.

Scatton, B., Simon, H., Moal, M.L., and Bischoff, S., 1980, Origin of dopaminergic innervation of the rat hippocampal formation, Neurosci. Lett., 18:125-131.

Schulz, D.W., Stanford, E.J., and Mailman, R.B., 1985a, Subcellular localization of the SCH 23390 receptor: Dissociation from dopamine-stimulated adenylate cyclase, Soc. Neurosci. Abstr., 11:888.

Schulz, D.W., Stanford, E.J., Wyrick, S.W., and Mailman, R.B., 1985b, Binding of [^{3}H] SCH 23390 in rat brain: Regional distribution and effects of assay conditions and GTP suggest interactions at a D$_1$-like dopamine receptor, J. Neurochem., 45:1601-1611.

Schulz, D.W., Wyrick, S.D., and Mailman, R.B., 1985c, [^{3}H] SCH 23390 has the characteristics of a dopamine receptor ligand in the rat central nervous system, Eur. J. Pharmacol., 106:211-212.

Schwarcz, R., Creese, I., Coyle, J.T., and Snyder, S.H., 1978, Dopamine receptors localized on cerebral cortical afferents to rat corpus striatum, Nature, 271:766-768.

Seeman, P., Ulpian, C., Grigoriadis, D., Pri-Bar, I., and Buchman, O., 1985, Conversion of dopamine D1 receptors from high to low affinity for dopamine, Biochem. Pharmacol., 34:151-152.

Setler, P.E., Sarau, H.M., Zirkle, C.L., and Saunders, H.L., 1978, The central effects of a novel dopamine agonist, Eur. J. Pharmacol., 50:419-430.

Shepperson, N.B., Duval, N., Massingham, R., and Langer, S.Z., 1982, Differential blocking effects of several dopamine receptor antagonists for peripheral pre- and postsynaptic dopamine receptors in the anesthetized dog, J. Pharmacol. Exp. Ther., 221:753-761.

Sidhu, A., and Kebabian, J.W., 1985, An iodinated ligand identifying the D-1 dopamine receptor, Eur. J. Pharmacol., 113:437-440.

Sokoloff, P., Brann, M., Redouane, K., Martres, M.P., Schwartz, J.C., Bouthenet, M.L., Sales, N., Mann, A., Hamdi, P., Wermuth, C.G., Roy, J., and Morgat, J.L., 1985, The use of [^{3}H](-)-DO 710 as a selective dopaminergic ligand for binding and autoradiographic studies, Eur. J. Pharmacol., 107:243-251.

Sokoloff, P., Martres, M.P., and Schwartz, J.C., 1980, Three classes of dopamine receptor (D-2, D-3, D-4) identified by binding studies with ^{3}H-apomorphine and ^{3}H-domperidone, Naunyn-Schmiedeberg's Arch. Pharmacol., 315:89-102.

Sumners, C., Dijkstra, D., DeVries, J.B., and Horn, A.S., 1981, Neurochemical and behavioral profiles of five dopamine analogues, Naunyn-Schmiedeberg's Arch. Pharmacol., 316:304-310.

Stoof, J.C., and Kebabian, J.W., 1981, Opposing roles for D-1 and D-2 dopamine receptors in efflux of cyclic AMP from rat neostriatum, Nature, 294:366-368.

Stoof, J.C., and Kebabian, J.W., 1984, Two dopamine receptors: Biochemistry, physiology and pharmacology, Life Sci., 35:2281-2296.

Stoof, J.C., Thieme, R.E., Vrijmoed-de-Vries, M.C., and Mulder, A.H., 1979, In vitro acetylcholine release from rat caudate nucleus: A model for testing drugs with dopamine receptor activity, Naunyn-Schmiedeberg's Arch. Pharmacol., 309:119-124.

Tassin, J.P., Simon, H., Herve, D., Blanc, G., LeMoal, M., Glowinski, J., and Bockaert, J., 1982, Non-dopaminergic fibers may regulate dopamine-sensitive adenylate cyclase in the prefrontal cortex and nucleus accumbens, Nature, 295:696-698.

Terai, M., Usuda, S., Kuroiwa, I., Noshiro, O., and Maeno, H., 1983, Selective binding of YM-09151-2, a new potent neuroleptic, to D-2 dopaminergic receptors, Jpn. J. Pharmacol., 33:749-755.

Theodorou, A., Crockett, M., Jenner, P., and Marsden, C.D., 1979, Specific binding of [^{3}H]-sulpiride to rat striatal preparations, J. Pharm. Pharmacol., 31:424-426.

Theodorou, A., Reavill, C., Jenner, P., and Marsden, C.D., 1981, Kainic acid lesions of striatum and decortication reduce specific [^{3}H]-sulpiride binding in rats, so D-2 receptors exist post-synaptically on corticostriate afferents and striatal neurons, J. Pharm. Pharmacol., 33:439-444.

Thierry, A.M., Tassin, J.P., and Glowinski, J., 1984, Biochemical and electrophysiological studies of the mesocortical dopamine system, in, "Monoamine Innervation of Cerebral Cortex," L. Descarries, T.R. Reader, and H.H. Jasper, eds., pp. 233-261, Alan R. Liss, Inc., New York.

Titus, R.D., Kornfeld, E.C., Jones, N.D., Clemens, J.A., Smalstig, E.B., Fuller, R.W., Hahn, R.A., Hynes, M.D., Mason, N.R., Wong, D.T., and Foreman, M.M., 1983, Resolution and absolute configuration of an ergoline-related dopamine agonist, trans-4,4a,5,6,7,8,8a,9-octahydro-5-propyl-1H(or 2H)-pyrazolo[3,4-g]quinoline, J. Med. Chem., 26:1112-1116.

Wamsley, J.K., and Palacios, J.M., 1983, Apposition techniques of autoradiography for microscopic receptor localization, in, "Current Methods in Cellular Neurobiology," J. Barker and J. McKelvy, eds., pp. 241-268, John Wiley and Sons, New York.

Wamsley, J.K., Zarbin, M.A., Birdsall, N.J.M., and Kuhar, M.J., 1980, Muscarinic cholinergic receptors: Autoradiographic localization of high and low affinity agonist binding sites, Brain Res., 200:1-12.

Wamsley, J.K., Zarbin, M.A., and Kuhar, M.J., 1984, Distribution of muscarinic cholinergic high and low affinity agonist binding sites: A light microscopic autoradiographic study, Brain Res. Bull., 12:233-243.

Wang, R.Y., 1981, Dopaminergic neurons in the rat ventral tegmental area. II. Evidence for autoregulation, Brain Res. Rev., 3:141-152.

Weiss, S., Sebben, M., Garcia-Sainz, J., and Bockaert, J., 1985, D_2-dopamine receptor-mediated inhibition of cyclic AMP formation in striatal neurons in primary culture, Mol. Pharmacol., 27:595-599.

White F.J., and Wang, R.Y., 1984a, A10 dopamine neurons: Role of autoreceptors in determining firing rate and sensitivity to dopamine agonists, Life Sci., 34:1161-1170.

White, F.J., and Wang, R.Y., 1984b, Pharmacological characterization of dopamine autoreceptors in the rat ventral tegmental area: Microiontophoretic studies, J. Pharmacol. Exp. Ther., 231:275-280.

Woodruff, G.N., and Freedman, S.B., 1981, Binding of [³H]-sulpiride to purified rat striatal synaptic membranes, Neurosci., 6:407-410.

Unnerstall, J.R., Niehoff, D.L., Kuhar, M.J., and Palacios, J.M., 1982, Quantitative receptor autoradiography using [³H] Ultrofilm: Application to multiple benzodiazepine receptors, J. Neurosci. Meth., 6:59-73.

Yamamura, H.I., Enna, S.J., and Kuhar, M.J., 1985, "Neurotransmitter Receptor Binding," Raven Press, New York.

Yamamura, H.I., Kuhar, M.J., and Snyder, S.H., 1974, In vivo identification of muscarinic cholinergic receptor binding in rat brain, Brain Res., 80:170-176.

Young, W.S., III, and Kuhar, M.J., 1979, A new method for receptor autoradiography: [³H]-opioid receptors in rat brain, Brain Res., 179:255-270.

Zahniser, N.R., and Dubocovich, M.L., 1983, Comparison of dopamine receptor sites labeled by [³H]S-sulpiride and [³H]-spiperone in striatum, J. Pharmacol. Exp. Ther., 227:592-599.

DOPAMINE D_1-RECEPTOR BINDING IN THE LIVING HUMAN BRAIN

Göran Sedvall[1], Lars Farde[1], Sharon Stone-Elander[2] and Christer Halldin[2]

Department of Psychiatry, Psychology[1] and Pharmacy[2], Karolinska Hospital
Stockholm, Sweden

The neurotransmitter dopamine, which plays a role in the pathophysiology of Parkinson's Disease and possibly also schizophrenia, mediates its actions in the brain by at least two types of receptors (Kebabian and Calne, 1979). By the activation of the dopamine D_1 receptor, dopamine stimulates the enzyme adenylate cyclase (Kebabian et al., 1972). Activation of the dopamine D_2 receptor is not, or is possibly negatively, coupled to a dopamine sensitive adenylate cyclase (Stoof and Kebabian, 1984). Many behavioural effects of dopamine seem to be mediated by D_2 receptors (Peroutka and Snyder, 1980). The analysis of D_2 receptors has been facilitated by the availability of selective drugs interacting with this receptor. The exploration of dopamine D_1 receptor characteristics and function has been hampered by the previous lack of such pharmacological tools.

Recently two halogenated benzazepines, SCH 23390 and SKF R-83566, have been described as potent dopamine D_1 receptor antagonists (Iorio et al., 1983, O'Boyle and Waddington, 1985). ^{3}H-SCH 23390 has been shown to bind selectively to D_1 receptors in membranes of the rat and human striatum (Raisman et al., 1985, Schultz et al., 1985). The distribution of ^{3}H-SCH 23390 binding in the rat brain has also been examined by in vitro autoradiography (Dawson et al., 1985).

The possibility of studying subtypes of dopamine receptors in the living human brain has been provided by positron emission tomography (PET) and the availability of dopamine D_2 selective ligands (Sedvall et al., 1983, Farde et al., 1985 a,b). An attempt to localize D_1 receptors to the striatum of a rhesus monkey has also been made using [76]Br SCH 23390 (Friedman et al., 1985). In this study, we used ^{11}C labelled SCH 23390 and PET to provide the first localization of dopamine D_1 receptor binding in the living human brain. ^{11}C-SCH 23390 was prepared by methylation of demethylated SCH 23390 using ^{11}C methyliodide (Halldin et al., 1986). ^{11}C-SCH 23390 (8 mCi, S.A. 300 Ci/nmol) was rapidly injected intravenously into a 32 year old male healthy volunteer. A four ring PET system (PC-384) was used to obtain quantitative data on the regional concentration of the ligand within seven sections of the brain (Farde et al., 1985 a). The study comprised 13 sequential scans of each section during a period of 63 minutes. Regional activity corrected for ^{11}C decay was measured in each region of interest and plotted versus time. After injection of ^{11}C-SCH 23390 there was a rapid accumulation of radioactivity in the brain. The highest level was obtained in the dopamine rich caudate putamen with a maximum reached within 10 min (Fig. 1). The radioactivity later declined with a half life of about 30 min. Within the dopamine poor cerebellum the radioactivity was substantially lower than in the caudate-putamen during the whole experiment. The maximal cerebellar activity was reached within 5 min and subsequently declined at a faster rate than the activity in the caudate-putamen. At 35 min after injection the radioactivity in the putamen was threefold higher than in the cerebellum. The caudate putamen was clearly delineated in the PET scan images by the conspicuous accumulation of radioactivity (Fig. 2). There was also a significantly higher amount of radioactivity in most neocortical areas than in the cerebellum. Prefrontal and limbic cortical areas apparently did not contain more radioactivity than the temporal and parietal cortical areas.

The present in vivo analysis in man demonstrated a heterogenous distribution of ^{11}C-SCH 23390 within the brain. The high accumulation of the ligand in the caudate putamen, a region known to contain a high level of dopamine stimulated adenylate cyclase activity indicates that this region has the highest density of dopamine D_1 receptors in the human brain. The distribution of ^{11}C-SCH 23390 within the caudate putamen was similar to the distribution of the selective D_2 receptor ligand raclopride (Farde et al., 1985a). With the low resolution technique used in this study this finding does not exclude the possibility that D_1 and D_2 receptors within the caudate-putamen belong to functionally different dopamine regulated systems. There was also a conspicuous distribution

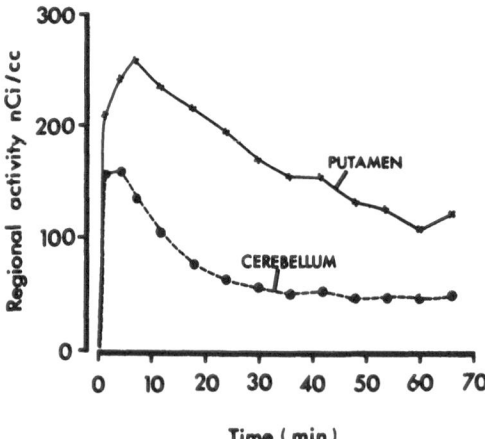

Figure 1. Time course for accumulation of radioactivity in the putamen and the cerebellum in a 32 years old healthy man after i.v. injection of 8 mCi ^{11}C-SCH 23390.

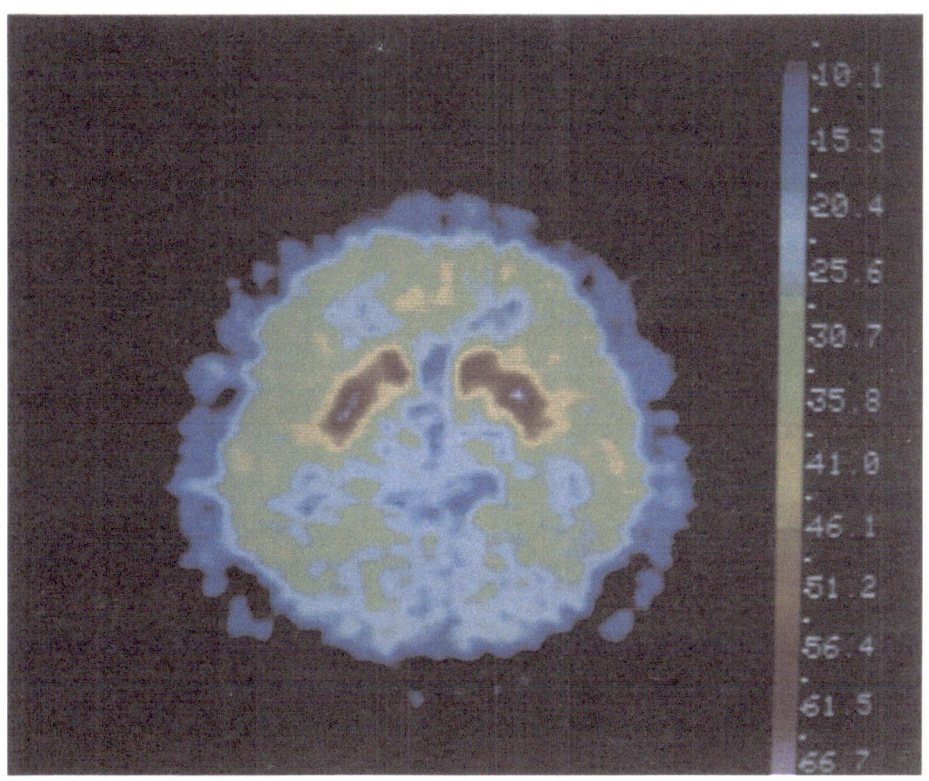

Figure 2. PET scan through the caudate putamen level, showing integrated radioactivity during the interval 10-69 min after the i.v. injection of 8 mCi ^{11}C-SCH 23390 into a healthy man. The scale shows the relationship between colour and relative amount of radioactivity.

of ^{11}C-SCH 23390 to neocortex but not cerebellar cortex. Whether this radioactivity reflects specific binding has to be further evaluated. SCH 23390 has been shown to have affinity for 5-HT$_2$-sensitive ^{3}H-spiperone binding sites in the rat brain and to antagonize effects of 5-HT in vascular smooth muscle and brain (Hyttel, 1983, Hicks et al., 1984). It is unlikely that the cortical accumulation of ^{11}C-SCH 23390 represents nonspecific binding since nonspecific binding of ^{3}H SCH 23390 in vitro was found to be similar in all regions of the rat brain (Schultz et al., 1985). The accumulation of ^{11}C-SCH 23390 in the neocortical areas differed markedly from the low degree of distribution of the D$_2$ receptor antagonist raclopride to these brain areas. If the accumulation of ^{11}C-SCH 23390 in the neocortical areas reflects D$_1$ receptor binding the results accordingly indicate different distribution patterns of D$_1$ and D$_2$ receptors in some regions of the human brain. In summary, the present results support the view that ^{11}C-SCH 23390 has a high affinity for D$_1$ receptors in the human caudate-putamen. The results indicate that ^{11}C-SCH 23390 and the previously described D$_2$ receptor ligand ^{11}C-raclopride will be useful as selective tools for the analysis of subtypes of dopamine receptors in the living human brain.

ACKNOWLEDGEMENTS

Demethylated SCH 23390 was kindly supplied by Dr. Allan Barnett, Schering Plough Co., Bloomfield, New Jersey, U.S.A. Britt-Marie Berggren, Kjerstin Lind, Birgit Lonn and Dr. Frits-Axel Wiesel supplied skillful technical assistance. Support by the Swedish Medical Research Council, The Bank Sweden Tercentenary Fund, Bergvalls Foundation, Jeansson's Foundation, the Soderstrom-Konigska Foundation and the Karolinska Institute.

REFERENCES

Dawson, T.M., Gehlert, D.R., Yamamura, H.I., Barnett, A. and Wamsley, J.K., 1985, D$_1$ dopamine receptors in the rat brain: Autoradiographic localization using ^{3}H SCH 23390, Eur. J. Pharmacol., 108:323-325.

Farde, L., Ehrin, E., Eriksson, L., Greitz, T., Hall, H. Hedstrom, C.G., Litton, J-E. and Sedvall, G., 1985, Substituted benzamides as ligands for visualization of dopamine receptor binding in the human brain by positron emission tomography, Proc. Natl. Acad. Sci., 82:3863.

Farde, L., Hall, H., Ehrin, E. and Sedvall, G., 1985, Quantitative analysis of dopamine D$_2$ receptor binding in the living human brain by PET, Science, 231:258.

Flaim, K.E., Gessner, G.W., Crooke, S.T., Sarau, H.M., and Weinstock, J., 1985, Binding of a novel dopaminergic agonist radioligand ^{3}H-fenlodopam (SKF 82526) to D$_1$ receptors in rat striatum, Life Sci., 36:1427-1436.

Friedman, A., Dejesus, O.T., Woolverton, W.L., van Moffaert, G., Goldberg, L.I., Prasad, A., Barnett, A. and Dinerstein, R., 1985, Positron tomography of radio-brominated analog of the D$_1$/DA$_1$ antagonist, SCH 23390, Eur. J. Pharmacol. 108:327.

Halldin, C., Stone-Elander, S., Farde, L., Ehrin, E., Fasth, K.J., Langstrom, B. and Sedvall, G., 1986, Preparation of ^{11}C labelled SCH 23390 for the in vivo analysis of dopamine D_1 receptors by positron emission tomography, J. Appl. Radiochem. Isotop, In press.

Hicks, P.E., Schoemaker, H. and Langer, S.Z., 1984, 5HT-receptor antagonist properties of SCH 23390 in vascular smooth muscle and brain, Eur. J. Pharmacol., 105:339-342.

Hyttel, I., 1984, Functional evidence of selective dopamine D_1 receptor blockade by SCH 23390, Neuropharmacol., 23:1395-1401.

Iorio, L.C., Barnett, A., Leitz, F.H., Houser, V.P., Korduba, C.A., 1983, SCH 23390, a potential benzazepine antipsychotic with unique interactions on dopaminergic systems, J. Pharmacol. Exp. Ther., 226:462-468.

Kebabian, J.W. and Calne, D.B., 1979, Multiple receptors for dopamine, Nature 277:93-96.

Kebabian, J.W., Petzold, G.L. and Greengard, P., 1972, Dopamine-sensitive adenylate cyclase in caudate nucleus of rat brain, and its similarity to the "dopamine receptor", Proc. Nat. Acad. Sci., 69, No. 8, 2145-2149.

Peroutka, S.J. and Snyder, S.H., 1980, Relationship of neuroleptic drug effects at brain dopamine, serotonin, alpha-adrenergic, and histamine receptors to clinical potency, Am. J. Psychiatry 173:12, 1518-1522.

Raisman, R., Cash, R., Ruberg, M., Javoy-Agid, F. and Agid, Y., 1985, Binding of ^{H}3-SCH 23390 to D_1 receptors in the putamen of control and parkinsonian subjects, Eur. J. Pharmacol., 113:467.

Sedvall, G., Blomqvist, G., dePaulis, S., Ehrin, E., Eriksson, L., Farde, L., Greitz, T. Hedstrom, C.G., Ingvar, D.H., Litton, J.E., Nilsson, J.L.G., Stone-Elander, S., Widen, L., Wiesel, F.A. and Wik, G., 1983, 11-C-labelled benzamides as ligands for imaging of dopamine receptors in the human brain, 1983 ACNP Annual Meeting, San Juan, December 12-16.

Stoof, J.C. and Kebabian, J.W., 1984, Two dopamine receptors: Biochemistry, physiology and pharmacology, Life Sci., 35:2281-2296.

ENANTIOMERIC ANALOGUES OF SCH 23390 AS NEW PROBES FOR
BEHAVIORAL INTERACTIONS BETWEEN D_1 AND D_2 DOPAMINERGIC
FUNCTION

John L. Waddington, Anthony G. Molloy, Kathy M.
O'Boyle and Marcellina Mashurano

Department of Clinical Pharmacology
Royal College of Surgeons in Ireland
St. Stephen's Green
Dublin 2, Ireland

INTRODUCTION

The recent identification of the first selective D_1
dopamine (DA) receptor antagonist, the l-phenyl-lH-3-
benzazepine derivative SCH 23390 (Iorio et al., 1983; Hyttel,
1983; Cross, et al., 1983; O'Boyle and Waddington, 1984a), was
an event eagerly awaited as the final piece in a psychopharmacological jigsaw that had for some time remained incomplete.
The now widely accepted designation of D_1 and D_2 subtypes of
DA receptor (Kebabian and Calne, 1979; Seeman, 1980; Leff and
Creese, 1983; Waddington, et al., 1986) arose in the absence
of selective D_1 antagonists. Therefore, such a drug was
clearly required to substantiate any functional distinctions
between these subtypes, in the classical manner of previous
schemes for heterogeneity in non-DAergic receptor populations.
In the years immediately preceding the introduction of SCH
23390, indirect and correlational data were interpreted as
indicating a pre-potent role for D_2 receptors in the mediation
of the majority of typical behavioral and neurochemical
actions of dopamine agonist and antagonist drugs, and the D_1
receptor relegated from such considerations (Kebabian and
Calne, 1979; Seeman, 1980; Leff and Creese, 1983; Creese et
al., 1983; Laduron, 1983).

Unfortunately, studies with SCH 23390 have failed to
reveal the double dissociation that might have been expected
in comparison with selective D_2 antagonists. For example, if
typical DA agonist-induced stereotyped behavior is indeed a
D_2-stimulated syndrome that is sensitive to blockade by
selective D_2 antagonists, then these responses might be
expected to show resistance to blockade by SCH 23390.
Numerous studies have now shown that SCH 23390 is a highly
potent antagonist of stereotyped behaviors such as sniffing
and locomotion induced by the typical DAergic agonists
apomorphine or amphetamine (Iorio et al., 1983; Molloy and
Waddington, 1984; Christensen et al., 1984; Mailman et al.,
1984). Indeed, SCH 23390 potently blocks stereotyped behavior

induced by the selective D_2 agonist RU 24213 (Pugh et al., 1985). This raises questions as to the selectivity of action of SCH 23390 <u>in vivo</u>, or prompts us to reconsider the functional role of D_1 receptors and whether D_1 and D_2 dopaminergic mechanisms invariably constitute functionally independent processes (Molloy and Waddington, 1984; Pugh et al., 1985).

SCH 23390 and its structural analogue the D_1 partial agonist SK&F 38393 (Setler et al., 1978; Waddington et al. 1982), have been the only tools available for influencing the D_1 receptor with any degree of selectivity. The purposes of this article are to describe the properties of some newer selective D_1 agents, and to characterize behavioral responses to a D_1 agonist in the intact adult rat.

R- AND S-SK&F 83566 AND OTHER NEW 1-PHENYL-1H-3-BENZAZEPINES AS SELECTIVE D_1 AGENTS

SK&F 38393 is a 7,8-dihydroxy-1-phenyl-2,3,4,5-tetrahydro-1H-3-benzazepine and SCH 23390 its 7-chloro, 3-methyl analogue. These two agents, a partial D_1 agonist and D_1 antagonist respectively, therefore differ only in the nature of their 7- and 3- substituents. We have investigated further a series of benzazepine analogues differing only in substituents at these apparently critical positions: SK&F 77174 (7-H-3-H); SKF&F 83692 (7-H-3-CH_3); SK&F 75670 (7-OH-3-CH_3); SK&F 85257 (7-CH_3-3-H) and SK&F 83566 (7-Br-3-CH_3). Additionally, as the 1-phenyl-1H-3-benzazepines are chiral compounds, we have also investigated the stereoselectivity of receptor interactions using the resolved <u>R</u>- and <u>S</u>- enantiomers of SK&F 83566.

These drugs were compared for their activity to displace the binding of ^{3}H-SCH-23390 to D_1 receptors in post-mortem human putamen (0.3-0.8nM ^{3}H-SCH 23390; specific binding defined by 100nM piflutixol, O'Boyle and Waddington,1985a). Results were contrasted with our previous measures of their affinities for rat striatal D_1 and D_2 receptors, assayed using ^{3}H-piflutixol and ^{3}H-spiperone respectively (O'Boyle and Waddington, 1984a,b; O'Boyle and Waddington, 1985b). K_i values for the benzazepines at these sites are presented in Table 1 together with values for typical reference compounds.

In human putamen, the binding of ^{3}H-SCH 23390 shows characteristics similar to those previously described for rat striatum (Billard et al., 1984); thus, it is displaced by unlabelled SCH 23390, by dopamine and by non-selective dopamine antagonists such as flupenthixol and fluphenazine, but negligibly by selective D_2 antagonists such as domperidone and sulpiride, or by a range of non-dopaminergic agents (O'Boyle and Waddington, 1985a). This D_1 profile for displacement of ^{3}H-SCH 23390 binding is very similar to that of ^{3}H-piflutixol (r = 0.84, p < 0.005) but distinct from that of ^{3}H-spiperone (r = 0.41, NS) over the range of compounds compared in Table 1. It is beyond the scope of this article to discuss the relationships between structure and affinity for D_1 receptors within this benzazepine series, other than in the most general terms. They have been discussed in detail elsewhere in relation to their displacement of ^{3}H-piflutixol vs ^{3}H-spiperone binding (O'Boyle and Waddington, 1984b,

Table 1. Displacement of ^{3}H-SCH 23390 from Human Brain
D$_1$ Receptors, in Comparison with Displacement
of ^{3}H-Piflutixol and ^{3}H-Spiperone

Displacing agent	K$_i$ (nM)		
	^{3}H-SCH 23390	^{3}H-PIF	^{3}H-SPIP
Flupenthixol	12	0.8	1.0
Fluphenazine	49	19	1.0
Domperidone	2,750	>5,000	0.3
Sulpiride	>50,000	>50,000	109
Dopamine	1,300	23,300	778
SK&F 77174	898	590	22,900
SK&F 38393	735	1,390	12,600
SK&F 83692	538	165	1,300
SK&F 75670	132	1,400	30,600
SK&F 85257	169	75	7,300
SCH 23390 (R)	1.3	0.7	1,080
SK&F 83566 (R)	2.7	1.4	1,200
SK&F 83566 (S)	1,470	425	5,100
3,4-DHNOM (R)	24,700	---	---
3,4-DHNOM (S)	3,600	---	---

Data are means of 2-5 separate estimations

1985b). The actions of these analogues to displace ^{3}H-SCH-
23390 were similar to those using ^{3}H-piflutixol, with the
exception that the 7-OH-3-CH$_3$ compound (SK&F 75670) was a
somewhat more potent displacer of the former than of the
latter. Generally, 7-substituents, particularly halogens,
were critical determinants of affinity for D$_1$ but not D$_2$
receptors, over a range of some three orders of magnitude.
Conversely, 3-substituents had somewhat less marked effects,
and their influence extended to affinity for D$_2$ as well as D$_1$
receptors.

We have previously reported that, in rat striatum, the D$_1$
affinity of the chiral benzazepine agonist SK&F 38393 (O'Boyle
and Waddington, 1984a) and antagonist SK&F 83566 (O'Boyle and
Waddington, 1984b) resides stereoselectively in the R- but not
the S- enantiomer; weak residual affinity for the D$_2$ receptor
showed negligible enantioselectivity. In human brain ^{3}H-SCH
23390 was potently and stereoselectively displaced by R- but
not by S- SK&F 83566, with more than 500-fold separation
between the enantiomers. There was some stereoselective
displacement of ^{3}H-SCH 23390 by the enantiomers of 3,4-
dihydroxynomifensine (3,4-DHNOM) (Dandridge et al., 1984),
with the greater activity residing in the S-antipode.

These structural and stereochemical considerations relate
not just to affinity, as revealed in ligand binding assays;
they extend, within the limited range investigated, to
intrinsic pharmacological activity in terms of transition from
partial agonist to full antagonist activity in appropriate
neurochemical assays (O'Boyle and Waddington, 1985b; Dandridge
et al., 1984; Itoh et al., 1984; Kaiser et al., 1982). Their
behavioral significance will be discussed below.

Table 2. Behavioral Counts For the Induction of Sn, Gr and Gr$_i$ by SK&F 38393

	mg/kg	Sn	Gr	Gr$_i$
Vehicle		3.0+0.8	1.2+0.3	0.1+0.1
SK&F 38393	2.5	2.0+0.6	1.4+0.7	1.8+1.1
	10.0	4.3+0.9	6.8+1.0[a]	3.1+0.8[a]
	40.0	6.0+0.4[a]	7.3±1.5[a]	2.7±0.5[a]

[a], $p < 0.05$ vs. vehicle; n=4-10

ENANTIOMERIC INDUCTION OF GROOMING AND OTHER BEHAVIORS BY R- AND S-SK&F 38393

The only available selective D$_1$ receptor stimulant, the partial agonist SK&F 38393, has been assumed to be essentially inert in terms of behavioral response in the intact adult rat; it fails to induce the stereotypies and locomotion of typical DA agonists (Setler et al., 1978; Waddington et al., 1982). Under particular experimental conditions, however, we have found SK&F 38393 to be behaviorally active. Following a period of prolonged habituation to the observation cage, and with the use of a rapid time sampling behavioral check list procedure for assessment, SK&F 38393 induced quantifiable episodes of fragmented, discontinuous and non-stereotyped sniffing, rearing and locomotor behavior, interpolated between episodes of a particularly prominent grooming response (Molloy and Waddington, 1984; Molloy and Waddington, 1985a). The locomotor response, like rearing, is generally fragile behavior, and some of its characteristics have been outlined previously (Molloy and Waddington, 1985a; Molloy et al., 1986). Described here are some of the characteristics of SK&F 38393-induced grooming, in comparison with sniffing (Sn) behavior; the term grooming (Gr) is used in a very general sense, while intense grooming (Gr$_i$) refers to a characteristic response whereby the snout may be washed with the front paws before vigorous grooming of the flank and/or trunk by plunging the snout into the body fur.

Table 2 shows the dose-dependent induction of Sn, Gr and Gr$_i$ in animals given 2.5-40.0 mg/kg s.c. racemic SK&F 38393, in comparison with vehicle-injected animals. Data are behavioral counts + S.E.M. derived by summing the number of 5 sec. observation windows in which the indicated behavior was noted, over the period of 30-60 min after challenge for Sn, and over 20-40 min after challenge for Gr and Gr$_i$; these procedures are described in more detail elsewhere (Molloy and Waddington, 1985, 1985a, 1986).

These responses to 40.0 mg/kg SK&F 38393 were subjected to a preliminary pharmacological characterization using 30 min s.c. pretreatments with haloperidol (HAL, 0.25 mg/kg), sulpiride (SULP, 100 mg/kg), naloxone (NAL, 10 mg/kg) and ketanserin (KET, 10 mg/kg). Each of the behaviors of Sn, Gr and Gr$_i$ was blocked by this dose of haloperidol. Sulpiride, however, potentiated Gr and GR$_i$ responses, while it reduced counts for Sn. Naloxone attenuated Gr and Gr$_i$ but spared Sn, while ketanserin attenuated Sn without influencing Gr and Gr$_i$ (Table 3).

	mg/kg	Sn	Gr	Gr_i
Vehicle		1.3+0.5	0.2+0.1	0.0+0.0
SK&F 38393	40.0	7.0+0.8[a]	3.2+0.6[a]	1.4+0.2[a]
+ HAL	0.25	0.3+0.2*	1.3+0.2*	0.3+0.2*
+ SULP	100.0	1.6+0.7*	5.2+0.2*	2.3+0.5
+ NAL	10.0	5.5+1.3	1.8+0.3	0.5+0.2*
+ KET	10.0	2.4+0.8*	3.3+0.6	2.0+0.4

a, p<0.05 vs. vehicle; *, p<0.05 vs. SK&F 38393; n=6-17

The comparative effects of 20 mg/kg of the R- and S-enantiomers of SK&F 38393, in terms of the induction of these behaviors, are shown in Table 4. There appeared to be little induction of Sn by S-SK&F 38393, with this effect residing in the R-enantiomer. While Gr was also induced by R-SK&F 38393, there was some activity in its S-antipode; this involved the induction of grooming of the face with the forepaws. The induction of Gr_i showed complete enantioselectivity, being induced by R- but not by S- SK&F 38393.

These responses to R-SK&F 38393 were characterized further using 30 min pretreatments with SCH 23390, the R- and S- enantiomers of the related D_1 antagonist SK&F 83566, and metoclopramide (MET). As shown in Table 4, all three of the behaviors of Sn, Gr and Gr_i were blocked by as little as 100 μg/kg SCH 23390. There was no such blockade associated with S-SK&F 83566, and Gr and Gr_i responses were in fact increased by this pretreatment. All three behaviors were dose-dependently blocked by 40-200 μg/kg R-SK&F 83566 with complete enantioselectivity. There was no significant effect of metoclopramide (1.0-5.0 mg/kg) on Sn or Gr, while the induction of Gr_i was antagonized.

Table 4. Behavioral Responses to R- and S- SK&F 38393
          and the Influence of Selective Antagonists

	mg/kg	Sn	Gr	Gr_i
Vehicle		2.4+0.5	1.2+0.3	0.1+0.1
S-SK&F 38393	20.0	4.1+0.8	3.2+0.6[a]	0.1+0.1
R-SK&F 38393	20.0	11.1+0.6[a]	4.0+0.3[a]	1.8+0.2[a]
+ SCH 23390	0.1	1.4+0.5*	1.7+0.5*	0.1+0.1*
+ S-SK&F 83566	0.2	10.2+1.6	7.3+1.7*	3.5+0.5
+ R-SK&F 83566	0.04	7.4+1.6	4.0+0.8	1.8+0.8
	0.2	1.2+0.4*	1.8+0.6*	0.6+0.2*
4+ MET	1.0	12.6+0.6	4.3+0.4	0.8+0.4*
	5.0	8.6+1.2	2.9+0.5	0.5+0.3*

a, p<0.01 vs. vehicle; *, p<0.05 vs. R-SK&F 38393; n=4-38.

PHARMACOLOGICAL CHARACTERIZATION OF BEHAVIORAL RESPONSES TO
SK&F 38393

The induction of Sn, Gr and Gr_i by the D_1 agonist SK&F
38393 was readily blocked by a moderate dose of the typical
neuroleptic haloperidol, an antagonist that preferentially
blocks D_2 receptors but which has some D_1 antagonist
activity (Seeman, 1980). This confirms an important general
DAergic component in these responses to SK&F 38393.
Sulpiride, a selective D_2 antagonist, enhanced the induction
of Gr and Gr_i, while Sn was reduced. This would suggest that
selective D_2 blockade has no consistent effect on the range of
behaviors induced by SK&F 38393. However, the elevated
induction of Gr and GR_i in the presence of sulpiride might
artefactually reduce counts for Sn by response competition,
and other possibilities will be discussed below. The action
of the opiate antagonist naloxone to attenuate Gr and Gr_i,
while at first sight unexpected, might in fact have been
predicted. Grooming is a behavior that can be induced by
environmental situations such as novelty (Jolles et al.,
1979), and by various neuropeptides such as ACTH (Isaacson et
al., 1983). Grooming induced by ACTH can be blocked by
fluphenazine and haloperidol, indicating a DAergic mechanism
in the expression of this response; it can also be blocked by
naloxone (Isaacson et al., 1983), suggesting a general
opiatergic influence on the expression of grooming that might
underlay the present effect. Such a process would be
consistent with the failure of naloxone to influence SK&F
38393-induced Sn. The action of the 5-HT_2 antagonist
ketanserin to attenuate SK&F 38393-induced Sn may be similarly
explained, as apomorphine-induced Sn is also attenuated by
this drug (Tricklebank et al., 1985). This suggests a general
serotonergic influence on the expression of Sn, consistent
with the ability of a range of serotonergic manipulations to
influence DA-mediated behaviors (Gerson and Baldessarini,
1980). Irrespective of these considerations, the double-
dissociation between the actions of naloxone and ketanserin on
Gr/Gr_i and Sn argues against a general opiatergic or
serotonergic action of SK&F 38393 in their induction.

There was significant and substantial separation between
the enantiomers of SK&F 38393 for the induction of Sn and Gr_i;
in the latter case, behavioral activity showed complete
enantioselectivity for R - but not S- SK&F 38393. This
parallels the D_1 agonist activity of the enantiomers, which
also resides stereoselectively in the R-configuration (O'Boyle
and Waddington, 1984a). Other actions of SK&F 38393 such as
residual D_2, 5-HT_1 and 5-HT_2 agonist activity show little or
no enantioselectivity (O'Boyle and Waddington, 1984a; Cross et
al., 1986). This is strong evidence that the present
behavioral effects have their basis in D_1 receptor
stimulation. The activity of S-SK&F 38393 to induce some
episodes of Gr need not contradict this analysis, as the
compound so designated is not enantiomerically pure and
contains a modest proportion of its R-antipode as contaminant
(Kaiser. et al., 1982); this would account for some behavioral
activity in the S-sample at such high doses, in terms of low
threshold Gr (and occasional Sn) responses, but its inactivity
to induce the high threshold Gr_i response.

The ability of as little as 100 μg/kg SCH 23390 to block all behaviors induced by R- SK&F 38393 further suggests a primary role for D_1 receptor stimulation in the genesis of these responses. Their antagonism by SK&F 83566 showed complete stereoselectivity for the R- but not the S-enantiomer, in which D_1 antagonist activity resides (O'Boyle and Waddington, 1984b); other actions of SK&F 83566 such as weak D-2, $5-HT_1$, and $5-HT_2$ antagonist activity show less or no enantioselectivity (O'Boyle and Waddington, 1984b; Cross et al., 1986). Thus, a primary role for D_1 receptors in the induction of these behaviors is again indicated.

Moderate doses of the selective D_2 antagonist metoclopramide (Seeman, 1980) had no effect on R-SK&F 38393-induced Sn and Gr, but antagonized Gr_i. Metoclopramide may have some activity to attenuate the overall severity of grooming, or else the Gr_i response may be pharmacologically distinct from these other behaviors. It is notable that sulpiride, another selective D_2 antagonist (Seeman, 1980), showed essentially opposite effects by potentiating grooming but attenuating Sn. There are many precedents for sulpiride and metoclopramide exerting conflicting effects on DAergic function (Jenner and Marsden, 1979; Robertson and MacDonald, 1985). Whether these reflect intrinsic differences in their actions at distinct DA (or other) receptor sub-populations, or regional effects, is unresolved. Irrespective of these considerations, the double dissociation between the actions of sulpiride and metoclopramide on Sn and Gr/Gr_i argues against any general D_2 agonist action of SK&F 38393 in their induction. One explanation is that D_1 and D_2 receptor mechanisms may not invariably constitute functionally independent processes (Molloy and Waddington, 1984), such that drug effects on D_2 activity may modulate the expression of behaviors induced by D_1 receptor stimulation. These notions will be discussed further below.

D_1: D_2 RECEPTOR SYSTEMS AND THE REGULATION OF DOPAMINERGIC BEHAVIORS

Selective D_1 agonists can, under particular experimental conditions, induce episodes of non-stereotyped behaviors, such as grooming, which are sensitive to blockade by selective D_1 antagonists. Stereochemical relationships, revealed using the enantiomers of SK&F 38393 and SK&F 83566, are particularly powerful evidence for a primary role of D_1 receptor stimula-tion in the initiation of these responses. These effects appear to complement the induction by selective D_2 agonists such as RU 24213 of different forms of behavior that are sensitive to blockade by selective D_2 antagonists such as (-)-piquindone (Pugh et al., 1985). However, these are clearly more complex processes than such a superficial analysis would indicate. The selective D_2 antagonists such as sulpiride and metoclopramide are able to influence responsiveness to SK&F 38393 (Molloy and Waddington, 1985a; Molloy et al., 1986) (see above) and the selective D_1 antagonists SCH 23390 and SK&F 83566 are able to influence responsiveness to RU 24213 (Pugh, et al., 1985; Molloy and Waddington, 1985b). One inter-pretation of these data is that there is only one brain DA receptor, such that behavioral responses do not show consistent selectivity for receptor antagonists; this would question the functional relevance of the D_1: D_2 subdivision that is usually made on in vitro considerations. However, selective D_1 and D_2 agonists do induce different forms of behavioral response, even though they are not doubly-dissociable in terms of selective D_1 and D_2 antagonists. Interestingly, the mixed DA agonist apomorphine induces grooming behavior only in animals pre-treated with modest doses of metoclopramide or sulpiride, perhaps by antagonizing prepotent D_2 activity and unmasking the D_1 component (Molloy and Waddington, 1985a; 1986).

It is such data that prompted the suggestion (Molloy and Waddington, 1984) that D_1 and D_2 receptor systems may not invariably constitute functionally independent processes. To concentrate on one of many examples, stereotypy induced by the selective D_2 agonist RU 24213 is sensitive to blockade not only by SCH 23390 (Pugh et al, 1985) but also by R- but not S-SK&F 83566 (Molloy and Waddington, 1985b). This is strong evidence that this 'paradoxical' effect genuinely has its basis in D_1 and not residual D_2 receptor blockade. The status of SCH 23390 and RU 24213 as selective agents, the possible generation of non-selective active metabolites, and the influence of possible non-dopaminergic actions have been discussed previously (Pugh et al., 1985) above, and cannot easily account for such results. In saturation studies of ^{3}H-piflutixol and ^{3}H-spiperone binding, SCH 23390 increases the Kd for the former at sub-nM concentrations, but increases the Kd for the latter only in the μM range; B_{max} values did not appear to change (O'Boyle et al., 1986). Thus SCH 23390 shows the properties of a potent, competitive D_1 antagonist with weak residual competitive D_2 antagonist activity. SCH 23390, at a concentration 5-fold greater than was necessary to so influence ^{3}H-piflutixol binding, fails to influence the potent displacement of ^{3}H-spiperone by RU 24213 (O'Boyle et al., 1986). Thus SCH 23390 does not appear to influence D_2 receptor characteristics at the level of the protein recognition site.

It is striking that SCH 23390 appears to be a selective D_1 antagonist in isolated, non-functional in vitro preparations or in vivo physiological test systems that contain only D_2 receptors, such as the regulation of emesis by the chemoreceptive trigger zone or of prolactin secretion by the pituitary (Waddington et al.; Pugh, et al., 1985). However, when the test procedure is one that contains both D_1 and D_2 receptors, such as in behavioral studies or in striatal slice preparations where functional integrity of local D_1 and D_2 systems is preserved, SCH 23390 appears to exert paradoxical antagonism of D_2 agonist responses (Waddington et al. 1986; Pugh, et al., 1985). This would suggest that in such situations , tonic D_1 dopaminergic activity is required for the expression of D_2 receptor-induced responses such as stereotyped behavior, i.e. that D_1 tone serves an 'enabling' function in relation to D_2-initiated processes (Pugh, et al., 1985; Molloy, et al., 1986).

If D_1 antagonists block D_2 agonist-induced responses in this way, a corollary would be that D_1 agonists might alter the form of response to such agents in the direction of fixated stereotypies. We have found it difficult to induce compulsive, fixated stereotyped behavior even with high doses of the selective D_2 agonist RU 24213 (Pugh et al., 1985), though these are a typical response to the mixed D_1/D_2 agonist apomorphine. Perhaps these distinctions reflect the absence and presence of D_1 agonist activity. In preliminary studies, we have found that a threshold dose of RU 24213 (2.5 mg/kg s.c.) for the induction of stereotyped behavior (peak score 2.4 $\pm$0.2), induces a greater stereotypy response when immediately preceded by 15 mg/kg SK&F 38393 (score 3.4$\pm$0.4, n=8; p<0.05); this dose of SK&F 38393 fails to induce stereotypy when given alone (score 1.8$\pm$0.2, n=6). In the combination group, 50% of animals showed the compulsive stereotypies of fixated sniffing, with or without licking, while these behaviors were not evident in any of the single treatment groups (p<0.05).

Putative mechanisms for how D_1 antagonists might influence D_2 agonist responses, such as those discussed above, are conjectural and supported only by indirect data; even less is known about how D_2 antagonists might influence behaviors initiated by D_1 receptor stimulation. Perhaps the situation is somewhat analogous conceptually to the effects of adrenergic antagonists on cardiovascular indices; both alpha and beta-receptor blockers can induce a reduction in blood pressure, but these effects are mediated via distinct receptor sub-types through which initially distinct mechanisms ultimately influence the same physiological process.

CONCLUSIONS AND CAVEATS

The introduction of these new specific and selective D_1 agonist and antagonist drugs, especially as enantiomeric pairs, has prompted new interest in D_1 receptor function. The notion of concerted D_1: D_2 interplay in the regulation of dopaminergic behaviors (Molloy and Waddington, 1984; Pugh et al, 1985) clearly requires mechanistic support at the neuronal level. Perhaps distinct D_1 and D_2 receptor systems can in some instances each exert an influence over what is ultimately the same efferent pathway, as in a neuronal logic gate.

However, any mechanism must be able to account for the ability of each receptor sub-type to select a particular mode of expression of the same behavior, e.g. non-stereotyped vs stereotyped sniffing, and also to initiate different behaviors such as grooming. Additionally, in animals in whom tonic DAergic function has been removed by 6-hydroxydopamine or reserpine/alpha-methyl-p-tyrosine pretreatment, and in whom adaptive receptor changes are likely, D_1 and D_2 receptors can then be doubly dissociated in terms of responses to D_1 or D_2 agonists and their differential responses to selective antagonists (Arnt and Hyttel, 1984; Arnt, 1985; Breese and Mueller, 1985). Thus the extent of tonic DAergic activity appears to be a crucial determinant of the behavioral profile of selective D_1 and D_2 agonists and antagonists. Also problematic is recent data indicating that catalepsy induced by SCH 23390 cannot be overcome by even quite high doses of SK&F 38393 (Morelli and Di Chiara, 1985), There is now preliminary data that at least some component of ^{3}H-SCH 23390 binding may be dissociable from DA-sensitive adenylate cyclase activity in terms of both sub-cellular fractionation (Schulz et al., 1985) and regional localization (Mailman et al., 1985).

It has been noted (Waddington, 1985) that novel pharmacological or technical procedures for neuroscience research produce exciting and startling results soon after their introduction. Subsequent studies usually reveal unappreciated problems and limitations, and often report contradictory data that challenge the new theoretical concepts. Eventually, review of all the data leads to a more pragmatic appreciation of the extent to which our knowledge may in fact have been advanced. In several years we will be able to look back and better evaluate the impact of SCH 23390, and hopefully of additional selective D_1 agents from other chemical classes, and the renascence of interest in the D_1 receptor which it has generated.

ACKNOWLEDGEMENTS

This work was supported by the Medical Research Council of Ireland, the Royal College of Surgeons in Ireland, the Irish Council for Overseas Students and by generous gifts of experimental agents from Schering and Smith Kline & French.

REFERENCES

Arnt, J., 1985, Hyperactivity induced by stimulation of separate dopamine D_1 and D_2 receptors in rats with bilateral 6-OHDA lesions, Life Sci., 37:717.

Arnt, J. and Hyttel, J., 1984, Differential inhibition by dopamine D_1 and D_2 antagonists of circling behavior induced by dopamine agonists in rats with unilateral 6-hydroxydopamine lesions, Eur. J. Pharmacol., 102:349.

Billard, W., Ruperto, V., Crosby, G., Iorio, L.C. and Barnett, A., 1984, Characterization of the binding of ^{3}H-SCH-23390, a selective D_1 receptor antagonist ligand in rat striatum, Life Sci., 35:1885.

Breese, G.R. and Mueller, R.A., 1985, SCH 23390 antagonism of a D_2 dopamine agonist depends upon catecholaminergic mechanisms, Eur. J. Pharmacol., 113:109.

Christensen, A.V., Arnt, J., Hyttel J., Larsen, J.J. and Svendsen, O., 1984, Pharmacological effects of a specific dopamine antagonist SCH 23390 in comparison with neuroleptics, Life Sci., 32:1529.

Creese, I., Sibley, D.R., Hamblin, M.W. and Leff, S.E., 1983, The classification of dopamine receptors: Relationship to radioligand binding, Ann. Rev. Neurosci., 6:43.

Cross, A.J., Mashal, R.D., Johnson, J.A. and Owen, F., 1983, Preferential inhibition of ligand binding to calf striatal dopamine D_1 receptors by SCH23390, Neuropharmacol., 22:1327.

Cross, A.J., Hewitt, L., Slater, P. and Waddington, J.L., Interactions of benzazepine derivatives with rat brain serotonin receptors. In preparation.

Dandridge, P.A., Kaiser C., Bremer, M., Gaitanopoulos, D., Davis, L.D., Webb, R.G., Foley, J.J. and Sarau, H.M., 1984, Synthesis, resolution, absolute stereochemistry, and enantioselectivity of 3',4'-dihydroxynomifensine, J. Med. Chem. 27:28.

Gerson , S.C. and Baldessarini,R .J., 1980, Motor effects of serotonin in the central nervous system, Life Sci. 27:1435.

Hyttel, J., 1983, SCH 23390: The first selective dopamine D_1 antagonist, Eur. J. Pharmacol. 91:153.

Iorio, L.C., Barnett, A., Leitz, F.H., Houser, V.P. and Korduba, C.A., 1983, SCH 23390, a potential benzazepine antipsychotic with unique interactions on dopaminergic systems, J. Pharmacol. Exp. Ther. 226:462.

Isaacson, R.L., Hannigan, J.H., Brakkee, J.H., and Gispen, W.H., 1983, The time course of excessive grooming after neuropeptide administration, Brain Res. Bull. 11:289.

Itoh, Y., Beaulieu, M. and Kebabian, J.W., The chemical basis for the blockade of the D-1 dopamine receptor by SCH23390, 1984, Eur. J. Pharmacol. 100:119.

Jenner, P. and Marsden, C.D., 1979, The substituted benzamides: A novel class of dopamine antagonists, Life Sci., 25:479.

Jolles, J., Rompa-Barendregt, J. and Gispen, W.H., 1979, Novelty and grooming behavior in the rat, Behav. Neural Biol., 25:563.

Kaiser, C., Dandridge, P.A., Garvey, E., Hahn, R.A., Sarau, H.M., Setler, P.E., Bass, L.S. and Clardy, J., 1982, Absolute stereochemistry and dopaminergic activity of enantiomers of 2,3,4,5-tetrahydro-7, 8-dihydroxy-1-phenyl-1H-3-benzazepine, J. Med. Chem., 25:687.

Kebabian, J.W. and Calne, D.B., 1979, Multiple receptors for dopamine, Nature 277:93.

Laduron, P., 1983, Dopamine sensitive adenylate cyclase as a receptor site, in: Dopamine Receptors, C. Kaiser, and J.W. Kebabian, eds., American Chemical Society, Washington.

Leff, S. and Creese, I., 1983, Dopamine receptors re-explained, Trends Pharmacol. Sci. 4:463.

Mailman, R.B., Schulz, D.W., Lewis, M.H., Staples, L., Rollema, H. and Dehaven, D.L., 1984, SCH 23390: A selective D_1 dopamine antagonist with potent D_2 behavioral actions, Eur. J. Pharmacol. 101:159.

Mailman, R.B., Schulz, D.W. and Kilts, C.D., 1985, D_1-like dopamine receptors: Recognition sites with selectivity for SCH 23390 that are not linked to adenylate cyclase, Soc. Neurosci. Abstr. 11:313.

Molloy, A.G. and Waddington, J.L., 1984, Dopaminergic behavior stereospecifically promoted by the D_1 agonist R-SK&F 38393 and selectively blocked by the D_1 antagonist SCH 23390, Psychopharmacol. 82:409.

Molloy, A.G. and Waddington, J.L., 1985a, Sniffing, rearing and locomotor responses to the D_1 dopamine agonist R-SK&F 38393 and to apomorphine: Differential interactions with the selective D_1 and D_2 antagonists SCH 23390 and metoclopramide, Eur. J. Pharmacol. 108:305.

Molloy, A.G. and Waddington, J.L., 1985b, The enantiomers of SK&F 83566, a new selective D_1 dopamine antagonist, stereospecifically block stereotyped behavior induced by apormorphine and by the selective D_2 agonist RU 24213, Eur. J. Pharmacol. 116:183.

Molloy, A.G., O'Boyle, J.M., Pugh, M.T. and Waddington, J.L., Locomotor behaviors in response to new selective D_1 and D_2 dopamine receptor agonists, and the influence of selective antagonists (In press), Pharmacol. Biochem. Behav..

Morelli, M. and DiChiara, G., 1985, Catalepsy induced by SCH 23390 in rats, Eur. J. Pharmacol., 117:179.

O'Boyle, K.M. and Waddington, J.L., 1984a, Selective and stereospecific interactions of R-SK&F 38393 with ^{3}H-piflutixol but not ^{3}H-spiperone binding to striatal D_1 and D_2 dopamine receptors: comparisons with SCH 23390, Eur. J. Pharmacol. 90:433.

O'Boyle, K.M. and Waddington, J.L., 1984b, Identification of the enantiomers of SK&f 83566 as specific and stereoselective antagonists at the striatal D_1 dopamine receptor: Comparisons with the D_2 enantioselectivity of Ro 22-1319., Eur. J. Pharmacol. 106:219.

O'Boyle, K.M. and Waddington, J.L., 1985a, Binding of ^{3}H-SCH 23390, a selective D_1 dopamine receptor antagonist in human brain, Brit. J. Pharmacol. 86:435P.

O'Boyle, K.M. and Waddington, J.L., 1985b, Structural determinants of selective affinity for brain D_1 dopamine receptors within a series of 1-phenyl-1H-3-benzazepine analogues of SK&F 38393 and SCH 23390, Eur. J. Pharmacol. 115:291.

O'Boyle, K.M., Molloy, A.G. and Waddington, J.L., Benzazepine derivatives: Nature of the selective and stereospecific interactions of SK&F 38393 and SCH 23390 with brain D_1 receptors in: "Dopaminergic Systems and their Regulation", G.N. Woodruff, ed., (In Press) Macmillan Press, London.

Pugh, M.T., O'Boyle, K.M., Molloy, A.G. and Waddington, J.L., 1985, Effects of the putative D_1 antagonist SCH 23390 on stereotyped behavior induced by the D_2 agonist RU 24213, Psychopharmacol. 87:308.

Robertson, A. and MacDonald, C., 1985, Opposite effects of sulpiride and metoclopramide on amphetamine-induced stereotypy, Eur. J. Pharmacol. 109:81.

Schulz, D.W., Stanford, E.J. and Mailman, R.B., Subcellular localization hte SCh23390 receptor: Dissociation from dopamine-stimulated adenylate cyclase, 1985, Soc. Neurosci. Abstr. 11:888.

Seeman, P., 1980, Brain Dopamine receptors, Pharmacol. Rev. 32:229.

Setler, P.E., Sarau, H.M., Zirkle, C.L. and Saunders, H.L , 1978, The central effects of a novel dopamine agonist, Eur. J. Pharmacol. 50:419.

Tricklebank, M.D., Forler, C., Middlemiss, D.N. and Fozard, J.R., 1985, Sub-types of the 5-HT receptor mediating the behavioral responses to 5-methoxy-N, N-dimethyltryptamine in the rat, Eur. J. Pharmacol., 117:15.

Waddington, J.L., 1985, Structural brain pathology and clinical features in schizophrenia: further clues on the neurobiology of psychosis, Trends Pharmacol. Sci. 8:374.

Waddington, J.L., Cross, A.J., Gamble, S.J. and Bourne, R.C., 1982, Functional heterogeneity of multiple dopamine receptors during six months treatment with distinct classes of neuroleptic drugs., Adv. Biosci. 37:143.

Waddington, J.L., Molloy, A.G., O'Boyle, K.M. and Pugh, M.T., Aspects of stereotyped and non-stereotyped behavior in relation to dopamine receptor subtypes. In "The Neurobiology of Behavioral Stereotypy", S.J. Cooper, and C.T. Dourish, eds., Oxford University Press, London (in press).

FUNCTIONAL INTERACTIVE EFFECTS OF D_1 AND D_2 DOPAMINE RECEPTOR
BLOCKADE

A. I. Salama and C. F. Saller

Department of Pharmacology
Stuart Pharmaceuticals, Div. of ICI Americas
Inc.
Wilmington, DE 19897

INTRODUCTION

Multiple types of dopamine (DA) receptors have been shown
to exist in the striatum (Seeman, 1980). These receptor
populations have been divided into those which stimulate the
enzyme adenylate cyclase (D_1 sites) and those which are not
directly linked to or suppress this enzyme (D_2 sites, Kebabian
and Calne, 1978; Stoof and Kebabian, 1984). Until now, the
functional effects of DA receptor activation in the brain have
been attributed to drug action at D_2 receptor sites. Thus,
good correlations exist between the ability of neuroleptic
drugs to displace ^{3}H-spiroperidol from specific binding sites
on D_2 receptors (Seeman, 1980) and their antipsychotic
activity (Seeman, 1977; Creese et al., 1979; Seeman, 1980).
Although no obvious physiological function for D_1 sites in
brain is known, recent evidence has suggested an interaction
between D_1 and D_2 sites. For example, SKF 38393, a D_1 agonist,
stimulates the efflux of cAMP from superfused striatal tissue
slices, and this stimulation is antagonized by LY 141865, a
selective D_2 agonist. Moreover, (-)-sulpiride, a D_2
antagonist, prevents the effect of LY 141865 (Stoof and
Kebabian, 1981). However, very recent evidence for behavioral
manifestations of D_1 receptor function has been observed and
are cited in this volume.

The major problem in determining a role for D_1 receptors
has been the lack of selective drugs for this site. However,
recently SCH 23390 has been described as a relatively
selective D_1 antagonist in vitro (Iorio et al., 1983; Hyttel,
1983), and it has provided the first tool to study the effects
of D_1 receptor blockade on dopaminergic transmission. This
compound has been found to displace ^{3}H-piflutixol from its
specific binding site to D_1 receptors (Hyttel, 1983; Boyce et
al., 1985), and it inhibited the DA stimulation of adenylate
cyclase activity but only weakly displaces either ^{3}H-
haloperidol or ^{3}H-spiroperidol from their binding sites on D_2
receptors on rat striatal membrane preparations (Mailman et
al., 1984; Pletje et al., 1984; Boyce et al., 1985; Saller and
Salama, 1986a).

Table 1. Inhibition of DA Stimulated Adenylate Cyclase
and Displacement of ^{3}H-Spiperone Binding to Rat
Striatal Membrane by Haloperidol and SCH 23390

	^{3}H-Spiperone Binding (K_i, nM)	DA-Stimulated Adenylate Cyclase (IC_{50}, nM)
Haloperidol	2.5	1,500
SCH 23390	>3,000	36

In this report, we will present evidence both in vitro
and in vivo to suggest that D_1 receptor blockade may attenuate
the effects of D_2 DA receptor blockade.

IN VITRO STUDIES

In these studies, adenylate cyclase activity and the K^+-
evoked release of ^{3}H-acetylcholine (Ach) in rat striatal
tissues were used as functional measures of DA receptor
activity (Stoof and Kebabian, 1982; Starke et al., 1983;
Lehman and Lange, 1983; Saller and Salama, 1986a).

The displacement of ^{3}H-spiroperidol binding from striatal
membrane preparations reveals that, unlike haloperidol, SCH
23390 is only weakly effective at the D_2 DA receptor site
(Table 1). On the other hand, SCH 23390 was a potent inhibitor
of adenylate cyclase in rat striatal membrane preparations
when stimulated by either DA (Table 1) or by the selective D_1
DA agonist, SKF 38393 (Fig. 1). These observations are in
agreement with those of Hyttel (1983, 1984) and Boyce et al.
(1985) which suggest that SCH 23390 is a relatively selective
D_1 DA receptor antagonist. Although haloperidol is a
relatively weak inhibitor of either DA or SKF 38393 stimulated
adenylate cyclase (Table 1, Fig. 1), low concentrations of
haloperidol, ranging between 0.1 to 10 μM, are capable of
enhancing the stimulation of adenylate cyclase elicited by SKF
38393 (Fig. 1). Similar observations were also obtained with
(-) sulpiride, a more selective D_2 DA antagonist (unpublished
observation). Dopamine, which stimulates both D_1 and D_2 DA
receptors, did not cause such enhancement of adenylate cyclase
activity. As expected, when D_1 receptors were blocked by SCH
23390, the haloperidol induced enhancement of SKF-stimulated
adenylate cyclase activity was abolished (Fig. 2). Thus, as
was suggested by Stoof and Kebabian (1981), it is possible to
facilitate the effects of D_1 receptor stimulation by actually
removing the tonic inhibitory control exerted on the D_2
subtype. Similarly, the inhibition by SCH 23390 of DA
stimulated cAMP formation in striatal homogenates was reversed
by sulpiride (Onali et al., 1984). Furthermore, the data
presented in Figure 2 suggest that haloperidol is also capable
of attenuating the inhibitory effects of SCH 23390 on D_1
receptors. In addition, as with low concentrations of SCH
23390, high concentrations of haloperidol, presumably by

blocking D_1 receptors, did prevent SKF 38393-induced increases in cAMP synthesis (Fig. 1).

Studies of the effects of SCH 23390 and haloperidol on the K^+-evoked release of ^3H-Ach from rat striatal tissue slices also suggest that a functional interaction exists between D_1 and D_2 DA receptors (Saller and Salama, 1985). Several studies (Scatton, 1982; Stoof and Kebabian, 1982; Starke et al., 1983) have suggested that haloperidol, at concentrations which appear to be selective for D_2 blockade, increases the release of ^3H-Ach from superfused striatal tissue slices (Table 2). Interestingly, SCH 23390 is capable of antagonizing the K^+-evoked ^3H-Ach release induced by 1 µM haloperidol (Saller and Salama, 1986a; Fig. 3). By itself, SCH 23390, at concentrations which are known to block D_1 receptors (1 to 50 nM), did not alter basal ^3H-Ach release (Boyce et al., 1985; Saller and Salama, 1986a). However, SCH 23390 reduces the ability of haloperidol to antagonize the inhibition of ^3H-Ach induced by apomorphine (Fig. 4). Moreover, it appears that SCH 23390 becomes less effective at attenuating haloperidol's antagonism of apomorphine as the concentration of haloperidol is increased. This suggests that the ratio of D_1 and D_2 receptor blockade may be an important determinant of the overall response to DA receptor blockade. These observations are consistent with the concept that D_1 receptor blockade attenuates the effects of D_2 receptor blockade in vitro. Furthermore, together with the observations

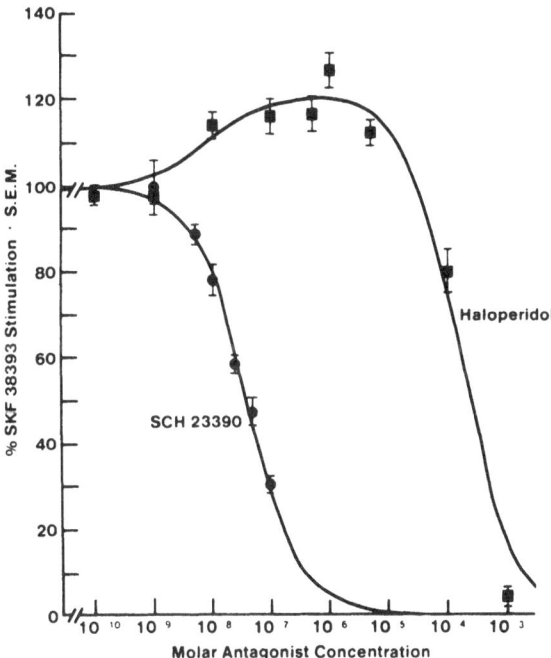

Fig. 1.   SKF 38393 (100 µM) stimulated adenylate cyclase activity in the presence of either SCH 23390 or haloperidol. Each value represents the mean of triplicate determinations. Points for SCH 23390 concentrations greater than 1 nanomolar are significantly different ($p < 0.05$) from the stimulation induced by SKF 38393.

Table 2. Effect of Haloperidol on the K^+-Evoked
Release of ^{3}H-Ach from Rat Striatal Slices

Haloperidol Concentration (M)	^{3}H-Ach Release (% Control $\pm$ S.E.M.)
10^{-8}	101.0 ± 5
5×10^{-8}	96.7 ± 6
10^{-7}	98.3 ± 5
5×10^{-7}	112.1 ± 6*
10^{-6}	131.4 ± 7
10^{-5}	122.6 ± 6*
10^{-4}	57.6 ± 3

Control S2/S1 ratio (0.88 ± 0.04) set at 100% was calculated as described by Saller and Salama, 1986a.
*Significantly different from control values ($p < .05$).

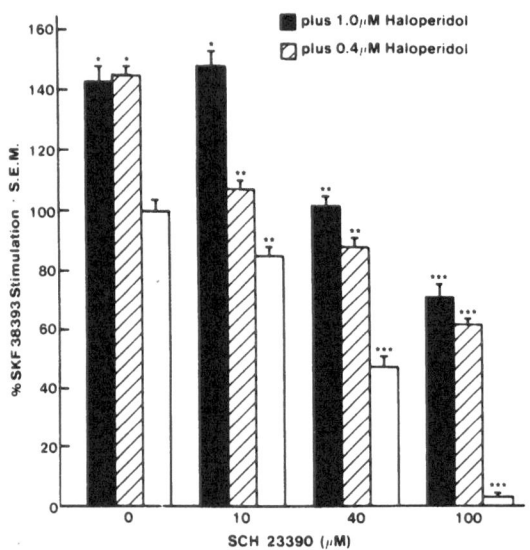

Fig. 2. Antagonism by SCH 23390 of the enhancement of
SKF 38393 (100 μM) stimulated adenylate cyclase
activity produced by haloperidol. Open bars
represent the effects of SKF 38393 and varying
doses of SCH 23390 in the absence of
haloperidol. Each value is the mean ($\pm$ S.E.M.)
of three determinations. *Significantly
different from SKF 38393 stimulated values in
the absence of SCH 23390 and haloperidol
($p < 0.05$.) **Significantly different from
haloperidol enhanced SKF 38393 stimulated
values in the absence of SCH 23390 ($p < 0.05$).
***Significantly different from haloperidol
enhanced and basal SKF 38393 stimulated values
in the absence of SCH 23390 ($p < 0.05$).

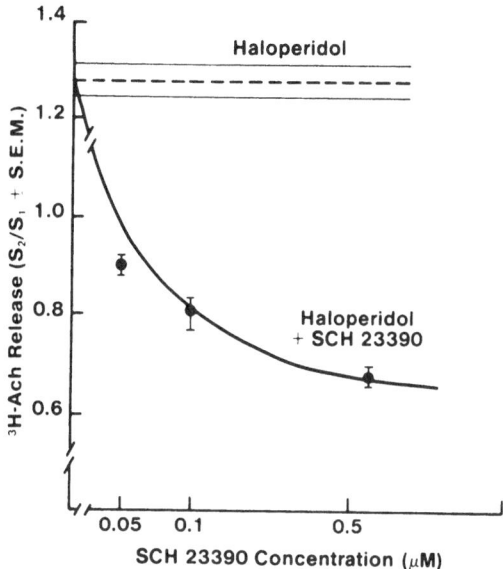

Fig. 3.   Antagonism of haloperidol (10 μM) induced
           release of ^{3}H-Ach by SCH 23390. The dashed line
           represents the increase in ^{3}H-Ach release
           induced by haloperidol. Each point represents
           the mean (± S.E.M.) of three determinations.

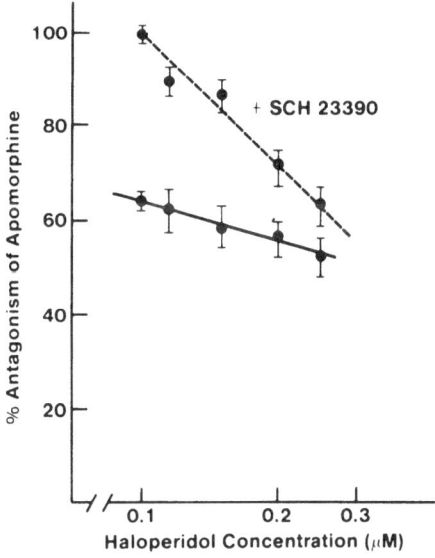

Fig. 4.   SCH 23390 (0.1 μM) reduces the ability of
           haloperidol to antagonize apomorphine-induced
           inhibition of ^{3}H-Ach release from striatal
           tissue slices. Each point represents that mean
           (± S.E.M.) of 4 determinations.

on the effects of SCH 23390 and haloperidol on cAMP synthesis, they suggest that the interaction of these compounds on adenylate cyclase activity and ^{3}H-Ach release may be closely related.

IN VIVO STUDIES

Rosengarten et al. (1983) have shown that low doses of spiperone which block D_2 receptors can induce abnormal perioral movements in rats. This behavior can be greatly potentiated by SKF 38393, suggesting that a reciprocal interaction may be occurring between the D_1 and D_2 DA receptor subtypes.

To investigate this possible interaction in vivo, the levels of the two major metabolites of DA, 3,4 dihydroxy-phenylacetic acid (DOPAC) and homovanillic acid (HVA) in rat striatum were used as indices of DA metabolism. In addition, plasma prolactin concentrations were also measured to obtain another index of the possible effects of D_1 receptor blockade on the response to D_2 receptor blockade (Saller and Salama, 1985, 1986a, and 1986b).

It is well known that the administration of spiperone and other D_2 antagonists will result in significant increases of both striatal DOPAC and HVA levels. At doses of spiperone (40 µg/kg), which produce large increases in both DOPAC and HVA, when they are co-administered with SKF 38393 (2.4 mg/kg), there was a tendency for a further increase in the levels of these DA metabolites (Saller and Salama, 1985; Fig. 5) although these effects were found to be not statistically significant. A lower dose of spiperone (25 µg/kg), which did not alter DOPAC or HVA levels by itself, but when administered in combination with SKF 38393 (2.4 mg/kg), did cause a significant increase (50%) in the levels of these DA metabolites (Fig. 5). The dose of SKF 38393 used did not alter levels of DA metabolite. This finding suggests that D_1 receptor stimulation can potentiate the effects of D_2 receptor blockade.

In another paradigm, when pergolide, a D_2 agonist, was administered to stimulate D_2 receptors, the co-administration of SKF 38393 markedly inhibited the response to pergolide on DA metabolites (Fig. 6). Similarly, decreases in levels of DOPAC and HVA observed following the selective D_2 agonist LY 171555 (100 µg/kg) were also attenuated by SKF 38393 (Saller and Salama, 1985). Thus, it appears that D_1 receptor stimulation can antagonize the response to D_2 receptor stimulation. Moreover, the observation that SKF 38393 does not, by itself, alter DA metabolites levels but does alter the response to both D_2 agonist and D_2 antagonist, suggests that D_1 receptors in the nigrostriatal DA system might serve to modulate ongoing D_2 receptor mediated changes on dopaminergic neurotransmission.

The effects of varying doses of SCH 23390 on DA metabolites was measured to explore whether after D_1 receptor blockade, D_2 receptor modulation might also exist, as was the case under in vitro conditions (Saller and Salama, 1986a). Depending on the dose range used, SCH 23390 at low doses (0.25-0.5 µg/kg) caused a small to moderate increase in DOPAC

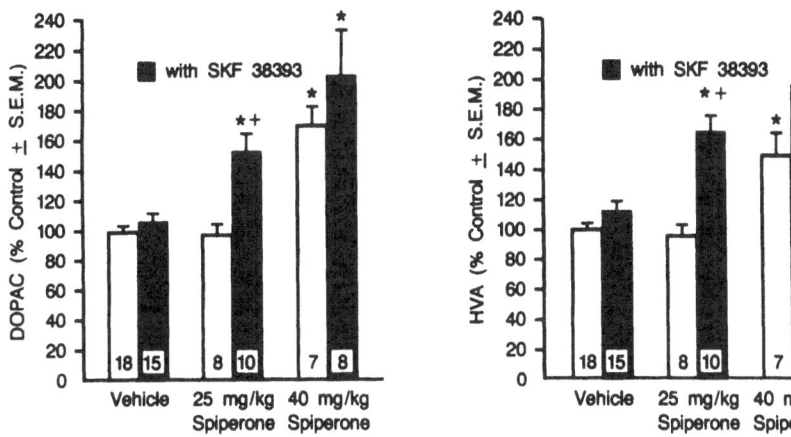

Fig. 5.   SKF 38393 induced potentiation of spiperone
induced increases in rat striatal DOPAC and HVA
concentrations. Spiperone-treated groups were
pretreated 1 hr prior to SKF 38393 (2.4 mg/kg
i.p.). All groups of rats were sacrificed 30
min later. Control values for DOPAC and HVA
were 0.63 ± 0.02 µg/gm and 0.52 ± 0.02 µg/gm,
respectively. *Significantly different from
control ($p < .05$). +Significantly different
from spiperone group ($p < .05$).

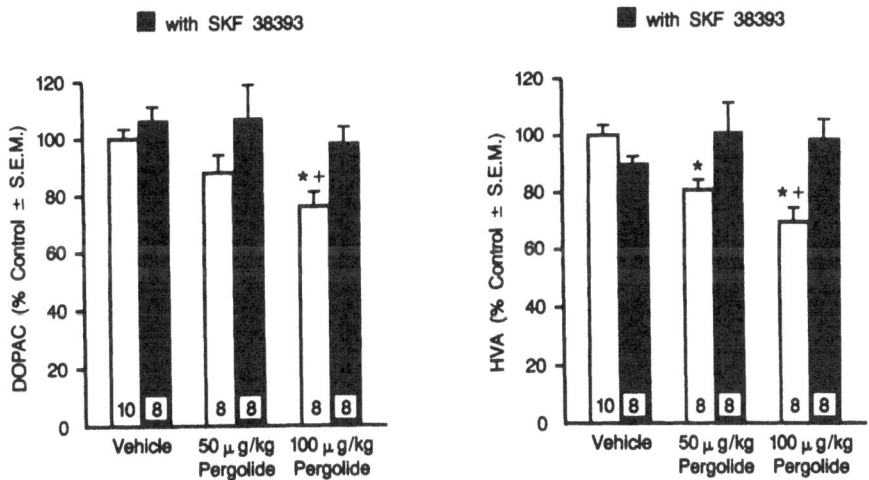

Fig. 6.   Attenuation of pergolide-induced decrease in
rat striatal DOPAC and HVA concentrations.
Pergolide and/or SKF 38393 were pretreated 30
min. prior to sacrifice. Control values of
DOPAC and HVA are the same as those on Fig. 5.
*Significantly different from control.
+Significantly different from pergolide with
SKF 38393 group ($p < 0.05$).

and HVA levels, whereas at higher doses (1-2.5 µg/kg), there was a significant increase in these levels (Table 3 and Fig. 7). Boyce et al. (1985) have also reported moderate increases in DA metabolite concentrations with some doses of SCH 23390. Similarly, Mereu et al. (1985) have reported that SCH 23390 increased the firing rates of nigrostriatal dopaminergic neurons in unanesthetized rats.

The effect of very low doses of SCH 23390 on the response to haloperidol administration revealed that within a dose range between 0.25 and 0.5 µg/kg of SCH 23390 there was an attenuation of the haloperidol-induced increase in striatal HVA and DOPAC levels (Fig. 7). Increasing the dose of SCH 23390 to 1 µg/kg seems to reduce its effectiveness in antagonizing the effects of haloperidol. Similar drug interactions between SCH 23390 and spiperone, and other D_2 antagonists, were also observed (Saller and Salama, 1986a). Interestingly, although the doses of SCH 23390 which attenuate haloperidol caused modest increases in DA metabolites, the increase produced by either haloperidol or spiperone were clearly not additive.

Dopamine released from tuberoinfundibular hypothalamic neurons tonically inhibits the secretion of prolactin (PRL) from the pituitary. This response to DA appears to be mediated by D_2 DA receptors which are negatively coupled to adenylate cyclase (Enjalbert and Bockaert, 1982; Swennen and Denef,

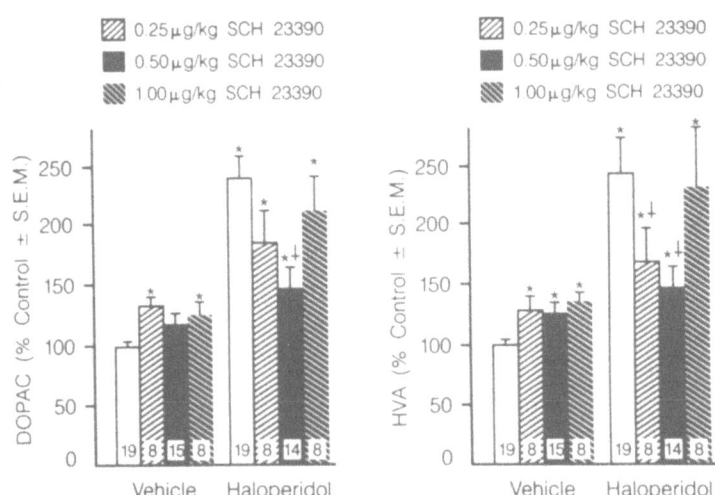

Fig. 7.   The attenuation of haloperidol-induced increases in rat striatal DOPAC and HVA levels by SCH 23390. Haloperidol (0.1 mg/kg, i.p.) was administered 1 hr prior to SCH 23390. All rats were sacrificed 30 min later. Control values for DOPAC and HVA were 0.87 $\pm$ 0.02 µg/gm and 0.57 $\pm$ 0.02 µg/gm, respectively. *Significantly different from control (p < 0.05). +Significantly different from haloperidol group (p < 0.05).

Table 3. Effects of SCH 23390 on Rat Striatal DOPAC and HVA
         Concentrations

SCH 23390	DOPAC	HVA
(μg/gm, i.p.)	(% Control + S.E.M.)	
0	100 + 4	100 + 4
5	125 + 5*	122 + 6*
50	128 + 9*	124 + 7*
250	145 + 14*	136 + 13*
2500	169 + 9*	174 + 7*

Control DOPAC and HVA concentrations were 0.65 + 0.03 μg/gm
and 0.48 + 0.02 μg/gm, respectively. SCH 23390 was pretreated
for 1 hour prior to death to groups of 6-8 rats.

1981). However, no role for D_1 DA receptors in the regulation
of PRL secretion has yet been demonstrated. To extend and to
further explore the interactive effects between D_1 and D_2
receptor blockade in another DA innervated system, plasma PRL
levels were measured (Saller and Salama, 1986b).

     The D_1 selective agonist SKF 38393 exerted a dose-
dependent increase in plasma PRL concentrations (Fig. 8), a
response which was several times greater from baseline control
levels. It should be noted that Setler et al. (1978) did not
observe an elevation in PRL levels following SKF 38393
administration. This may have been due to the use of
polyestradiol primed rats in their study. This treatment would
likely have produced near maximal increases in plasma PRL
levels, masking any further increases arising from SKF 38393.
On the other hand, doses ranging between 25 to 250 μg/gm of
the D_1 antagonist SCH 23390 tended to lower PRL levels below
control values (Saller and Salama, 1986b). Higher doses of SCH
23390 did not alter PRL levels, in agreement with Iorio et al.
(1983). However, pretreatment of rats with SCH 23390
completely abolished the SKF 38393-induced increase in PRL
levels (Table 4). The possible involvement of D_1 receptor
mediated increases in cAMP in the SKF 38393 stimulation
of PRL secretion is supported by the observation that
caffeine, a phosphodiesterase inhibitor, potentiated the
PRL response to SKF 38393. By itself, caffeine (50 mg/kg) did
not alter plasma PRL appreciably (Saller and Salama, 1986b).
Thus, prevention of cAMP breakdown seems to potentiate the PRL
response to the D_1 agonist SKF 38393. It is of interest to
note that compounds which increase intracellular cAMP
concentrations (i.e., dibutyrl cAMP and isobutyl-
methylxanthine) appear to interfere with the ability of D_2 DA
receptor stimulation (which inhibits cAMP formation) to
inhibit the secretion of PRL from cultured anterior pituitary
cells (Swennen and Denef, 1982). Putting these observations
together, it would appear that D_1 receptors may be involved in
the stimulation of PRL secretion. Furthermore, the expected

Table 4. Antagonism of SKF 38393 Induced Increases in Plasma PRL Concentrations

| SCH 23390 (μg/gm, i.p.) | Plasma PRL Concentrations (ng/ml ± S.E.M.) | |
	Plus Saline	Plus SKF 38393
0	5.9 ± 0.8	16.1 ± 1.6*
1	5.8 ± 1.7	18.5 ± 3.2*
5	8.1 ± 1.5	17.9 ± 1.8*
50	4.1 ± 0.9	5.4 ± 1.4
250	6.1 ± 2.8	8.2 ± 1.1

SCH 23390 was pretreated 30 min before SKF 38393 (5 mg/kg, i.p.) administration, and all rats were decapitated 30 min later.   N = 8-10 in each group. *Significantly different from control (p < .05).

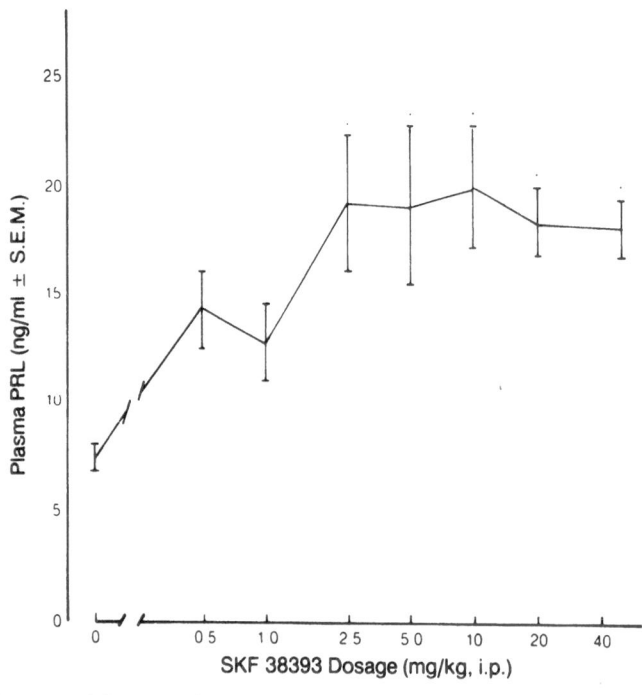

Fig. 8.   Effect of SKF 38393 on rat plasma PRL concentrations 30 min after administration. *Significantly different from control values (p < 0.05).

increases in PRL induced by haloperidol were attenuated by low doses (0.5 μg/kg) of SCH 23390 (Fig. 9). Thus, responses to D_2 receptor blockade which mediate dopaminergic neurotransmission in striatum and PRL secretion by pituitary cells appear to be attenuated by D_1 receptor blockade. Conversely, the increases in plasma PRL elicited by neuroleptics may be at least in part due to a disinhibition of a response to D_1 receptor stimulation.

Several behavioral paradigms (Mailman et al., 1984; Meller et al.,1985) have indicated that SCH 23390, at the doses tested, possesses D_2 antagonist-like properties. On the other hand, the ability of SCH 23390 to inhibit motor behaviors (e.g., stereotypy) in the rat was suggested to be due to its action on D_1 receptors by Boyce et al. (1985). However, SCH 23390, at doses up to 2 mg/kg, fails to inhibit apomorphine-induced inhibition of DA cell firing (Mereu et al., 1985). In addition, SCH 23390, at doses as high as 250 μg/kg, does not affect the ability of the selective D_2 agonist LY 171555 to reduce either striatal DA metabolite concentrations or plasma prolactin levels (unpublished observations). The basis for the observation that only very low doses of SCH 23390 are effective in attenuating responses to D_2 receptor blockade in vivo should be investigated further.

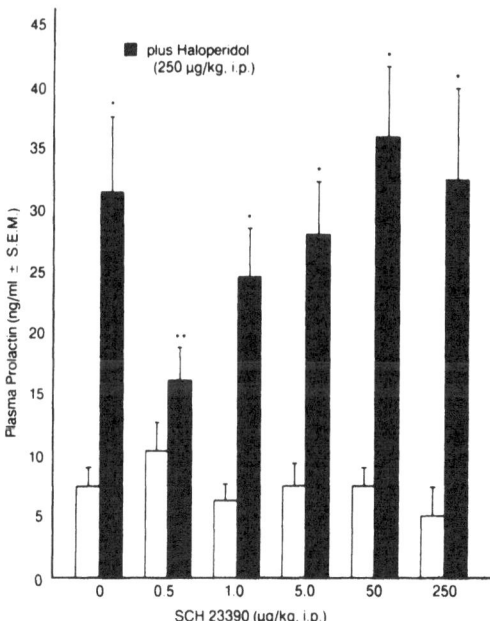

Fig. 9.   Attenuation of haloperidol-induced elevations in rat plasma PRL concentrations by SCH 23390. Haloperidol-treated groups were pretreated 1 hr prior to SCH 23390. All groups of animals were sacrificed 30 min later. *Significantly different from control ($p < 0.05$). **Significantly different from haloperidol group ($p < 0.05$).

The interaction between D_1 and D_2 receptor mediated functions under in vivo conditions seems to be more complex than from mere extrapolation from in vitro studies. In addition to its DA receptor blocking properties, SCH 23390 possesses significant $5HT_2$ and α_2-adrenergic blocking activity (Hyttel, 1983 and Hicks et al., 1985), which might account for some of the unexplained effects of SCH 23390 administration in vivo.

CONCLUSIONS

The reciprocal interaction between D_1 and D_2 DA receptors in the regulation of cAMP synthesis has been observed in rat striatum (Stoof and Kebabian, 1981; Onali et al., 1984; Weiss et al., 1985). Additional support and extension of these interactions has been described both in vitro and in vivo in this review.

These investigations have shown that D_1 receptor stimulation is capable of potentiating the response to D_2 receptor blockade. This is evidenced by the observation that SKF 38393, which by itself produces negligible changes in the concentrations of striatal DA metabolites, potentiates the increase in DA metabolites elicited by spiperone in the striatum. Similarly, the lowering of DA metabolites induced by either pergolide or LY 171555 is prevented by SKF 38393 administration.

Conversely, it appears that D_1 receptor blockade can attenuate responses to D_2 receptor blockade. In support of this hypothesis, the D_1 receptor antagonist SCH 23390 reduces the increases in striatal DA metabolites and plasma PRL concentrations elicited by D_2 receptor blockade with haloperidol and spiperone. Similarly, under in vitro conditions, SCH 23390 antagonizes the release of ^{3}H-Ach in striatal slices induced by haloperidol. Moreover, SCH 23390 also antagonizes the SKF 38393-stimulated enhancement of cAMP synthesis produced by haloperidol. Furthermore, SCH 23390 reduces the ability of haloperidol to antagonize the inhibition of ^{3}H-Ach release produced by apomorphine. However, SCH 23390 becomes less effective as the concentration of haloperidol is increased, suggesting that the ratio between D_1 and D_2 receptor blockade may be an important determinant of DA neurotransmission.

The precise localization and nature of the interaction of these receptors has yet to be determined. Nevertheless, one might speculate that pharmacological manipulation of D_1 and D_2 receptor interactions might have useful clinical implications.

REFERENCES

Boyce, S., Kelly, E., Davis, A., Fleminger, S., Jenner, P., and Mardsden, C. D., 1985, SCH 23390 may alter dopamine-mediated motor behavior via striatal D-1 receptors, Biochem. Pharmacol., 34:1665.
Creese, I., Burt, D. R., and Snyder, S. H., 1979, Biochemical actions of neuroleptic drugs: Focus on the dopamine receptor, in: "Handbook of Psychopharmacology," L. L. Iversen, S. D. Iversen, and S. H. Snyder, eds., Plenum Press, New York.

Enjalbert, A., and Bockaert, J., 1983, Pharmacological characterization of the D2 dopamine receptor negatively coupled with adenylate cyclase in rat anterior pituitary, Mol. Pharmacol., 23:576.

Hicks, P. E., Shoemaker, H., and Langer, S. Z., 1984, 5HT-receptor antagonist properties of SCH 23390 in vascular smooth muscle and brain, Eur. J. Pharmacol., 105:339.

Hyttel, J., 1983, SCH 23390 - The first selective D_1 antagonist, Eur. J. Pharmacol., 91:153.

Hyttel, J., 1984, Functional evidence for selective dopamine D_1 receptor blockade by SCH 23390, Neuropharmacol., 23:1395.

Iorio, L. C., Barnett, A., Leitz, F. H., Hower, V. P., and Korduba, C. A., 1983, SCH 23390, a potential benzazepine antipsychotic with unique interactions on dopaminergic systems, J. Pharmacol. Exp. Ther., 226:462.

Kebabian, J. W., and Calne, D. B., 1978, Multiple receptors for dopamine, Nature, 277:93.

Lehman, J., and Langer, S. Z., 1983, The striatal cholinergic interneurons: Synaptic target of dopaminergic terminals? Neurosci., 10:1105.

Mailman, R. B., Schulz, D. W., Lewis, M. H., Staples, L., Rolloma, H., and Dehaven, D. L., 1984, SCH 23390: A selective D_1 antagonist with potent D_2 behavioral actions, Eur. J. Pharmacol., 101:159.

Meller, E., Kuga, S., Friedhoff, A., and Goldstein, M., 1985, Selective D_2 dopamine receptor agonists prevent catalepsy induced by SCH 23390, a selective D_1 antagonist, Life Sci., 36:1857.

Mereu, G., Collu, M., Ongini, E., Biggio, G., and Gessa, G. L., 1985, SCH 23390, a selective dopamine D_1 antagonist, activates dopamine neurons but fails to prevent their inhibition by apomorphine, Eur. J. Pharmacol., 111:393.

Onali, P., Olianas, M. C., and Gessa, G. L., 1984, Selective blockade of dopamine D_1 receptors by SCH 23390 discloses striatal dopamine D_2 receptors mediating the inhibition of adenylate cyclase in rats, Eur. J. Pharmacol., 99:127.

Plantje, J. F., Daus, F. J., Hansen, H. A., and Stoof, J. C., 1984, SCH 23390 blocks D_1 and D_2 dopamine receptors in rat neostriatum in vitro, Nauyn-Schmiedeberg's Arch Pharmacol., 327:180.

Rosengarten, H., Schweiter, J. W., and Friedhoff, A. J., 1983, Induction of oral dyskinesias in naive rats by D_1 stimulation, Life Sci., 33:2479.

Saller, C. F., and Salama, A. I., 1985, Dopamine receptor subtypes: In vivo biochemical evidence for functional interaction, Eur. J. Pharmacol., 109:297.

Saller, C. F., and Salama, A. I., 1986a, D_1 and D_2 dopamine receptor blockade: Interactive effects in vitro and in vivo, J. Pharmacol. Exptl. Therap., 236:714.

Saller, C. F., and Salama, A. I., 1986b, D_1 dopamine receptor stimulation elevates plasma prolactin levels, Eur. J. Pharmacol., 122:139.

Scatton, B., 1982, Further evidence for the involvement of D_2, but not D_1 dopamine receptors in dopaminergic control of striatal cholinergic transmission, Life Sci., 31:2883.

Seeman, P., 1977, Anti-schizophrenic drugs: Membrane receptor sites of action, Biochem. Pharmacol., 26:1741.

Seeman, P., 1980, Brain dopamine receptors, Pharmacological Reviews, 32:230.

Setler, P. E., Sarau, H. M., Zirkle, C. L., and Saunders, H. L., 1978, The central effects of a novel dopamine agonist, Eur. J. Pharmacol., 50:419.

Starke, K., Spach, L., Lang, J. D., and Adelung, C., 1983, Further functional in vitro comparison of pre- and postsynaptic dopamine receptors in the rabbit caudate nucleus, Nauyn-Schmiedeberg's Arch Pharmacol., 323:298.

Stoof, J. C., and Kebabian, J. W., 1981, Opposing roles for D_1 and D_2 dopamine receptors in efflux of cAMP from rat neostriatum, Nature, 294:366.

Stoof, J. C, and Kebabian, J. W., 1982, Independent in vitro regulation by D_2 dopamine receptor of dopamine-stimulated efflux of cyclic AMP and K+-stimulated release of acetylcholine from rat neostriatum, Brain Res., 250:263.

Stoof, J. C., and Kebabian, J. W., 1984, Two dopamine receptors: Biochemistry, physiology and pharmacology, Life Sci., 35:2281.

Swennen, L., and Denef, C., 1982, Physiological concentrations of dopamine decrease adenosine 3'5' monophosphate levels in cultured rat anterior pituitary cells and enriched populations of lactotrophs: Evidence for casual relationship to inhibition of prolactin release, Endocrinology, 111:398.

INTERACTION OF D_1 AND D_2 DOPAMINE RECEPTORS IN THE EXPRESSION OF DOPAMINE AGONIST INDUCED BEHAVIORS

Allen R. Braun, Paolo Barone, and Thomas N. Chase

Experimental Therapeutics Branch, National Institute of
Neurological and Communicative Disorders and Stroke
National Institutes of Health, Building 10, Room 5C103
9000 Rockville Pike, Bethesda, MD 20892

INTRODUCTION

The study of behaviors induced by centrally acting dopaminergic
agents is a classical means of investigating the pharmacology of the
dopamine system and the pathophysiology of human neuropsychiatric
diseases for which these behaviors serve as animal models.
Observation and quantification of stereotypic and nonstereotypic
behaviors has been a standard research protocol since the earliest
work on the central activity of amphetamine and related agents
(Randrup and Munkvad, 1967; Kelly and Iversen, 1975). Quantification
of rotational behavior in lesioned rats (Ungerstedt and Arbuthnott,
1970) has more recently become an established means of investigating
the activity of dopaminergic agents within the CNS. The
compartmentalization of dopamine receptors on the basis of their
ability to stimulate (D_1 receptors) or not stimulate (D_2 receptors)
adenylate cyclase (Kebabian and Calne, 1979) and the introduction of
agents selective for these receptor subtypes have provided the means
with which to extend the classical behavioral observations and to
utilize these techniques to more comprehensively characterize the
pharmacology of the central dopamine system.

The conventional notion has been that all dopamine agonist
induced behaviors are mediated by the D_2 receptor (Creese, et al.,
1983). This conclusion largely derives from studies which used
relatively selective D_2 antagonists to inhibit all classes of
behavior induced by nonselective dopamine agonists such as apomorphine
or amphetamine. The D_1 receptor was for a considerable period of time
dismissed as a "receptor in search of a function". Nevertheless the
selective D_1 agonist SKF 38393 has been shown to induce behaviors such
as nonstereotypic grooming, sniffing and locomotion in a dose
dependent manner (Molloy and Waddington, 1984, 1985), and the
selective D_1 antagonist SCH 23390 has been found to block behavioral
effects of both apomorphine and amphetamine (Mailman et al 1984;
Christensen et al 1984), as well as those induced by the selective D_2
agonist RU 24213 (Pugh et. al, 1985). These data suggest that a
functional interaction between dopamine receptor subtypes may underly
the expression of agonist related behaviors. The series of
experiments from our own laboratory which we report here (Barone et

al, 1986; Braun et al, submitted) demonstrates and further clarifies the nature of this interaction.

We sought first to characterize the behavioral consequences of independant D_1 receptor stimulation and to contrast this with the effects of independent stimulation of the D_2 receptor. Secondly, behaviors associated with concurrent stimulation of the D_1 and D_2 receptor systems were examined in order to deliniate any specific behavioral consequences of D_1/D_2 receptor interaction. We then utilized selective dopamine antagonists and catecholamine depleting agents to determine whether such an interaction might not in fact be necessary for the generation of motor behaviors in the intact animal.

The pharmacologic agents utilized were the selective D_1 agonist SKF 38393 and antagonist SCH 23390, and the selective D_2 agonist LY 171555 and antgonist Ro 22-1319. We used two different behavioral models, each providing a unique means of studying the effects of these agents in animals with normosensitive dopamine receptors. Behavioral effects of dopamine receptor activation were studied in rats with unilateral striatal lesions induced by 1 microliter of a 300 nanomolar solution of quinolonic acid. This endogenous excitotoxin, resembling kainic acid, destroys the striatal neurons sparing the axons projecting into the nucleus (Schwarcz et. al 1983). In such a model the ispilateral rotation evoked by dopamine agonists is generally attributed to an unbalanced stimulation of the two sides without involving the phenomenon of dopamine receptor supersensitivity. Lesions were placed unilaterally in the center of the anterior caudatoputamen (cordinates according to Pellogrino-Cushman Atlas: A = 8.2, L = 2.6, V = 4.8). Two weeks were allowed for recovery postoperatively. Rotational behavior was recorded in automated rotometer bowls.

Unconditioned behaviors were quantified in unlesioned rats utilizing a behavioral check list similar to that described by Fray et al., (1980). This allowed independent quanitification of locomotion, grooming and rearing as well as posture and movements of the head mouth trunk and limbs. Stereotyped behavior was rated independently and stereotypy scores, using a modification of the Ernst Scale, could be derived using data taken directly from the check list as well. Behavior was observed over a period of over 2 to 10 hours by raters unaware of the animal treatments. Orientation, approach and duration of investigation of a novel object introduced in the animals home cage was quanitified as was the intensity of the initial response and the duration of immobility following presentation of a noxious stimulus. Duration of pursuit of a moving object and exploratory behavior/locomotor activity in an open field situation were also rated for each animal.

RESULTS

Behavioral effects of D_1 receptor stimulation

The behavioral effects of the selective D_1 agonist SKF 38393 were initially evaluated in rats treated with this agent alone. In the unilateral quinolinic acid lesioned rat (Figure 1), SKF 38393 did not induce rotation at any of the doses employed. Instead of turning, these rats displayed grooming and sniffing behaviors as seen in the intact animal (see below). There was no lateralization in relation to the side of brain lesion. In contrast, the D_2 agonist LY 171555 induced ipsilateral rotation in a dose dependent manner. A pattern characterized by bursts of turning alternating with short intervals (5

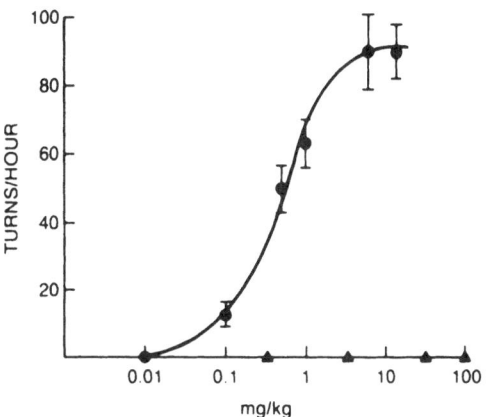

Fig. 1: Ipsilateral rotation induced by LY 171555 (●) and SKF
38393 (▲) in rats with unilateral, quinolinic acid induced
striatal lesion. Each value indicates the mean ± S.E.M. of data from
8-10 rats. (Barone, et al., 1986; modified).

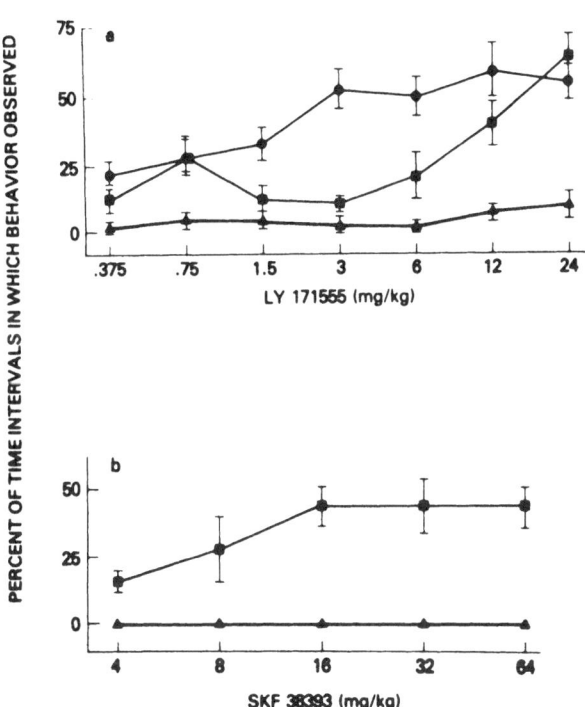

Fig. 2: Effects of independantly administered D_1 and D_2 agonists on
motor function. Scores for grooming (■), locomotion (●) and
stereotypic behavior (▲) following varying doses of LY 171555 (A)
and SKF 38393 (B) are illustrated; N = 5 for all groups of animals.

to 10 minutes) of rest was consistently observed. The number of
bursts reflected the total duration of turning and therefore was dose
dependent. During rotation, occasional licking behavior was also
observed. Intense licking, biting or gnawing was not seen.

In the unlesioned rat, SKF 38393 produced a dose dependent
increase in intensive grooming (figure 2). Although sniffing,
locomotion, and rearing occured, none of these individual behaviors
varied in a dose dependent fashion. Overall motor activity, however,
measured as the percentage of intervals in which any behavior was
recorded, increased in a dose dependent manner. No stereotypic
behavior was observed. The D_1 agonist produced dose dependent
decreases in investigation of a novel stimulus and exploratory
activity in an open field situation. An 18 hour fast prior to testing
failed to alter the frequency of behaviors elicited by a fixed dose of
the agonist.

In contrast, the D_2 agonist LY 171555 (figure 2) produced a dose
dependent increase in sniffing and locomotion as well as grooming.
Animals tended to express either grooming or locomotor/exploratory
activity in response to the drug. The frequencies of these behaviors
were inversely correlated within each animal at all doses employed.
Overall motor activity increased in a dose response fashion. The
agonist also produced dose dependant increases in exploratory posture
(straight legs, arched back) retropulsion and ballistic locomotion.
The highest doses elicited spontaneous unilateral rotation.
Stereotypic behavior was observed but was, however, rare occurring in
less than 5% of observational intervals overall; it did not increase
in a dose dependent fashion. Stereotypies when present, consisted of
brief, intermittant bursts of licking or biting, consistently
interrupted by grooming or exploratory activity. Licking, biting and
gnawing syndromes or complex head and limb stereotypies elicited by
mixed D_1 D_2 agonists such as apomorphine or amphetamine were not seen.
Separate experiments utilizing doses up to 96 mg/kg demonstrated no
increase in the frequency of these discontinuous sterotypies nor the
appearance of intense apomorphine or amphetamine-like stereotypic
behavior. The D_2 agonist also produced a dose dependent increase in
the active investigation of a novel object and pursuit of a moving
stimulus and a concommitant decrease in the duration of response to a
noxious stimulus. An overnight fast altered the response to a fixed
dose of this agent, with fasted rats showing significantly more
sniffing and locomotor activity and non fasted rats significantly more
grooming behavior, while total overall motor activity did not differ
between the two groups.

Behavioral effects of combined D_1 and D_2 stimulation

The interaction of D_1 and D_2 agonists was studied in the
unilateral quinolinic lesioned animals by injecting LY 171555 at a
fixed effective dose and SKF 38393 at varying doses as illustrated in
figure 3. The D_1 agonist, which elicited no rotational behavior when
administered alone, increased the number of rotations induced by LY
171555 in a dose dependent manner, without modifying the duration of
turning. The combined administration of drugs produced a tight
rotational pattern accompanied by intense stereotypic gnawing and
licking, while LY 171555 alone elicited less tight rotation with
infrequent licking.

D_1/D_2 receptor interactions were studied in intact rats utilizing
a dose response matrix in which levels of both the D_1 and D_2 agonists

were varied (figure 4). Doses were in the range used in the individual dose response curves; a dose of either agonst which produced no significant behavioral response in the intact animal was included as well. At all doses of the D_2 agonist, concurrent stimulation of the D_1 receptor elicited classical stereotypic behaviors in a dose dependent fashion (figure 4c). These did not resemble the relatively infrequent, discontinous stereotypies seen in animals treated with LY 171555 alone, but were in each case identical to the well-recognized intense and invariant stereotypic syndromes elicited by apomorphine or amphetamine. While the full expression of

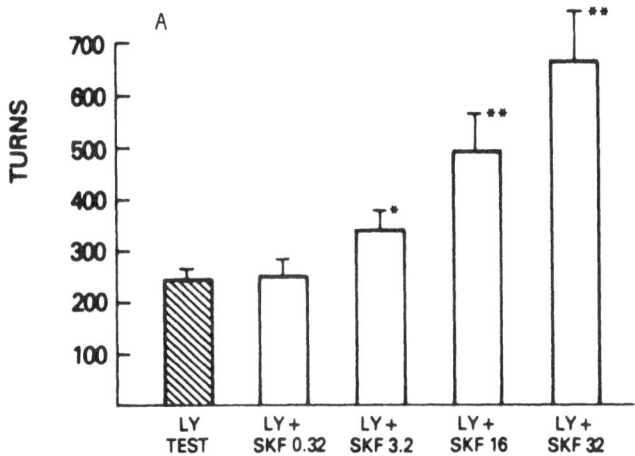

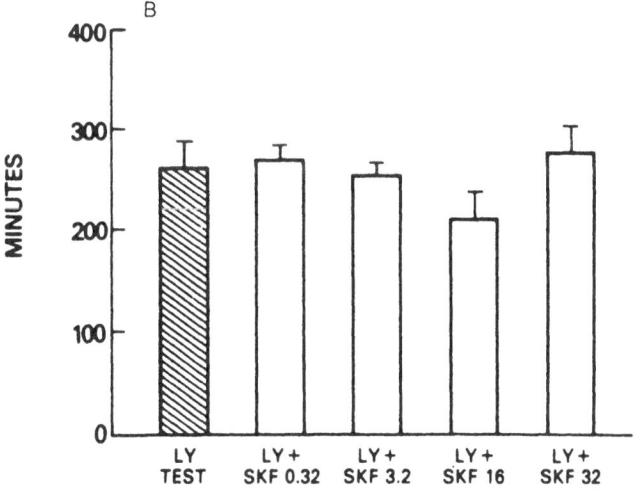

Fig. 3: Effect of SKF 38393 (mg/kg) on ipsilateral turning induced by LY 171555 (1 mg/kg). The D_1 agonist potentiates the total rotation (A) but not the duration (B). Values are expressed as Mean ± S.E.M. Dose effects were analyzed using ANOVA N = 9; * = P < 0.05; ** = P < 0.01. (Barone et al., 1986; modified).

Ly 171555 (mg/kg)

SKF 38393 (mg/kg)	a. .1	.75	3	12	x̄	b. .1	.75	3	12	x̄	c. .1	.75	3	12	x̄	d. .1	.75	3	12	x̄
0	.36	.63	.72	.68	.60	.10	.36	.52	.56	.39	0	0	.08	0	.02	.17	.33	.40	1.00	.48
2	.57	.84	.76	.96	.78	.23	.40	.68	.48	.45	0	.04	.08	.04	.04	.33	.40	1.00	.80	.63
8	.67	1.00	1.00	1.00	.92	.27	.04	.07	0	.10	0	.64	.75	.76	.54	0	.40	.33	.17	.23
32	.97	.87	1.00	1.00	.96	.30	.12	0	.04	.11	.30	.67	.86	.90	.68	0	0	0	0	0
x̄	.64	.84	.87	.91		.23	.23	.32	.27		.08	.34	.44	.43		.13	.28	.43	.49	
	TOTAL MOTOR ACTIVITY NS = .27					NON STEREOTYPIC GROOMING NS = .20					STEREOTYPIC BEHAVIOR NS = 0					RESPONSE TO NOVEL OBJECT NS = .25				

Fig. 4: Behavioral effects of combined administration of D_1 and D_2 agonists. Numbers represent mean frequency of intervals in which a specific behavior was observed at each dose combination. Data were analyzed using ANOVA and Duncan's multiple range tests. (A) illustrates that both LY 171555 and SKF 38393 significantly increase total motor activity ($P < .001$ in either instance). (B) illustrates that the higher doses of LY 171555 elicit increased frequencies of grooming behavior only at the lower doses of SKF 38393. ($P < .01$ for all three doses). Higher doses of the D_1 agonist significantly reduced grooming behavior at these same doses of LY 171555 ($P < .001$). (C) illustrates that SKF 38393 induces sterotypic behavior at all doses of LY 171555. ($P < .001$) Both LY 171555 and SKF 38393 contribute in dose response fashion to frequencies of stereotypic behavior at the higher doses of SKF 38393 ($P < .001$ for both drugs), while LY 171555 will not elicit sterotypic behavior in combination with the lower doses of SKF 38393. (D) illustrates that LY 171555 elicits a dose response increase in the active investigation of a novel object at lower levels of D_1 receptor stimulation ($P < .001$). The higher doses of SKF 38393 produce sensory unresponsiveness in combination with all doses of LY 171555 ($P < .001$). N = 5-7, each group.

stereotypic behavior appears to require an adequate level of D_1 receptor stimulation, both the nature and the frequency of these stereotypies appears to depend upon the degree of both D_1 and D_2 receptor activation once this threshold is reached. Lower levels of the agonists are associated with apomorphine-like licking, biting or gnawing syndromes; higher doses elicit behaviors characteristic of high doses of amphetamine such as unvarying lateral to and fro movements of the head and limbs, and stereotyped fragments of grooming movements resulting in self mutalation. At doses of LY 171555 which elicit conspicious locomotor activity and grooming in the intact animal, concurrent administration of the D_1 agonist produced dose dependent decreases in these behaviors as stereotypic behaviors intervened (figure 4b). At all doses of the D_2 agonist, concommitiant adminstration of SKF 38393 produced a dose-dependant increase in the frequency of intervals during which the animal's head remained down and fixed in a single position at the floor. At all doses of LY 171555, the D_1 agonist produced a dose dependent decrease in responsiveness to a noxious stimulus, decreased investigation of a novel object (with preservatation of the orientation reaction) (figure 4d) and decreased exploratory behavior in the open field.

The effects of increasing D_2 receptor stimulation, on the other hand, were not the same throughout the matrix but depended upon the underlying degree of D_1 receptor tone. At lower doses of the D_1 agonist, D_2 receptor stimulation, as in the intact animal, elicited complex motor programs such as grooming, locomotion and exploratory activity and a dose dependent increase in responsiveness to environmental stimuli. At higher doses of the D_1 agonist - when the expression of more complex endogenous behaviors is reduced and overall sensory responsiveness diminished - increasing D_2 receptor stimulation, as outlined above, appears principally to modify the nature of the stereotypies expressed. In a spearate experiment, the injection of SKF 38393 was delayed for an hour after administration of LY 171555.   Animals that were predominantly engaged in either grooming or locomotor activity prior to the second injection consistently displayed grooming and locomotor (head and limb) stereotypies respectively.

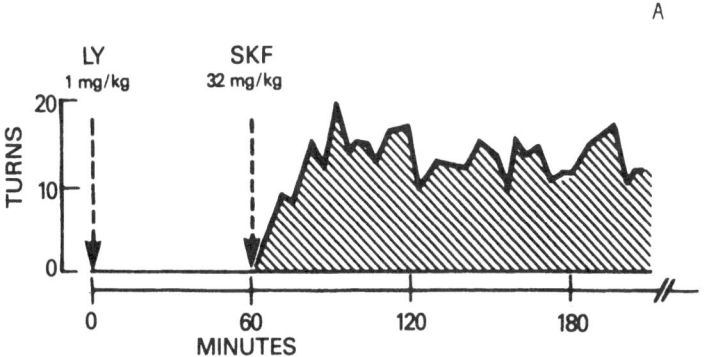

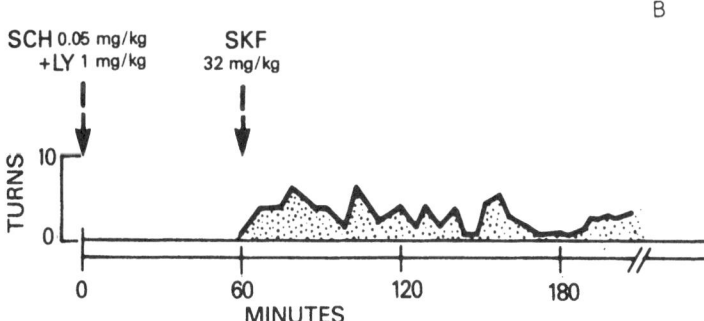

Fig. 5: Effect of AMPT pretreatment (A) and SCH 23390 (B) on rotation induced by LY 171555 (1 mg/kg). AMPT (200 mg/kg) was injected four and again two hours before LY 171555. SCH 23390 (0.05 mg/kg) was injected at the same time as LY 171555. SKF 38393 (32 mg/kg), injected one hour after LY 171555, restored turning. Shaded areas represent the mean of the rotations recorded in 4 rats. (Barone, et al., 1986; modified).

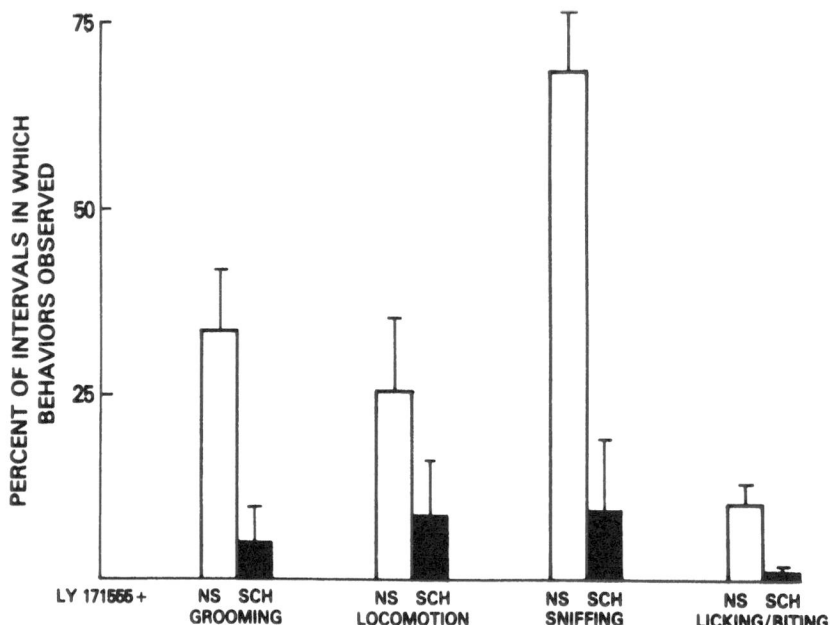

Fig. 6: Effects of the selective D_1 antagonist SCH 23390 on behaviors elicited by the D_2 agonist LY 171555. Mean frequencies of observed behaviors and the standard errors of these means are illustrated. SCH 23390 (0.1 mg/kg, I.P.) delivered 30 minutes prior to the injection of LY 171555 significantly reduced the frequencies of grooming, locomotor activity, sniffing and licking/biting. ($P < .01$ in each instance, Student's T test with Bonferroni correction). $N = 6-7$, each group.

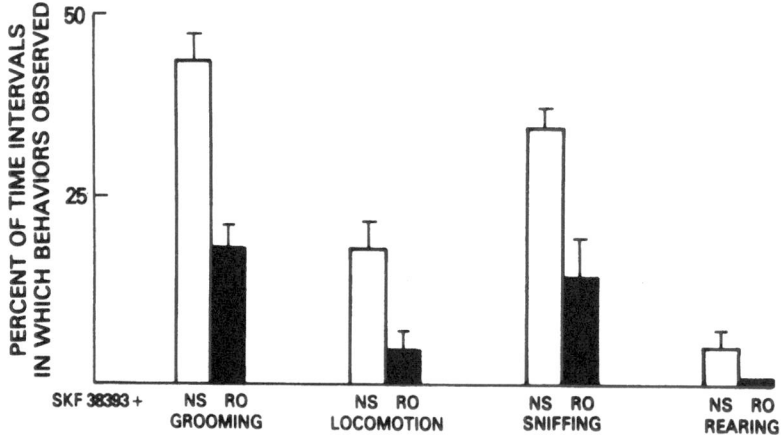

Fig. 7: Effects of the selective D_2 agonist RO 22-1319 on behaviors elicited by the D_1 agonist SKF 38393. Mean frequencies and standard errors are illustrated for individual behaviors. Injection of RO 22-1319 (0.4 mg/kg, I.P.) 30 minutes prior to injection of SKF 38393 significantly reduced grooming, locomotion and sniffing ($P < .01$, Student's T tests with Bonferroni correction) and produced a non-significant decrease in rearing behavior. $N = 7-8$, each group.

The effects of selective dopamine antagonists and catecholamine depletion upon agonist induced behaviors

Rotation induced in the quinolic acid lesioned rat by the selective D_2 agonist was totally inhibited by concurrent administration of the selective D_1 antagonist SCH 23390 (figure 5b). One hour after the injection of these agents, subsequent injection of a fixed dose of SKF 38393 (32 mg/kg) was able to restore rotational behavior. Similarly, pretreatment with AMPT, which depletes endogenous dopamine and thus precludes dopamine receptor stimulation by endogenous amines, prevented the rotational behavior elicited by LY 171555. Again, rotation could be restored by injecting SKF 38393 (figure 5a).

In the intact animals a low dose of the D_1 antagonist significantly reduced all behaviors elicited by LY 171555 (figure 6.) while low doses of the selective D_2 antagonist Ro 22-1319 significantly reduced the behaviors elicited by SKF 38393 (figure 7). Higher doses of the selective antagonists blocked all the behavioral effects of either dopamine agonist administered alone or in combination.

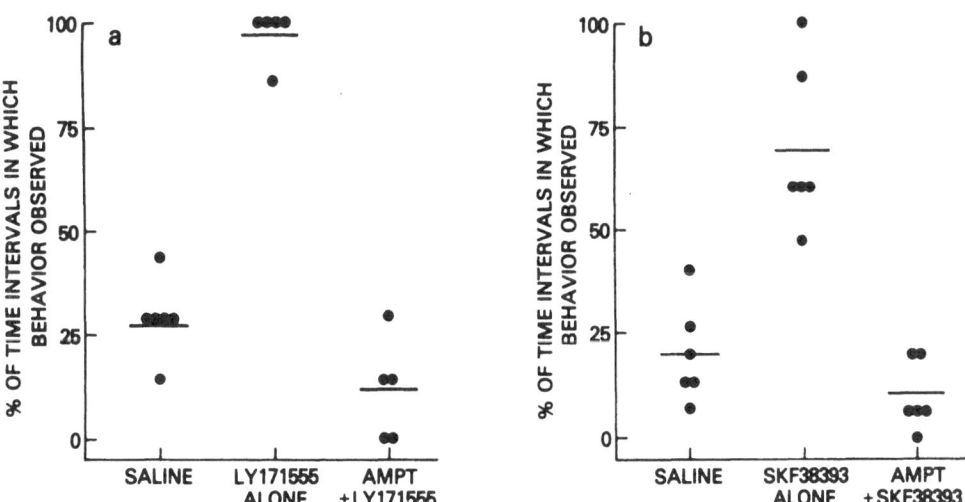

Fig. 8: Effects of catecholamine depletion on agonist induced behaviors. The behavioral activity of saline treated animals is compared with activity elicited by administration of 3 mg/kg LY 171555 (A) or 8 mg/kg SKF 38393 (B) in intact and AMPT pretreated rats; n = 6 for all groups. Points represent individual animals and denote the percentage of intervals in which any motor behavior (including locomotion, grooming, sniffing, rearing, licking, biting or gnawing) was observed. Bars represent the means for each treatment group. AMPT pretreated and saline groups differ from non-depleted animals in either instance (p < .001, ANOVA, Duncan's multiple range test).

AMPT pretreatment inhibited the behaivoral response to either LY 171555 or SKF 38393 when these drugs were administered alone (figure 8). However, the full range of behaviors seen previously could be restored in these animals by concurrent administration of the D_1 and D_2 agonist in the same ratios which elicited the behaviors in untreated animals (figure 9). Similarly, the characteristic patterns of responses to environmental stimuli observed in the dose response matrix could be restored by concurrent adminstration of the agonists in the appropriate ratios.

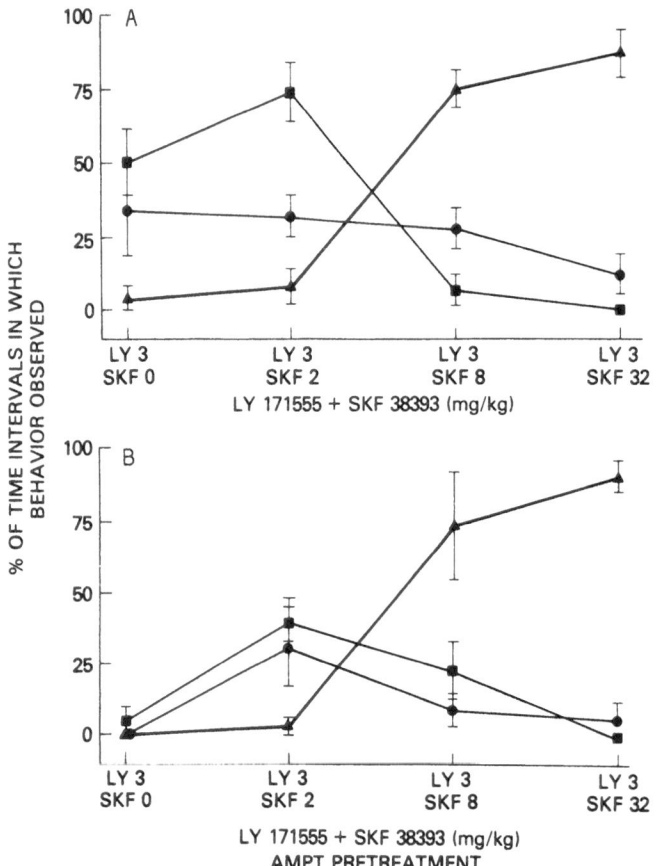

Fig. 9: Behavioral effects of concurrent administration of a fixed dose of LY 171555 and varying doses of SKF 38393 in (A) intact rats and in (B) rats pretreated with AMPT (300 mg/kg i.p. 4 hours and 200 mg/kg i.p. 2 hours prior to agonist administration). Scores for grooming (■), locomotion (●), and stereotypic behavior (▲) are displayed. Points indicate the mean percentage of intervals in which the behaviors were observed, bars denote the standard errors. The frequency of behaviors elicited by the 3 different dose combinations was statistically congruent in intact and AMPT pretreated animals (curves overlap and are parallel for each behavior, 2 way ANOVA). N = 5-7 animals in each group.

CONCLUSIONS

D_1/D_2 receptor synergy in the expression of motor behaviors

The results of these experiments suggest that a complex
functional interaction between D_1 and D_2 receptors is involved in the
generation of certain behaviors. What is initially apparent is that
the D_1 receptor exerts its most profound behavioral effects when the
D_2 receptor is stimulated concurrently. The D_1 agonist will not
produce rotation in quinolinic acid lesioned animals but will
augment and significantly alter the nature of the rotational response
to the D_2 agonist, producing a shift from a wide to a tight rotational
pattern. In the intact animal, the D_1 agonist administered alone does
produce a significant, although relatively nonspecific, behavioral
response. When coadministered with the D_2 agonist, however, it
produces a substantial alteration in the animals' responsiveness to
environmental stimuli and elicits classical stereotypic behaviors
which are not seen when either agonist is administered alone. These
intense stereotypic behaviors, classically associated with apomorphine
and amphetamine, are produced only at relatively high levels of D_1
receptor stimulation. This is consistent with the characteristic dose
response relationships of these mixed agonists, in which stereotypic
behavior emerges only at what may be doses which are high enough to
adequately stimulate the lower affinity D_1 receptor.

Obligatory D_1/D_2 interaction in the generation of motor behavior

The foregoing results not only document an interaction between DA
receptor subtypes but, in the experiments utilizing catecholamine
depleted or antagonist pretreated animals, also suggest that such an
interaction is essential. In the quinolinic acid lesioned animal, the
selective D_1 antagonist blocks the rotational response to the D_2
agonist. In the intact animal either selective antagonist effectively
inhibits behaviors elicited by D_1 or D_2 agonists administered alone
or in combination. Both D_1 and D_2 agonists are devoid of behavioral
effects in AMPT depleted animals, suggesting that their effects in
nondepleted animals may be due to stimulation of the complementary
receptor by endogenous dopamine. The restoration of all behaviors and
patterns of response to environmental stimuli in catecholamine
depleted animals by combined administration of the agonists, suggests
that in the normal animal all such unconditioned dopamine agonist
induced behaviors depend upon concurrent activation of D_1 and D_2
receptors. These results are consistent with previous work utilizing
selective antagonists (Christensen, et al., 1984; Molloy and
Waddington, 1984, 1985; Pugh, et al., 1985) and catecholamine depleted
preparations (Gershanik, et al., 1983). It should be stressed that
what appears to be the obligatory nature of D_1 and D_2 receptor
interaction may be the case only in the animal with normosensitive
dopamine receptors. In animals lesioned with 6-hydroxy-dopamine or in
which supersensitivity is induced by chronic reserpine pretreatment,
this interaction is apparently uncoupled. In these preparations both
agonists are capable of inducing either rotation or stereotypic
behavior, and the selective antagonists no longer effectively block
behaviors elicited by stimulation of the complementary receptor (Arnt,
1985; Arnt and Hyttel, 1984; Gershanik, et al., 1983; Breese and
Mueller 1985). In the future it may prove useful to test new
putative dopamine agonists in both 6 - hydroxydopamine and quinolinic
acid lesioned rats: the former model would generally identify the
agonist-like response of the drug, the latter could discriminate
between D_1 and D_2 agonist effects.

Nature of the D_1/D_2 receptor interaction

The tonic/phasic nature of D_1/D_2 receptor interaction

The results outlined here also suggest, given the obligatory nature of D_1 and D_2 receptor interaction, a qualitative difference in the roles played by these receptors in the generation of motor behavior. In quinolinic acid lesioned rats, D_1 receptor stimulation, while incapable of eliciting rotation by itself, is necessary for the induction of rotation by stimulation of the D_2 receptor. D_1 receptor stimulation may therefore provide a "tonic" background activation which allows the "phasic" component of D_2 stimulation to become effective (Barone, et al., 1986). D_2 receptor stimulation is necessary to trigger motor behavior, but only upon a requisite level of D_1 receptor tone. Further evidence of a phasic action of the D_2 receptor system derives from the observation that endogenous dopamine was unable to evoke any rotational behavior under resting conditions in rats two weeks after recovery from quinolic acid lesions. Spontaneous turning could be observed during periods of stress. Since rotation reflects dopamine receptor stimulation on the intact side (Schwartz et al., 1979), it is possible that in the absence of stress or pharmacologic stimulation, the rate of endogenous dopamine release in the intact striatum is insuffient to stimulate D_2 receptors. In fact, a significant reduction in dopamine turnover has been described on the intact side for weeks following the unilateral kainic acid lesion (Andersson, 1980).

The role of the D_1 receptor in mechanisms of attention and arousal: behavioral states associated with high and low levels of D_1 receptor stimulation

The results of the combined administration of agonists in intact animals support and extend the concept of D_1 receptor tone as critical in underlying and regulating the behavioral response to D_2 receptor stimulation. The data suggest that two distinct behavioral states exist which are largely a function of the degree of tonic activation of the D_1 receptor and are in each case modified by the degree of D_2 receptor activation. Once again it should be stressed that administration of the D_2 agonist produces essentially no behavioral response without concurrent activation of the D_1 receptor. At low levels of D_1 receptor stimulation (i.e. that produced by endogenous dopamine or restored by the administration of low doses of SKF 38393 to the AMPT depleted animal) D_2 receptor activation elicits complex motor responses such as grooming, locomotion and exploratory activity which are part of the animals' endogenous behavioral repertoire, seen for example when normal animals are placed in a novel environment. These behaviors are accompanied by organized, apparently goal directed responses to exteroceptive stimuli. In this case, D_2 receptor stimulation produces a dose dependent decrease in the response to a noxious stimulus and an increase in intense investigation of a discrete novel stimulus and pursuit of a moving object. This apparent transition from avoidance to approach behavior is accompanied by increased active exploration in an open field. The frequency of behaviors elicited by the D_2 agonist is altered following an overnight fast which may be interpreted as a similar modification of the behavioral response by an enteroceptive stimulus.

In contrast, higher levels of D_1 receptor stimulation are, at all doses of the D_2 agonist employed, associated with diminished responsiveness to environmental stimuli. Behaviors such as grooming and locomotor activity are invariably reduced in frequency and replaced by stereotypic behaviors which represent fragmentation and purposeless repetition of elements of these same behaviors. At higher doses of D_1 receptor activation the level of D_2 receptor stimulation appears to determine in part the nature of the stereotypies expressed. This relationship is more clearly demonstrated when the injection of SKF is delayed. The predominant behavior observed 1 hour after administration of LY 171555 consistantly determines the type of stereotypic behavior expressed after the injection of the D_1 agonist. Increasing D_1 receptor tone appears capable of "fragmenting" an ongoing behavior elicited by D_2 receptor stimulation.

The behaviors expressed at a low level of D_1 receptor tone can then be seen as purposeful, goal-oriented, and associated with efficient motor responsiveness to a variety of sensory stimuli. Contrasting sharply with this sort of integrated sensorimotor performance, the stereotypies expressed at higher levels of D_1 receptor stimulation are by definition purposeless, and are associated with a dramatic reduction in responsiveness to environmental stimuli. The transition between these behavioral states is consistent with the classical "inverted U" relationship between levels of arousal and behavioral response, in which low to moderate levels of arousal are associated with behavioral efficiency and high levels of arousal with behavioral disorganization (Duffy, 1957). This model has also been used to characterize the effect of dopamine agonists upon both conditioned and unconditioned behaviors in laboratory animals (Lyon and Robbins, 1975). Analysis of the dose-response matrix (figure 4) reveals that both D_1 and D_2 receptor stimulation contribute significantly, in dose response fashion, to overall arousal as measured by levels of motor activity per se. It appears, however, that it is increased stimulation of the D_1 receptor which is responsible for this major qualitative change in behavioral state, playing the critical role in the transition from functional to behaviorally dysfunctional levels of arousal.

A number of diseases, in which dopaminergic mechanisms have been implicated, have been characterized as states of hyperarousal associated with attentional deficits and behavioral disorganization. These include acute mania, attentional deficit disorders with hyperactivity in children, Lesch-Nyan disease, Gilles de la Tourette Syndrome and certain types of schizophrenia. Stereotypic behaviors are not infrequently observed in many of these conditions. The role of the D_1 receptor in the pathogenesis of these diseases bears further investigation.

D_1/D_2 receptor interaction: anatomical considerations

The anatomical substrate of D_1 and D_2 receptor interaction can only be a matter of speculation at this time. There is evidence that such interactions may take place at several levels along the neuraxis. Certain results suggest that D_1 and D_2 receptors may be located on the same postsynaptic cells in striatum (Stoof and Kebabian, 1981). On the other hand, unique and nonsuperimposable topographical distributions of D_1 and D_2 receptors within the basal ganglia have been demonstrated (Altar et al., 1985; Dubois and Scatton 1985; Dawson et al., 1986). In the cortex, D_1 and D_2 binding sites are located in different lamina and show different topographical distributions as well, with some regions (antreomedial frontal and suprahinal corticies) having only D_1 binding sites. In general, there appears to be significantly more D_1 than D_2 binding in the cortical areas to which the mesencephalic dopamine system projects (Dawson et al., 1985). D_1/D_2 receptor interactions responsible for the generation of behavior could therefore involve coactivation of receptors at the level of a single neuron, within distinct subcortical regions, or might represent concurrent stimulation of cortical and striatal receptor mechanisms. There is at present no way of relating the pharmacologic distinctions between goal directed locomotor activity and stereotypic behavior which we report here to the anatomical distribution of D_1 and D_2 receptors in a way that is consistent with the well established association of these behaviors with ventral and dorsal striatal mechanisms respectively (Kelly and Iversen, 1975). Further experiments using metabolic imaging techniques, selective ablations, or local injections of selective agonists may help clarify this issue.

In conclusion, our studies suggest that the most profound behavioral effects of D_1 receptor stimulation occur when the D_2 receptor is stimulated concurrently. This synergistic interaction between receptor subtypes appears, furthermore, to be essential. In animals with normosensitive dopamine receptors all unconditioned behaviors such as locomotor activity and stereotypy classically associated with postsynaptic activity of dopamine agonists, as well as the rotational behavior induced by these agents, appear to depend upon concurrent activation of D_1 and D_2 receptors. Activation of the D_1 receptor may represent a tonic background upon which a phasic component of D_2 stimulation operates. Increasing activation of the D_1 receptor reduces attention and organized motor responsiveness to environmental stimuli, and appears to be necessary for the generation of stereotypic behavior. The D_1 receptor may play a role in the transition from levels of arousal associated with behavioral efficiency to states of hyperarousal associated with behavioral disorganization.

REFERENCES

Altar, C.A., S. O'Neil, R.J. Walter and J.F. Marshall, 1985, Brain dopamine and serotonin receptor sites revealed by digital subtraction autoradiography, Science, 228: 597.

Andersson, K., R. Schwarcz, K. Fuxe, 1980, Compensatory bilateral changes in dopamine turnover after striatal kainate lesion, Nature, 283: 94.

Arnt, J., 1985, Behavioral stimulation is induced by separate D_1 and D_2 receptor sites in reserpine-pretreated but not in normal rats, European J. Pharmacol., 113: 79.

Arnt J. and J. Hyttel, 1984, Differential inhibition by dopamine D_1 and D_2 antagonists of circling behaviour induced by dopamine agonists in rats with unilateral 6-hydroxydopamine lesions, European J. Pharmacol., 102: 349.

Barone, P., T.A. Davis, A.R. Braun, and T.N. Chase, 1986, Dopaminrgic mechanisms and motor function: Characterization of D_1 and D_2 receptor interactions, European J. Pharmacol., in press.

Braun, A.R., P. Barone, and T.N. Chase, D_1 D_2 receptor interaction in the generation of dopamine agonist related behaviors, submitted.

Breese, G.R. and R.A. Mueller, 1985, SCH 23390 antagonism of a D2 dopamine agonist depends upon catecholaminergic neurons. European J. Pharmacol., 113: 109.

Christensen A.V., J. Arnt, J. Hyttel, and O. Svendsen, 1984, Behavioral correlates to the dopamine D_1 and D_2 antagonists, Pol. J. Pharmacol. Pharm., 36: 249.

Creese, I., D.R. Sibley, M.W. Hamblin, and S.E. Leff, 1983, The classification of dopamine receptors: Relationship to radioligand binding, Ann. Rev. Neurosci., 6: 43.

Dawson, T.M. D.R. Gehlert, R.T. McCabe, A. Barnett and J.K. Wamsley, 1986, D_1 dopamine receptors in the rat brain: A quantitative autoradiographic analysis, J. Neuroscience, in press.

Dubois, A., and B. Scatton, 1985, Heterogeneous distribution of dopamine D_2 receptors within the rat striatum as revealed by autoradiography of (^3H)N-n-propylnorapomorphine binding sites, Neurosci. Lett., 57: 7.

Duffy, E., 1957, The psychological significance of the concept of "arousal" or "activation", Psychol. Rev., 64(5): 265.

Fray, P.J., B.J. Sahakian, T.W. Robbins, G.F. Koob, and S.D. Iversen, 1980, An observational method for quantifying the behavioral effects of dopamine agonists: Contrasting effects of d-amphetamine and apomorphine, Psychopharmacology, 69: 253.

Gershanik, O., R.E. Heikkila, and R.C. Duvoisin, 1983, Behavioral correlates of dopamine receptor activation, Neurology, 33: 1489.

Kebabian, J.W., and D.B. Calne, 1979, Multiple receptors for dopamine, Nature, 277: 93.

Kelley, P.H., and S.D. Iversen, 1975, Amphetamine and apomorphine responses in the rat following 6-OHDA lesions of the nucleus accumbens septi and corpus striatum, Brain Res., 94: 507.

Lyon, M., and T. Robbins, 1975, The action of central nervous system stimulant drugs: A general theory concerning amphetamine effects, Current Developments in Psychopharmacology, 2: 79.

Mailman, R.B., D.W. Schultz, M.H. Lewis, L. Staples, J. Rollema, and D.L. Dehaven, 1984, SCH 23390: A selective D_1 dopamine antagonist with potent D_2 behavioral actions, European J. Pharmacol., 101: 159.

Molloy, A.G., and J.L. Waddington, 1984, Dopaminergic behavior stereospecifically promoted by the D_1 agonist R-SK&F 38393 and selectively blocked by the D_1 antagonist SCH 23390, Psychopharmacology, 82: 409.

Molloy, A.G., and J.L. Waddington, 1985, Sniffing, rearing and locomotor responses to the D_1 dopamine agonist R-SK&F 38393 and to apomorphine: Differential interactions with the selective D_1 and D_2 antagonists SCH 23390 and metoclopramide, European J. Pharmacol., 108: 305.

Pugh, M.T., K.M. O'Boyle, A.G. Molloy, and J.L. Waddington, 1985, Effects of the putative D_1 antagonist SCH 23390 on stereotyped behavior induced by the D_2 agonist RU 24213, <u>Psychopharmacology</u>, 87: 308.

Randrup, A., and I. Munkvad, 1967, Stereotyped activities produced by amphetamine in several animal species and man, <u>Psychopharmacologia</u>, 11(4): 300.

Stoof, J.C., and J.W. Kebabian, 1981, Opposing roles for D_1 and D_2 dopamine receptors in efflux of cyclic AMP from rat neostriatum, <u>Nature</u>, 294: 366.

Schwarcz, R., K. Fuxe, L.F. Agnati, T. Hokfelt and J.T. Coyle, 1979, Rotational behaviour in rats with striatal kainic acid lesions: A behavioral model for studies on intact dopamine receptors, <u>Brain Res.</u>, 170: 485.

Schwarcz, R., W.O. Whetsell, Jr., R.M. Mangano, 1983, Quinolinic Acid: An endogenous metabolite that produces axon-sparing lesion in rat brain, <u>Science</u>, 219: 316.

Ungerstedt, U. and G. Arbuthnott, 1970, Quantitative recording of rotational behaviour in rats after 6-hydroxydopamine lesions of the nigrostriatal dopamine system. <u>Brain Res.</u>, 24: 485.

ELECTROPHYSIOLOGICAL ASSESSMENT OF DOPAMINE RECEPTOR SUBTYPES

T. Celeste Napier and George R. Breese*

Neuropharmacology, *Departments of Psychiatry and Pharmacology, Biological Sciences Research Center, University of North Carolina at Chapel Hill, School of Medicine, Chapel Hill, North Carolina

INTRODUCTION

Scientific approaches to the characterization of brain systems can be globally classified into those approaches which demonstrate the presence of a phenomenon, and those which attribute a function to the described phenomenon. These approaches are interdependent and both are essential for understanding the whole organism. Previous chapters in this volume provide reviews of the presence and distribution of subtypes of central dopamine (DA) binding sites. Behavioral function has now been correlated with each of these proposed receptor groups. The present review is concerned with electrophysiological consequences of DA receptor activation. Electrophysiology provides assessment of function at the single cell level and allows for discrimination among neuronal systems. Therefore, electrophysiology serves as a bridge between the identification and anatomical location of a receptor, and the characterization of whole animal behaviors resulting from receptor activation. The purpose of the present chapter is to review current observations of neuronal responses to exogenously administered dopaminergic agents which are purported to be specific for identified subpopulations of DA recognition sites.

ANATOMY OF MESOTELENCEPHALIC DOPAMINE PATHWAYS

The rapidly increasing knowledge of the organization of central DA-containing neurons has provided great detail concerning the localization of dopaminergic fibers and their cell bodies. The mesotelencephalic system refers to the ascending projection of mesencephalic DA neurons which terminate in telencephalic structures. This system is comprised of two major divisions; (1) mesocortical and (2) mesostriatal. The mesocortical division includes A9 and A10 projections to both allocortical and neocortical areas. These projections terminate in the olfactory tubercle, septum, stria terminals, amygdala, piriform cortex, hippocampus, entorhinal cortex and frontal cortex (see Lindvall and Bjorklund, 1981 for review). The <u>mesostriatal division</u> consists of the traditionally denoted nigrostriatal system (A8 & A9) (nomenclature according to Anden et al., 1966; Ungerstedt, 1971) as well as mesolimbic (A10) fibers. The striatum and nucleus accumbens receive afferents (in disproportional amounts) from both the ventral tegmental region (A10) and the substantia nigra zona compacta (A8 & A9; as reviewed by Lindvall and Bjorklund, 1981) and are densely innervated with DA-containing fibers (Fuxe, 1965). The globus pallidus contains a sparse plexus of DA-containing terminals which are likely collaterals of ascending nigral dopaminergic projections (Lindvall and Bjorklund, 1979).

NEUROANATOMICAL LOCATION OF DOPAMINE RECEPTORS

A correlation between the anatomical locale of specific ligand binding and innervation of terminals which release a neurotransmitter possessing high affinity for the same binding sites lends considerable credence to possible physiological significance of that receptor population. Early binding studies using tritiated DA agonists and antagonists demonstrated a central distribution which overlapped nicely with known dopaminergic inputs (Burt, et al., 1976). Of the multiple binding sites which have been identified for dopaminergic drugs (for review see Seeman, 1981) perhaps the two most likely to demonstrate a physiological function are the D_1- and D_2-DA receptor subtypes. As originally defined by Kababian and Calne (1979), D_1-receptors are binding sites which are positively linked to adenylate cyclase activation. D_2-binding sites are either unassociated or negatively linked with cyclic AMP formation (Kababian and Calne, 1979; Stoof and Kababian, 1981). The recent development of both agonists and antagonists possessing good specificity for each receptor subtype has provided a means for determining the unique responses produced by activating subpopulations of DA receptors.

Morphological location of DA receptors influences the response which results from activation of a given subtype. At least three types of DA receptors can be identified by morphological locale: postsynaptic receptors which lie transsynaptically to a dopaminergic terminal, presynaptic receptors which occur on nerve terminals of efferents which may or may not contain DA as its neurotransmitter, and autoreceptors which are located on somas or dendrites of DA-containing cells (see Roth 1981 for review).

Dendrites of the DA-containing cells of the <u>substantia nigra</u> synthesize (Pickel, et al., 1975; Hokfelt et al., 1975), store (Geffen et al., 1976) and release DA (Geffen et al., 1976; Nicoullon et al., 1977); therefore, it is logical to predict that dopaminergic binding sites would also be located here. D_2-DA receptor binding has been demonstrated for the substantia nigra by several laboratories (for review see Creese et al., 1982). These binding sites are predominately located on the DA-containing neurons (Quik et al., 1979; Murrin et al., 1979) and likely correspond to the well characterized dopaminergic autoreceptors. Substantial concentrations of specific binding sites for ^{3}H-SCH 23390 (a D_1-DA antagonist) are also found in rat substantia nigra tissue (Dawson et al., 1985; Schulz et al., 1985; Napier et al., 1986c). Dawson and colleagues (1985) demonstrated very dense autoradiographic grains for ^{3}H-SCH 23390 in the substantia nigra zona reticulata (a terminal region for striatal-nigral projections), with minuscule concentrations in the zona compacta. This corresponds with studies demonstrating that nigral DA-stimulated adenylate cyclase predominately resides on terminals of striatal- and/or pallidal-nigral fibers (Premont et al., 1976; Gale et al., 1977; Phillipson et al., 1977; Quik et al., 1979).

The ventral tegmental area has considerable binding at sites characterized as D_2. However, even though several laboratories have investigated the possibility, no DA-sensitive adenylate cyclase activity has been detected in this region (Bockaert et al., 1977; Phillipson et al., 1977; Lorez and Burkard, 1979a&b), indicating a lack of D_1-sites in this brain region.

Dopaminergic receptor characteristics of the striatum have been extensively studied, but conflicting results hinder agreement concerning physiological significance of these receptors (for an in depth discussion the reader is referred to Stoof, 1983). Only a brief overview of the general observations will be presented here. Binding indicative of D_2-sites is dense in the caudate-putamen; however, the precise location of this binding remains an enigma. A portion of striatal D_2-binding sites are postsynaptic to dopaminergic afferents (Schwarcz et al., 1978; Govoni et al., 1978) and located on intrinsic neurons. DA-containing terminals make synaptic contact with the cholinergic interneurons of the striatum and activation of striatal D_2-DA receptors inhibit the release of acetylcholine. This inhibition is not observed with the D_1-agonist, SKF 38393, and is blocked by neuroleptics which have a high affinity for D_2-sites. Significant discussion still remains whether or not binding indicative of D_2-sites occurs on presynaptic terminals of afferent fibers from the cortex and/or from the substantia nigra (see Stoof, 1983). Kainic acid-induced lesions of intrinsic striatal neurons nearly eliminates striatal DA-activated adenylate cyclase activity (Govoni et al., 1978; Schwarcz et al., 1978), which suggests an intrinsic location for striatal D_1-binding.

Binding sites indicative of D_2-DA receptors have been reported for the nucleus accumbens (Beart and McDonald, 1982; Jastrow et al., 1984). DA-stimulated adenylate cyclase activity (Clement-Cormier et al., 1974; Horn et al., 1974), as well as SCH 23390 binding (Schulz et al., 1985), has been demonstrated for homogenates of nucleus accumbens. The D_1-sites are postsynaptic to tegmental innervation (Tassin et al., 1982).

Although the globus pallidus has not been traditionally considered to be monosynaptically associated with ascending DA fibers, this region contains DA and its major metabolites in concentrations which are approximately 10% of that observed for the striatum (Napier et al., 1986b). The pallidum also contains both D_1- (Schulz et al., 1985, Napier and Breese, 1986) and D_2-binding sites (Fields et al., 1977; DeKeyser et al., 1985; Napier and Breese, 1986). Immunocytochemical studies using DARPP-32 have revealed that high levels of adenylate cyclase, which correspond to D_1-receptor sites, are located in nerve terminals and axons within the globus pallidus (Ouimet et al., 1984).

DA-stimulated adenylate cyclase has been identified in the <u>cerebral cortex</u> by several investigators (for review see Thierry et al., 1984b) and is situated postsynaptic to cortical dopaminergic terminals (Tassin et al., 1982). D_1-binding sites are also located in cortical tissue (Schulz et al., 1985). Binding to sites characterized as D_2 is also observed for cortical tissue with a topographical distribution that is distinct from DA receptors coupled to adenylate cyclase (Tassin et al., 1982).

ELECTROPHYSIOLOGICAL PHARMACOLOGY OF DOPAMINERGIC SYSTEMS

This review will be concerned with only those studies which describe the electrophysiological responses to drugs considered specific for D_1- and D_2-DA receptor subtypes as defined above. The reader is referred to the excellent reviews of Clark, Hjorth and Carlsson (1985a&b) for a detailed description of the purported DA autoreceptor agonist 3-(3-hydroxyphenyl)-N-n-propyliperidine (3-PPP); and to Chiodo and Bunney (1984), and York (1979), for in depth overviews of electrophysiological pharmacology for dopaminergic cells and striatal cells, respectively, before the advent of specific D_1-acting drugs.

Responses of Dopamine-Containing Cells to Activation of Dopamine Receptors

The electrophysiological identification of midbrain DA-containing cells (Bunney et al., 1973b; Guyenet and Aghajanian, 1978) has provided investigators a valuable tool for studying this brain area. It is well established that activation of autoreceptors located on the dendrites or soma of DA-containing cells of the substantia nigra results in a profound depression of firing (Bunney et al., 1973a&b; Bunney and Aghajanian, 1976; Baring et al., 1980). This depression is readily blocked by antagonists thought to act at D_2-DA receptors (for review see Chiodo and Bunney, 1984). Increases in firing rates are observed with systemically administered "D_2-neuroleptics". However, maximum rate increases observed in anesthetized rats are about 50% of those increases observed with systemically administered D_2-neuroleptics in unanesthetized, paralyzed animals (Bunney et al., 1973b). Like D_2-neuroleptics, systemic administration of SCH 233390 increases firing rate in both anesthetized and unanesthetized rats (Napier et al., 1986c and Mereu et al., 1985, respectively). Also similar to D_2-neuroleptics, the maximum response to SCH 23390, as well as the dose necessary to increase rate by 50%, is attenuated with anesthesia (Napier et al., 1986c). However, when the ability of SCH 23390 to attenuate DA agonist-induced responses is compared to that seen with D_2-neuroleptics, striking differences are revealed. Haloperidol, a DA antagonist with high affinity for D_2-binding sites, reverses apomorphine-induced suppressions of DA cell firing (fig. 1) in doses that also block amphetamine- or apomorphine-induced increases in locomotion or stereotopies. SCH 23390, administered i.p. in doses of 0.05 to 0.5 mg/kg,

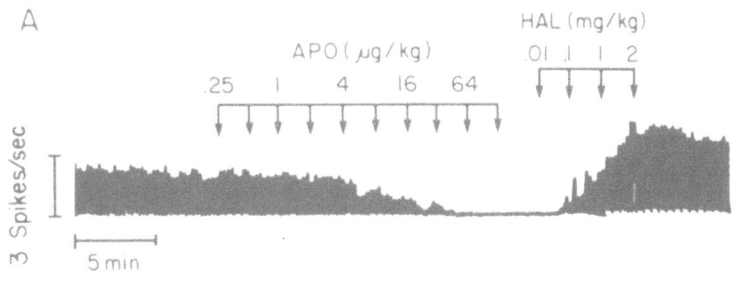

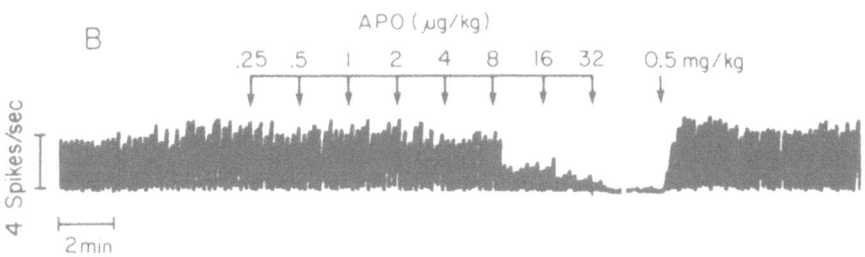

Fig. 1. Typical rate histograms obtained from dopaminergic
neurons located within the substantia nigra zona compacta.
These histograms illustrate the ability of haloperidol (HAL)
to reverse apomorphine (APO)-induced suppression and even to
supersede pretreatment baseline rates. A, frequency responses
to cumulative doses of APO up to 128 μg/kg, followed by
cumulative doses of HAL. B, responses to cumulative doses of
APO up to 32 μg/kg, followed by a single HAL injection. (From
Napier et al., 1986c, with permission.)

blocks behaviors resulting from the aforementioned DA
agonists, (Christensen et al., 1984) but antagonism of
apomorphine-induced decreases in dopaminergic cell firing are
not observed until much larger doses are administered (fig.
2). Another test for potential antagonism of responses caused
by agonist administration is the ability of antagonist
pretreatment to shift the agonist dose/response curve to the
right, i.e. to make the agonist less efficient in producing a
response. We also tested SCH 23390 in this paradigm and
discovered that D_1-blockade did not statistically alter the
apomorphine dose needed to produce 50% depression of
firing (fig. 3). However, an unexpected phenomenon was
observed. The ability of apomorphine to maximally suppress
firing was inhibited (fig. 3). These observations support a
theory proposed by Skirboll and colleagues (1979) which
suggests that low doses of apomorphine (<50 μg/kg i.v.)
preferentially affect DA receptors located on nigral
dopaminergic cells and that larger injections of apomorphine
are necessary before comparable suppressions are seen with
many striatal neurons. Apomorphine-induced changes in
striatal cells directly alter neuronal activity of nigral
dopaminergic cells (Scarnati et al., 1980). Since DA-
stimulated adenylate cyclase and SCH 23390 binding are located

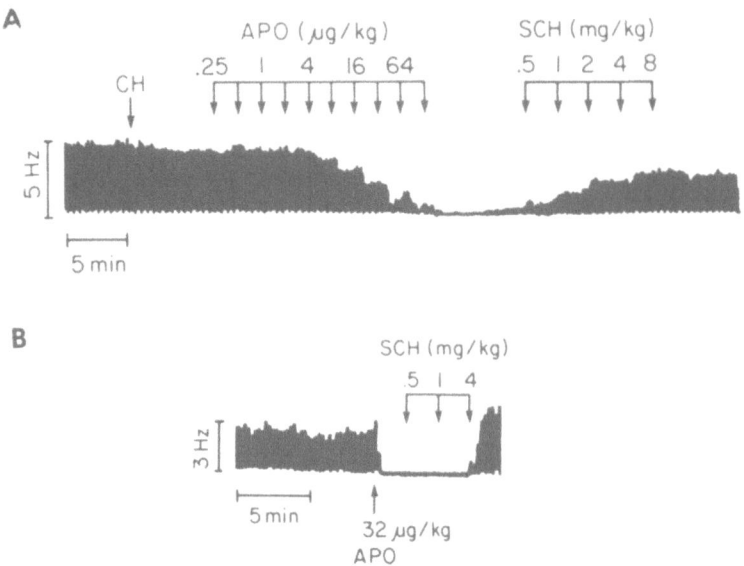

Fig. 2. Representative rate histograms demonstrating the
effects of SCH 23390 (SCH) and apomorphine (APO) on
spontaneous unit activity recorded from nigral dopaminergic
neurons. Drug concentrations represent the cumulative dose
administered. A, a histogram illustrating the suppression of
dopaminergic neuronal activity subsequent to APO
administration in doses up to 128 µg/kg i.v. B, partial
recovery of neuronal rate suppression produced by a single 32-
µg/kg dose of APO was observed with SCH. Neuronal activity
was not totally inhibited by APO; therefore, the cell was
monitored throughout the experiment. PreAPO baseline rates
were regained with larger doses of SCH. (From Napier et al.,
1986c, with permission.)

in the striatum, perhaps the ability of SCH 23390 pretreatment
to attenuate responses of dopaminergic cells to only the
higher doses of apomorphine reflect a blockade of D_1-receptors
within the striatum. Different striatal efferents may
regulate different DA receptor types (Herrera-Marschitz and
Ungerstedt, 1984) and subpopulations of DA cells have been
described (Skirboll et al., 1981); therefore, it is possible
that SCH 23390 administration delineates a group of nigral
neurons postsynaptic to striatal D_1-receptors from those which
are affected by striatal efferents containing D_2-receptors.
Certainly further experimentation is necessary to decipher the
exact mechanism of these connections, but resolving the
integration of dopaminergic cells with their receptor subtypes
will allow more sophisticated approaches to treating the
specific functional deficiencies observed in neurological
disorders while leaving other receptor subtypes intact to
minimize undesirable side effects.

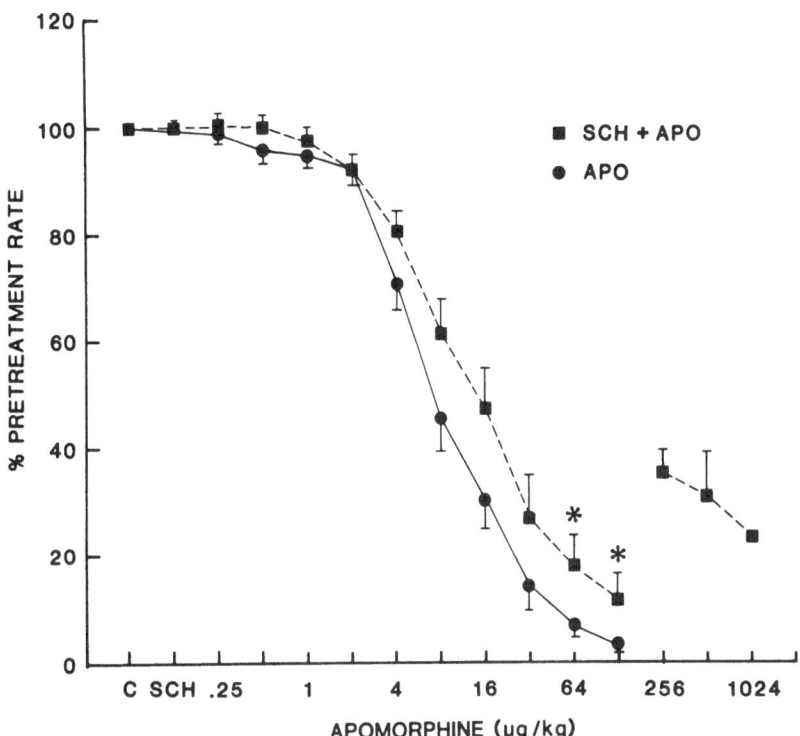

Fig. 3 A semilog plot of the cumulative dose-response curve
obtained for firing rates recorded from spontaneously active
dopaminergic cells after intravenous apomorphine
administration. The abscissa reflects cumulative doses with
two min lapsing between injections. Pretreatment baseline
control levels were standardized as 100% (illustrated on the
abscissa as C). Eighteen cells were recorded with apomorphine
(APO) alone, 15 cells were recorded with SCH 23390 (SCH)
followed by APO. SCH refers to rate obtained with 0.1 mg/kg
i.v. of SCH 23390. The number of cells tested with 256 and
512 µg/kg of APO equaled three, one cell was tested with 1024
µg/kg. *Significant differences (P<.05) between groups using
t-test comparisons. (From Napier et al., 1986c, with
permission.)

Autoreceptors which are sensitive to DA agonists are also
present on some DA-containing cells of the ventral tegmental
region (Wang 1981b). The ED_{50} dose for apomorphine-induced
depression of firing is the same as that reported for DA-
containing cells of the substantia nigra (Wang, 1981a).
Systemic administration of LY 141865, (a D_2-agonist), has a
dose response curve which is superimposable upon that observed
for apomorphine (Wang et al., 1984). Responses to both
apomorphine and to LY 141865 are completely antagonized by D_2-
neuroleptics. Iontophoretically applied LY 141865 is a potent
inhibitor of A10 cell firing and this response is blocked by
co-iontophoresing the D_2-antagonist, sulpiride (White and
Wang, 1984). Locally applied SKF 38393 is ineffective in
reducing DA cell activity, and SCH 23390 is unable to block
the depressant effects of DA agonists (White and Wang, 1984).
These experiments support the theory that autoreceptors
located on ventral tegmental dopaminergic neurons are, like
those of nigral DA-containing cells, of the D_2 type.

Responses of Neurons Located in Dopaminergic Terminal Regions to Dopamine Receptor Activation

A wealth of literature is available concerning the effects of DA neurotransmission on striatal neuronal communication. Intravenously administered apomorphine decreases firing of striatal cells (Skirboll et al., 1979), but microiontophoretic applications of DA are reported to increase as well as to decrease activity of these cells (e.g. Bloom et al., 1965; Woodruff et al., 1976; Norcross and Spehlmann, 1978; Skirboll et al., 1979). Iontophoresis of D_2-neuroleptics attenuate spike generation in the striatum which is produced by electrical activation of the substantia nigra (Ohno, et al., 1985). Similar application of SCH 23390 is ineffective with the majority of striatal cells tested (Ohno et al., 1985). These results indicate that nigrally evoked activity in the striatum is 'self-regulated' by presynaptic D_2-DA receptors. Iontophoretically applied D_2-antagonists are also reported to enhance greatly (Brown and Arbuthnott, 1983), as well as to not effect (Ohno et al., 1985), the excitation of striatal neurons subsequent to cortical stimulation. The reason for the disparity between these studies is unknown. However, there is biochemical evidence to suggest that DA activation of D_2-receptors located presynaptically on terminals of corticostriatal fibers decrease the release of the excitatory neurotransmitter glutamate (Mitchell and Doggett, 1980). This decrease is blocked by haloperidol and by spiperone but is not mimicked by cyclic AMP (Mitchell and Doggett, 1980), a product of adenylate cyclase activation. In support of this observation, rats with unilateral lesions of the ascending dopaminergic system demonstrate a decrease in the threshold for cortically-evoking striatal activity on the lesioned side (Arbuthnott et al., 1984). Although other interpretations of such data are possible, the majority of the present literature suggests that at least some of the excitatory cortical inputs to the striatum are under a tonic inhibition by DA being released from nigrostriatal fibers and acting at presynaptic D_2-receptors. The pharmacological profile of possible electrophysiological responses to striatal D_1-activation has not been systematically addressed. Striatal cells are known to be suppressed with iontophoretic applications of cyclic AMP (Siggins et al., 1974; Woodruff et al., 1976) which provides a functional correlate to the D_1-binding sites described for this brain region.

Activity of neurons located within the nucleus accumbens is often inhibited by locally applied DA (fig. 4; Woodruff et al., 1976; Akaike et al., 1984) and by stimulating the ventral tegmentum (Akaike et al., 1984). These responses are blocked by haloperidol. Firing of nucleus accumbens cells is inhibited with microiontophoretic applications of dibutyryl cAMP (Woodruff et al., 1976) and SKF 38393 (fig. 4), as well as following i.v. injections of the D_1-agonist (White and Wang, 1986). The effects of SKF 38393 are blocked by SCH 23390 and not by sulpiride (White and Wang, 1986). Microiontophoresis of LY 141865 also inhibits many nucleus accumbens cells but i.v. injections often produce biphasic (increase-decrease) responses (White and Wang, 1986). The inhibitory responses of each treatments are attenuated by sulpiride but not SCH 23390 (White and Wang, 1986). White and Wang (1986) explained the biphasic nature of rate changes

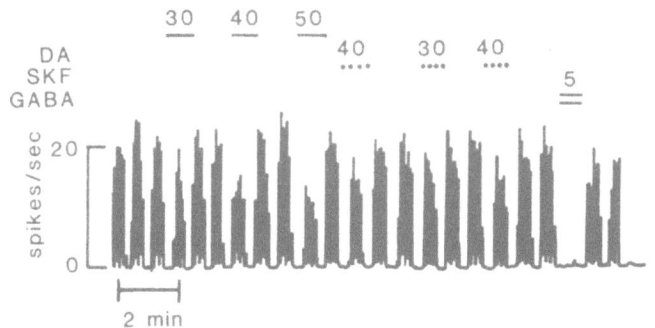

Fig. 4. A representative rate histogram of the responses observed in the nucleus accumbens with microiontophoretically applied DA and SKF 38393. The activity of this cell was evoked by pulsing on glutamate at 10 nA for 30 sec followed by a 10 sec interval where a 10 nA retaining current was applied to the glutamate containing barrel. Napier and Breese, 1986.

produced by systemically administered Ly 141865 as reflecting a higher affinity of this D_2-agonist for autoreceptors located on dopaminergic cells of the ventral tegmentum. Activation of these autoreceptors reduces the firing of DA-containing cells and results in a disinhibition of nucleus accumbens neurons. Therefore, low doses of LY 141865 causes an indirectly mediated increase of accumbens activity, whereas higher doses directly inhibit these cells. It is also important to note that the lack of nucleus accumbens neurons to demonstrate such a biphasic response to systemically administered SKF 38393 agree with reports which failed to demonstrate a D_1-induced response of ventral tegmental cells.

Systemically administered d-amphetamine (Bergstrom and Walters, 1981) and apomorphine (Bergstrom et al., 1982; Napier et al., 1984) increase firing frequency of the majority of cells recorded from the rat globus pallidus. The ED_{50} dose for apomorphine-induced increases (Table 1; Bergstrom et al., 1982) is in the range that produces substantial decreases in a subclass of striatal cells (Skirboll et al., 1979). The globus pallidus serves as a major output for striatal GABAergic (Nagy et al., 1978; Staines et al., 1980) and enkephalinergic neurons (Staines et al., 1980; Napier et al., 1983b) both of which are inhibitory to pallidal cells (for review of pallidal GABA-Waszcak et al., 1981; for opiates-Napier et al., 1983a; Frey and Huffman, 1985). Therefore, at least a part of the responses seen with pallidal neurons to systemically administered apomorphine may reflect a disinhibitory phenomenon. Decreases in firing of pallidal cells have also been observed following apomorphine injections. These cells demonstrated a maximum suppression of

Table 1. Responses of Spontaneously Firing Pallidal Cells in Chloral Hydrate Anesthetized Rats to Systemically Administered Apomorphine.

Response to apomorphine	Number of cells	ED_{50}[@] $(\bar{x}\pm SEM$ μg/kg)	Haloperidol reversal[$] (percent of cells tested)
Inhibition	4	12 ± 1.4	33%
Excitation	13	70 ± 10**	100%
Biphasic	4[#]	--	75%+
No effect	4	--	no change

** Significant at p<.05.
[$] The dose of haloperidol was 0.1 or 0.5 mg/kg i.v.
[@] ED_{50} value determined for each cell's dose-response curve and averaged for all cells within each response group.
[#] Activity of two cells was initially decreased and then increased with apomorphine and two cells demonstrated the opposite effect.
[+] Cells whose last apomorphine-induced response was reversed by haloperidol administration.

70% from pretreatment control rates, and an ED_{50} dose of apomorphine which is in the same range as that reported to decrease midbrain DA-containing cells (Table 1). Haloperidol administration to behaving monkeys (1-4 mg/kg i.m.) does not alter the firing frequency of globus pallidus cells (Filion 1979) but is reported to increase pallidal activity in acute experiments with rats (total cumulative dose of 1.6 mg/kg i.v.; Bergstrom et al., 1982). Using the criterion that return to pretreatment baseline rates defines antagonism, haloperidol injections were able to reverse apomorphine-induced increases in only 33% of pallidal cells tested in our laboratory (Table 1; fig. 5). However, more frequent blockade of both apomorphine- and amphetamine-induced increases has been observed (Bergstrom et al., 1982; Bergstrom and Walters, 1981, respectively). As illustrated in Table 1, haloperidol readily reversed apomorphine-induced suppressions. Systemic administration of lisuride or pergolide (potent D_2-agonists) increases firing rates of pallidal cells, but only the effects of pergolide are attenuated by subsequent haloperidol administration (Walters et al., 1982). The confusing responses of pallidal neurons to systemically administered drugs which presumably affect D_2-receptors is further confounded by recent investigations concerning D_1-sites. The stimulatory effect of apomorphine administration is reported to be blocked by SCH 23390 (1 mg/kg i.v.; Walters et al., 1984). However, intravenous injections of SKF 38393 (10-24 mg/kg) do not alter pallidal firing rates (Walters et al., 1982).

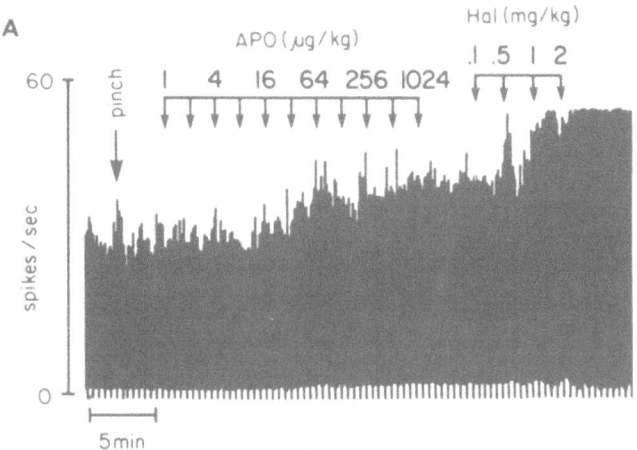

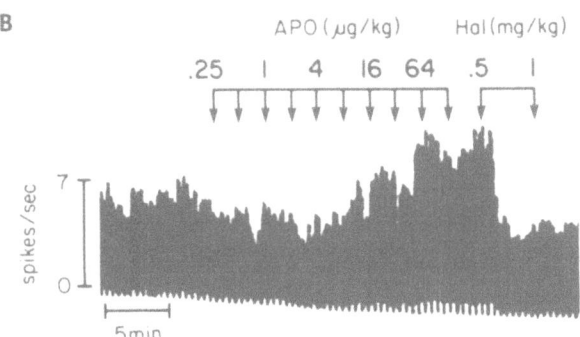

Fig. 5 Representative strip chart recordings illustrating pallidal cells that demonstrated an increase in firing rates (>20% of pretreatment baseline) with systemically administered apomorphine (cumulative doses of up to 1 mg/kg i.v.). A, the activity of this cell increased further following haloperidol injections. B, increases in rates caused by apomorphine were reversed by subsequent haloperidol administration.

Microiontophoretically applied DA has been reported to increase and also to decrease firing rates of pallidal activity (fig. 6; York, 1970; Yoshida and Obata, 1978; Bottger and Schmidt, 1980; Bergstrom and Walters, 1984; Napier and Breese, 1984). In experiments presently ongoing in our laboratory, DA-induced alterations of pallidal activity do not seem to be antagonized by systemically administered haloperidol (fig. 6); however, intravenous injections of cis-flupentixol (a DA antagonist with a propensity for D_1-receptors), as well as SCH 23390, do attenuate DA effects (fig. 6). We have also encountered pallidal cells whose excitations were not affected by systemically administered SCH 23390 but with subsequent injections of haloperidol reversal did occur (Napier and Breese, 1986). Supporting a role for D_1-receptors within the globus pallidus, Yoshida and Obata (1978) report inhibitory responses by pallidal cells with iontophoretically applied cAMP.

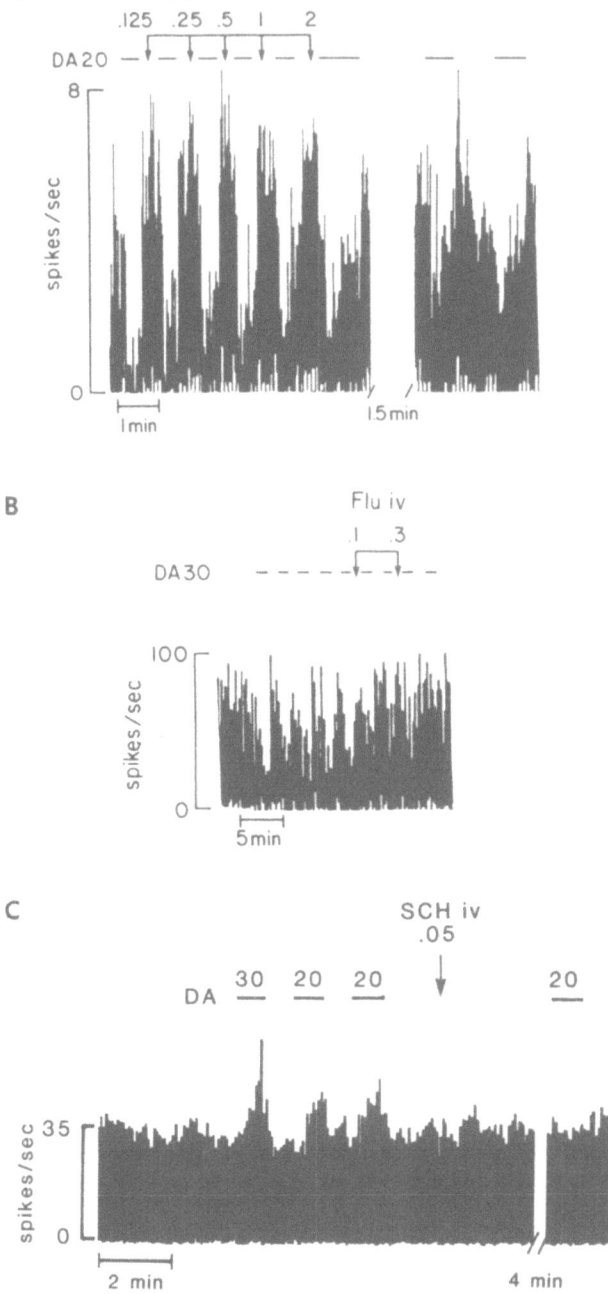

Fig. 6. Representative rate histograms of pallidal neuronal responses to iontophoretically applied DA before and after systemic injections of various DA antagonists. A, the DA-induced decreases in rate were not blocked by haloperidol (Hal), attenuation of response was observed with the 2 mg/kg dose. B, DA-induced suppressions were antagonized by intravenous injections of cis-flupentixol (Flu). C, SCH 23390 (SCH) also blocked the rate increases caused by iontophoretically applied DA (Napier et al., 1985; Napier and Breese, 1986).

These studies reveal the complexity of the proposed role of dopaminergic receptors in electrophysiological events of the globus pallidus. A conservative interpretation dictates that one assumes both D_1- and D_2-DA receptors influence pallidal neuronal activity; however, the precise mechanism of dopaminergic-induced responses remains to be elucidated.

Iontophoresis of DA results in both inhibition and excitation of cortical neurons (for review see Phillis, 1984). Both types of DA-induced responses are blocked by iontophoretically applied haloperidol and cis-flupentixol (Bevan et al., 1978). However, in layers V and VI of the prefrontal cortex, the layers with the heaviest dopaminergic innervation (Berger et al., 1976; Lindvall et al., 1978), DA generally suppresses activity and this suppression is antagonized by co-iontophoresing trifluoperazine (Bunney and Aghajanian, 1976). Stimulation of the ventral tegmentum evokes an inhibition of cortical neurons which is attenuated by i.p. administration of sulpiride (100 mg/kg; Thierry et al., 1984a). DA-induced excitations are observed for the rat somatosensory cortex (Bradshaw et al., 1983, 1985). This excitation is mimicked by locally applied LY 171555 and reversed by haloperidol but not by cis-flupentixol. No cortical response is demonstrated with iontophoretically ejected SKF 38393.

WHOLE ANIMAL CORRELATIONS TO ELECTROPHYSIOLOGICAL OBSERVATIONS

DA agonists and antagonists which seem specific for subpopulations of binding sites have only recently been characterized; therefore, pharmacological characterization of neuronal electrical events is in its infancy for DA receptor subtypes. The sparsity of available literature makes conclusive interpretations difficult; however, certain phenomena have been reported by enough investigators to merit a general acceptance. The areas of conflicting results underscores the complexity of the dopaminergic system and forces formulation of novel theories concerning the function of DA as a neurotransmitter. New facts and new theories are necessary to allow the correlation of electrophysiological consequences of DA receptor activation with the behavioral abnormalities associated with disturbances of brain DA communication.

The electrophysiological experiments reviewed in this chapter demonstrate that D_1- and D_2-DA binding sites are functionally distinct and that both are involved in neuronal communication of the central nervous system. Electrophysiological studies of DA-containing cells agree with earlier biochemical investigations showing that somatodendritic autoreceptors are of the D_2 type. If D_1-receptors are involved in communicative processes of dopaminergic neurons, this involvement is most likely via striatal or pallidal feedback loops, including D_1-receptor influences on GABAergic inputs to the substantia nigra zona reticulata. This suggestion is supported by behavioral studies; haloperidol microinjected into the substantia nigra zona compacta blocks behaviors induced by amphetamine (Jackson and Kelly, 1983) whereas zona compacta injections of SCH 23390 fail to alter apomorphine-induced behaviors (Napier et al., 1986c). Therefore, it appears that the ascending midbrain DA system is modulated at the dopaminergic cell body level by D_2-receptors, whereas descending outputs from the basal ganglia are modulated at the level of the substantia nigra zona reticulata by D_1-DA receptors.

The heterogeneous nature of responses to selective D_1- and D_2-receptor activation by cells located postsynaptic to dopaminergic inputs suggests that these receptor subtypes are involved in a variety of components of DA neurotransmission. This variety is also observed behaviorally (see other chapters). In attempting to interpret these findings it is necessary to realize the level of integration that is present in terminal regions of DA fibers. Neuronal firing changes resulting from systemically administered agonists likely reflect mutual regulation of DA receptor subtypes, even though a particular subset is directly activated. This theory is supported by biochemical studies which demonstrate that D_1-receptors play a permissive role in the ability of D_2-antagonists to increase rat striatal DA metabolite concentrations (Saller and Salama, 1985). Behavioral studies also indicate a functional integration between DA receptor subtypes. For example, circling behaviors in rats with unilateral lesions of the substantia nigra can be elicited by both D_1- and D_2-DA-agonists (Arnt and Hytell, 1984). Administration of D_1- or of D_2-agonists alone are ineffective in attenuating the akinesia produced by reserpine treatments in rats; but simultaneous activation of both DA receptor subtypes block the reserpine-induced motor dysfunction (Gershanik, et al., 1983). Therefore, both DA receptor subtypes are likely involved in normal animal behaviors; however, the morphological level at which each of these types of receptors exert their specific influence remains speculative.

It does appear that D_2-receptors of midbrain DA-containing cell bodies are more sensitive to D_2-agonists than cells recorded from DA terminal regions. However, both the striatum (Skirboll et al., 1979) and the globus pallidus (Table 1) demonstrate subpopulations of cells which exhibit the similar sensitivity to DA agonists as that observed for dopaminergic cell bodies. It is interesting that neuronal responses to systemically administered DA agonists are quite different among the various DA terminal regions. For example, the majority of cells encountered in the striatum are inhibited by apomorphine whereas the globus pallidus is more consistently excited with similar apomorphine treatments. Cells of the nucleus accumbens are inhibited by D_1-agonist administration but exhibit a biphasic response to systemically administered D_2-agonists. Since dose-response effects of striatal or pallidal cells to systemically administered SKF 38393 or LY 141865 have not been thoroughly studied it is difficult to know if a disinhibition of midbrain DA-containing cells contributes to the responses seen in these DA terminal areas. The ventral tegmentum communicates monosynaptically with nucleus accumbens cells (DeFrance and Yoshihara, 1975). Since a majority of the GABAergic terminals synapse with zona reticulata cells instead of directly onto dopaminergic neurons of the substantia nigra, perhaps the influences of nigral interneurons are responsible for effects observed in the globus pallidus and striatum following systemically administered DA-agonists. This phenomenon would explain the differences seen in these areas as compared to that observed for the nucleus accumbens with similar treatments. Behavioral responses to microinjection of dopaminergic drugs into the nucleus accumbens or the globus pallidus also reveal differences in DA-receptor subtypes between the two brain regions. For example low doses of haloperidol injected directly into the nucleus accumbens blocks the increased locomotion produced by pretreatments with intra-accumbens DA injections (Pijnenburg et al., 1975). Similar doses of haloperidol microinjected unilaterally into the globus pallidus does not induce circling behaviors in amphetamine-treated rats, whereas circling is produced with comparable injections of cis-flupentixol or SCH 23390 (Napier and Breese, 1984). These observations indicate that locomotor functions of the nucleus accumbens, but not of the globus pallidus, involve D_2-DA receptors.

Further investigation is obviously necessary before the physiological intricacies of DA receptor subtypes can be delineated. Understanding the complexities of behaviors involving central dopaminergic systems will require astute integration of electrophysiological observations with results gathered from anatomical, biochemical and pharmacological studies. With this multidiciplinary perspective approach, new methods will certainly be devised which will improve on today's pharmacological approaches to the treatments of central dopaminergic dysfunctions.

REFFERENCES

Akaike, A. Masashi, S. and Takaori, S., 1984, Microiontophoretic studies of the dopaminergic inhibition from the ventral tegmental area to the nucleus accumbens neurons, J. Pharm. Exp. Therap., 229:859-864.

Anden, N.-E., Dahlstrom, A., Fuxe, K., Olsson, K., and Ungerstedt, U., 1966, Ascending monoamine neurons to the telecephalon and diencephalon, Acta Physiol. Scand., 67:313-326.

Arbuthnott, G.W., Brown, J.R., Kapoor, V., and Whale, D., 1984, Presynaptic actions and dopamine in the neostriatum, in: "The Basal Ganglia, Structure and Function," J.S. McKenzie, R.E. Kemm and L.N. Wilcock, eds., pp. 173-203, Plenum Press, New York.

Arnt, J., and Hytell, J., 1984, Differential inhibition by dopamine D-1 and D-2 antagonists of circling behavior induced by dopamine agonists in rats with unilateral 6-hydroxydopamine lesions, Eur.J. Pharmacol., 102:349-354.

Baring, M.D., Walters, J.R., and Eng, N., 1980, Action of systemic apomorphine on dopamine cell firing after neonatal kainic acid lesion. Brain Res., 181: 214-218.

Beart, P.M., and McDonald, D., 1982, Neurochemical studies of the mesolimbic dopaminergic pathway: ^{3}H-spiperone labels two binding sites in homogenates of the nucleus accumbens of rat brain, J. Neurochem., 39: 1452-1460.

Berger, B., Thierry, A.M., Tassin, J.P., and Moyne, M.A., 1976, Dopaminergic innervation of the rat prefrontal cortex: A fluorescence histochemical study, Brain Res., 106:133-145.

Bergstrom, D.A., Bromley, S.D., and Walters, J.R., 1982, Apomorphine increases the activity of rat globus pallidus neurons, <u>Brain Res.</u>, 238:266-271.

Bergstrom, D.A., and Walters, J.R., 1981, Neuronal responses of the globus pallidus to systemic administration of d-amphetamine: Investigation of the involvement of dopamine, norephinephrine, and serotonin, <u>J. Neurosci.</u>, 1:292-299.

Bergstrom, D.A., and Walters, J.R., 1984, Dopamine attenuates the effects of GABA on single unit activity in the globus pallidus, <u>Brain Res.</u>, 310:23-33.

Bevan, P., Bradshaw, C.M., Pun, R.Y.K., Slater, N.T., and Szabadi, E., 1978, Responses of single cortical neurones to noradrenaline and dopamine, <u>Neuropharmacology</u>, 17:611-617.

Bloom, F.A., Costa, E., and Salmoiraghi, G.C., 1965, Anesthesia and the responsiveness of individual neurons of the caudate nucleus of the cat to acetylcholine, norepinephrine and dopamine administered by microelectrophoresis, <u>J. Pharmacol. Exp. Therap.</u>,

Bockaert, J., Premont, J., Glowinski, J., Tassin, J.P., and Thierry, A.M., 1977, Topographical distribution and characteristics of dopamine and B-adrenergic sensitive adenylate cyclase in the rat frontal cerebral cortex, striatum and substantia nigra. <u>Advan. Biochem. Psychopharmacol.</u>, 16: 29-37.

Bottger, G., and Schmidt, J., 1980, Der einflub von striatumreizung and mikroiontophoretisch appliziertem dopamin und azetylcholin auf die neuronale aktivitat im globus pallidus, <u>Acta biol. med. germ.</u>, 39:123-131.

Bradshaw, C.M., Pun, R.Y.K., Slater, N.T., Stoker,M.J., and Szabadi, E., 1983, Differential antagonistic effects of haloperidol on excitatory responses of cortical neurones to phenylephrine, noradrenaline and dopamine. <u>Neuropharmac.</u>, 22:945-952.

Bradshaw, C.M., Sheridan, R.D. and Szabadi, E., 1985, Excitatory neuronal responses to dopamine in the cerebral cortex: Involvement of D_2 but not D_1 dopamine receptors, <u>Br. J. Pharmac.</u>, 86:483-490.

Brown, J.R., and Arbuthnott, G.W., 1983, The electrophysiology of dopamine (D_2) receptors: A study of the actions of dopamine on corticostriatal transmission, <u>Neurosci.</u>, 10:349-355.

Bunney, B.S., and Aghajanian, G.K., 1976, d-Amphetamine-induced inhibition of central dopaminergic neurons: Mediation by a striato-nigral feedback pathway, <u>Science</u>, 192:391-393.

Bunney, B.S., and Aghajanian, G.K., 1976, Dopamine and norepinephrine innervated cells in the rat prefrontal cortex: Pharmacological differentiation using microiontophoretic techniques, <u>Life Sci.</u>, 19:1783-1792.

Bunney, B.S., Aghajanian, G.K., and Roth, R.H., 1973a, Comparison of effects of L-DOPA, amphetamine and apomorphine on firing rate of rat dopaminergic neurons. <u>Nature</u> 245: 123-125.

Bunney, B.S., Walters, J.R., Roth, R.H., and Aghajanian, G.K., 1973b, Dopaminergic neurons: Effect of antipsychotic drugs and amphetamine on single cell activity, <u>J. Pharmacol. Exp. Ther.</u>, 185: 560-571.

Burt, D.R., Creese, I., and Snyder, S.H., 1976, Properties of [^{3}H]haloperidol and [^{3}H]dopamine binding associated with dopamine receptors in calf brain membranes, <u>Mol. Pharmacol.</u>, 12:800-812.

Chiodo, L.A., and Bunney, B.S., 1984, Effects of dopamine antagonists on midbrain dopamine cell activity, <u>in</u>: "Catecholamines: Neuropharmacology and Central Nervous System-Theoretical Aspects," Vol. 8A, Neurology and Neurobiology, E. Usdin, A. Carlsson, A. Dahlstrom and J. Engel, eds., pp. 369-391, Alan R. Liss, Inc. New York.

Christensen, A.V., Arnt, J., Hyttel, J., Larsen, J.J., and Sverdsen, O., 1984, Pharmacological effects of a specific dopamine D-1 antagonist SCH-23390 in comparison with neuroleptics, <u>Life Sci.</u>, 334:1529-1540.

Clark, D., Hjorth, S., and Carlsson, A., 1985a, Dopamine-receptor agonists: Mechanisms underlying autoreceptor selectivity I. Review of the evidence, <u>J. Neural Trans.</u>, 62:1-52.

Clark, D., Hjorth, S., and Carlsson, A., 1985b, Dopamine-receptor agonists: Mechanisms underlying autoreceptor selectivity II. Theoretical considerations, <u>J. Neural Trans.</u>, 62:171-207.

Clement-Cormier, Y.C., Kebabian, J.W., Petzold, G.L., and Greengard, P., 1974, Dopamine-sensitive adenylate cyclase in mammalian brain: A possible site of action of antipsychotic drugs. <u>Proc. Nat. Acad. Sci.</u>, 71:113-117.

Creese,I., Morrow, A.L., Leff, S.E., Sibley, D.R., and Hamblin, M.W., 1982, Dopamine receptors in the central nervous system, <u>Inter. Rev. Neurobiol.</u>, 23: 255-301.

Dawson, T.M., Gehlert, D.R., Yamamura, H.I., Barnett, A., and Wamsley, J.K., 1985, D-1 dopamine receptors in the rat brain: Autoradiographic localization using ^{3}H-SCH 23390, <u>Eur. J. Pharmacol.</u>, 108: 323-325.

DeFrance, J.F. and Yoshihara, H., 1975, Fibria input to the nucleus accumbens septi, <u>Brain Res.</u>, 90:159-163.

De Keyser, J., De Backer, J-P, Convents, A., Ebinger, G. and Vauquelin, G., 1985, D_2 dopamine receptors in calf globus pallidus: Agonist high- and low-affinity sites not regulated by guanine nucleotide, <u>J. Neurochem.</u>, 977-979.

Fields, J.Z., Reisine, T.D., and Yamamura, H.I., 1977, Biochemical demonstration of dopaminergic receptors in rat and human brain using [^{3}H]spiroperidol, <u>Brain Res.</u>, 136:578-584.

Filion, M., 1979, Effects of interruption of the nigrostriatal pathway and of dopaminergic agents on the spontaneous activity of globus pallidus neurons in the awake monkey, <u>Brain Res.</u>, 178:425-441.

Frey, J.M. and Huffman, R.D., 1985, Effects of enkephalin and morphine on rat globus pallidus neurons, <u>Brain Res. Bul.</u>, 14:251-259.

Fuxe, K., 1965, Distribution of the monoamine nerve terminals in central nervous system, <u>Acta Physiol. Scand.</u>, 64(Suppl.247):39-85.

Gale, K., Guidotti, A., and Costa, E., 1977, Dopamine-sensitive adenylate cyclase location in substantia nigra, <u>Science</u>, 195: 503-505.

Geffen, I.B., Jessel, T.M., Cuello, A.C., and Iversen, I.I., 1976, Release of dopamine from dendrites in rat substantia nigra, <u>Nature</u>, 260:258-260.

Gershanik, O., Heikkila, R.E., and Duvoisin, R.C., 1983, Behavioral correlations of dopamine receptor activation, <u>Neurology</u>, 33:1489-1492.

Govoni, S., Olgiati, V.R., Trabucchi, M., Garau, L., Stefanini, E., and Spano., P.F., 1978, [^{3}H]haloperidol and [^{3}H]spiroperidol receptor binding after striatal injection of kainic acid, <u>Neurosci. Lett.</u>, 8:207-210.

Guyenet, P.G. and Aghajanian, G.K., 1978, Antidromic identification of dopaminergic and other output neurons of the rat substantia nigra, <u>Brain Res.</u>, 150: 69-84.

Herrera-Marschitz, M., and Ungerstedt, U., 1984, Evidence that striatal efferents relate to different dopamine receptors, <u>Brain Res.</u>, 323: 269-278.

Hokfelt, T., Halasz, N., Ljungdahl, A., Johansson, O., Goldstein, M., and Park, D., 1975, Histochemical support for a dopaminergic mechanism in the dendrites of certain periglomerular cells in the rat olfactory blub, <u>Neurosci. Lett.</u>, 1:85-90.

Horn, A.S., Cuello, A.C., and Miller, R.J., 1974, Dopamine in the mesolimbic system of the rat brain: Endogenous levels and the effects of drugs on the uptake mechanism and stimulation of adenylate cyclase activity, <u>J. Neurochem.</u>, 22:265-270.

Jackson, E.A., and Kelly, P.H., 1983, Role of nigral dopamine in amphetamine-induced locomotor activity, <u>Brain Res.</u>, 278:366-369.

Jastrow, T.R., Richfield, E., and Gnegy, M.E., 1984, Quantitative autoradiography of ^{3}H-sulpiride binding sites in rat brain, <u>Neurosci. Lett.</u>, 51:47-53.

Kebabian, J.W. & Calne, D.B., 1979, Multiple receptors for dopamine, <u>Nature</u>, 227:93-96

Lindvall, O., and Bjorklund, A., 1979, Dopaminergic innervation of the globus pallidus by collaterals from the nigrostriatal pathway, <u>Brain Res.</u>, 172: 169-173.

Lindvall, O., and Bjorklund, A., 1981, Neuroanatomy of central dopamine pathways: Review of recent progress, <u>in</u>: "Advances in Dopamine Research", M. Kohsaka, T. Shohmori, Y. Tsukada and G.N. Woodruff, eds., pp. 297-311, Pergamon Press, NY.

Lindvall, O., Bjoklund, A., and Divac, I., 1978, Organization of catecholamine neurons projecting to the frontal cortex in the rat, <u>Brain Res.</u>, 142:1-24.

Lorez, H.P., and Burkard, W.P., 1979a, Absence of dopamine sensitive adenylate cyclase in the A10 region: The origin of mesolimbic dopamine neurons, <u>Experientia</u> (Basel), 35:744-745.

Lorez, H.P., and Burkard, W.P., 1979b, Specific binding of ^{3}H-spiroperidol in the absence of dopamine-sensitive adenylate cyclase in the A10 cell region of the rat brain, <u>Experientia</u> (Basel), 35:938.

Mereu, G., Collu, M. Ongini, E., Biggio, G., and Gessa, G.L., 1985, SCH 23390, a selective dopamine D$_1$ antagonist, activates dopamine neurons but fails to prevent their inhibition by apomorphine, <u>Eur. J. Pharmacol.</u>, 111:393-396.

Mitchell, P.R., and Doggett, N.S., 1980, Modulation of striatal [^{3}H]-glutamic acid release by dopaminergic drugs, <u>Life Sci.</u>, 26:2073-2081.

Murrin, L.C., Gale, K., and Kuhar, M.J., 1979, Autoradiographic localization of neuroleptic and dopamine receptors in the caudate-putamen and substantia nigra: Effects of lesions, <u>Eur. J. Pharmacol.</u>, 60:229-235.

Nagy, J.I., Carter, D.A., and Fibiger, H.C., 1978, Anterior striatal projections to the globus pallidus,

entopeduncular nucleus and substantia nigra in the rat:
The GABA connection, Brain Res., 158:15-29.

Napier, T.C., and Breese, G.R., 1984, Dopamine functions of
the rodent globus pallidus: Effects of neurotensin and
neuroleptics, Neurosci. Abstr., 10:412.

Napier, T.C. and Breese, G.R., 1986, unpublished results.

Napier, T.C., Gay, D.A., Hulebak, K.L., and Breese, G.R.,
1985, Behavioral an biochemical assessment of time
related changes in globus pallidus and striatal dopamine
induced by intranigrally administered neurotensin,
Peptides, 6:1057-1068.

Napier, T.C., Givens, B.S., and Breese, G.R., 1986b,
unpublished results.

Napier,T.C., Givens, B.S., Schulz, D.W., Bunney, B.S., Breese,
G.R., and Mailman, R.B., 1986c, SCH23390 effects on
apomorphine-induced responses of nigral dopaminergic
neurons, J. Pharmacol. Exp. Therap., in press.

Napier, T.C., Pirch, J.H., and Peterson, S.L., 1983a,
Spontaneous unit activity in the globus pallidus
following cumulative injections of morphine in
phenobarbital- or chloral hydrate-anesthetized rats,
Neuropharmacology, 22:165-171.

Napier, T.C., Pirch, J.H., and Strahlendorf, H.K., 1983b,
Naloxone antagonizes striatally-induced suppression of
globus pallidus unit activity, Neuroscience, 9:53-59.

Napier, T.C., Simson, P.E., and Breese, G.R., 1985,
Systematically administered apomorphine increases and
microiontophoretically applied dopamine decreases
neuronal activity in rodent globus pallidus, Fed. Proc.
5:1387.

Nicoullon, A., Cheramy, A., and Glowinski, J., 1977, Release
of dopamine in vivo from rat substantia nigra, Nature
(London), 266:375-377.

Norcross, K., and Spehlmann, R., 1978, A quantitative analysis
of the excitatory and depressant effects of dopamine on
the firing of caudatal neurons: Electrophysiological
support for the existence of two distinct dopamine-
sensitive receptors, Brain Res., 156:168-174.

Ohno, Y., Sasa, M., and Takaori, S., 1985, Dopamine D-2
receptor-mediated excitation of caudate nucleus neurons
from the substantia nigra, Life Sci., 37:1515-1521.

Onali, P., Mereu, G., Olianas, M.C., Bunse, B., Rossetti, Z.,
and Gessa, G.L., 1985, SCH 23390, a selective D_1 dopamine
receptor blocker, enhances the firing rate of nigral
dopaminergic neurons but fails to activate striatal
tyrosine hydroxylase, Brain Res., 340:1-7.

Ouimet, C.C., Miller, P.E., Hemmings, Jr., H.C., Walaas, S.I.,
and Greengard, P., 1984, DARPP-32, a dopamine- and
adenosine 3':5'-monophosphate-regulated phosphoprotein
enriched in dopamine-innervated brain regions. III.
Immunocytochemical localization, J. Neurosci., 4:111-124.

Phillipson, O.T., Emson, P,C., Horn, A.S., and Jessell, T.,
1977, Evidence concerning the anatomical location of the
dopamine stimulated adenylate cyclase in the substantia
nigra, Brain Res., 136:45-58.

Phillis, J.W., 1984, Microiontophoresis of the cortical
biogenic amines, in: "Monoamine Innervation of Cerebral
Cortex", L. Descarries, P.R. Reader and H.H. Jasper,
eds., pp. 175-194, Alan R. Liss, Inc., New York.

Pijnenburg, A.J.J., Honig, W.M.M. and Van Rossum, J.M., 1975,
Effects of antagonists upon locomotor stimulation induced

by injection of dopamine and noradrenaline into the nucleus accumbens of nialamide-pretreated rats, Psychopharmacol., 41:175-180.

Pickel, N.M., Joh, T.H., Field, P.M., Becker, C.F., and Reis, D.J., 1975, Cellular localization of tyrosine hydroxylase by immunohistochemistry, J. Histochem. Cytochem., 23:1-12.

Premont, J., Thierry, A.M., Tassin, J.P., Glowinski, J., Blanc, G., and Bockaert, J., 1976, Is the dopamine sensitive adenylate cyclase in the substantia nigra coupled with "autoreceptors"?, FASEB Lett., 68:99-104.

Quik, M., Emson, P.C., and Joyce, E., 1979, Dissociation between the presynaptic dopamine-sensitive adenylate cyclase and ^{3}H-spiperone binding sites in rat substantia nigra, Brain Res., 167:355-365.

Roth, R.H., 1981, Dopamine autoreceptors: Pharmacology, function and comparison with postsynaptic dopamine receptors, Comm. Psychopharmacol., 3:429-445.

Saller, C.F., and Salama, A.I., 1985, Dopamine receptor subtypes: In vivo biochemical evidence for functional interaction, Eur. J. Pharmacol., 109:297-300.

Scarnati, E., Forchetti, C., Ciancarelli, G., Pacitti, C., and Agnoli, A., 1980, Responsiveness of nigral neurons to the stimulation of striatal dopaminergic receptors in the rat, Life Sci., 26:1203-1209.

Schulz, D. W., Stanford, E.J., Wyrick S.W, and Mailman, R.B., 1985, Binding of [^{3}H]SCH23390 in rat brain: Regional distribution and effects of assay conditions and GTP suggest interactions at a D_1-like dopamine receptor, J. Neurochem., 45: 1601-1611.

Schwarcz, R., Creese, I., Coyle, J.T., and Snyder, S.H., 1978, Dopamine receptors localized on cerebral cortical afferents to rat corpus striatum, Nature , 271:766-768.

Seeman, P., 1981, Brain dopamine receptors, Pharmac. Rev., 32:229-313.

Siggins, G.R., Hoffer, B.J., and Ungerstedt, U., 1974, Electrophysiological evidence for involvement of cyclic adenosine monophosphate in dopamine responses of caudate neurones, Life Sci., 15:779-792.

Skirboll,,L.R., Grace, A.A., and Bunney, B.S., 1979, Dopamine auto- and postsynaptic receptors: Electophysiological evidence for differential sensitivity to dopamine agonists, Science, 206:80-82.

Skirboll, L.R., Grace, A.A., Hommer, D.W., Rehfeld, J., Goldstein, M., Hokfelt, T., and Bunney, B.S., 1981, Peptide-monoamine coexistence: Studies of the actions of the cholecystokinin-like peptide on the electrical activity of midbrain dopamine neurons, Neuronscience, 6:2111-2124.

Staines, W.A., Nagy, J.I., Vincent, S.R. and Fibiger, H.C., 1980, Neurotransmitters contained in the efferents of the striatum, Brain Res., 194:391-402.

Stoof, J.C., 1983, Dopamine receptors in the neostriatum: Biochemical and physiological studies, in: "Dopamine Receptors," C. Kaiser and J.W. Kebabian, eds., pp. 117-145, American Chemical Society Symposium Series No. 224, Washington D.C.

Stoof, J.C., and Kababian, J.W., 1981, Opposing roles for D-1 and D-2 dopamine receptors in efflux of cyclic AMP from rat neostriatum, Nature 294:366-368.

Tassin, J.P., Simon, H., Herve, D., Blanc, G., LeMoal, M., Glowinski, J., and Bockaert, J., 1982, Non-dopaminergic fibres may regulate dopamine-sensitive adenylate cyclase in the prefrontal cortex and nucleus accumbens. Nature, 295:696-698.

Thierry, A.M., LeDouarin, C., Ferron, A. and Glowinski, J., 1984a, Influence of the mesocortical DA system of the activity of prefrontal cortical neurons in the rat, Clin. Neuropharmacol., 7(suppl.1):76-77.

Thierry, A.M., Tassin, J.P., and Glowinski, J., 1984b, Biochemical and electrophysiological studies of the mesocortical dopamine system, in: "Monoamine Innervation of Cerebral Cortex," Vol.10 Neurology and Neurobiology, L. Descarries, T.R. Reader and H.H. Jasper, eds., pp. 233-261, Liss, New York.

Ungerstedt, U., 1971, Stereotaxic mapping of the monoamine pathways in the rat brain., Acta Physiol. Scand., 367:1-48.

Walters, J.R., Berstrom, D.A., Bromley, S.D., Waszczak, B.L., and Jackson, D.M., 1982, Neurophysiological effects of dopamine agonists in the substantia nigra and globus pallidus, in: "Dopamine Receptor Agonists," A. Carlsson and J.L.G. Nilsson, eds., pp. 186-199, Swedish Pharmaceutical Press, Stockholm.

Walters, J.R., Carlson, J.H., Bergstrom, D.A., and Waszczak, B.L., 1984, Effects of SCH 23390-induced blockade of D-1 dopamine (DA) receptors on single unit activity in substantia nigra and globus pallidus, Neurosci. Abstr. 10:412.

Wang, R.Y., 1981a, Dopaminergic neurons in the rat ventral tegmental area. I. Identification and characterization, Brain Res. Rev., 3: 123-140.

Wang, R.Y., 1981b, Dopaminergic neurons in the rat ventral tegmental area. II. Evidence for autoregulation, Brain Res. Rev., 3:141-152.

Wang, R.Y., White, F.J., and Voigt, M.M., 1984, Effects of dopamine agonists on midbrain dopamine cell activity, in: Catecholamines: Neuropharmacology and Central Nervous System-Theoretical Aspects, eds., Alan R. Liss, Inc., New York, NY,pp.359-367.

Waszczak, B.L., Bergstrom, D.A., and Walters, J.R., 1981, Single unit responses of substantia nigra and globus pallidus neurons to GABA agonist and antagonist drugs, in: "GABA and the Basal Ganglia," ed., G. DiChiara and G.L. Gessa, pp. 79-94, Raven Press, New York.

White, F.J., and Wang, R.Y., 1984, Pharmacological characterization of dopamine autoreceptors in the rat ventral tegmental area: Microiontophoretic studies, J. Pharmacol. Exp. Ther. 231:275-280.

White, F.J., and Wang, R.Y., 1986, Electophysiological evidence for the existence of both D-1 and D-2 dopamine receptors in the rat nucleus accumbens, J. Neurosci., 6:274-280.

Woodruff, G.N., McCarthy, P.S., and Walker, R.J., 1976, Studies on the pharmacology of neurons in the nucleus accumbens of the rat, Brain Res., 115:233-242.

York, D.H., 1970, Possible dopaminergic pathway from substantia nigra to putamen, Brain Res., 20:233-249.

York, D.H., 1979, The neurophysiology of dopamine receptors, in: "The Neurobiology of Dopamine", A.S. Horn, J. Korf and B.H.C. Westerink, eds., pp. 395-415, Academic Press, New York.

Yoshida, M., and Kunihiko, O., 1978, Actions of putative neurotransmitters on cat pallidal neurons, in: "Iontophoresis and Transmitter Mechanism in the Mammalian Central Nervous System," Ryall and Kelly eds., pp.71-74, Elsevier; North-Holland Biomedical Press.

THE PATHOPHYSIOLOGICAL FUNCTIONS MEDIATED BY D_1 DOPAMINE RECEPTORS

Menek Goldstein, Shigeki Kuga, Yoji Shimizu and
Emanuel Meller

Department of Psychiatry
Neurochemistry Research Laboratories
New York University Medical Center
New York, New York   00016   USA

Pharmacological and biochemical studies have established the presence of at least two types of central dopamine (DA) receptors. The D_1 DA receptors are positively linked to the DA sensitive adenylate cyclase system, whereas the D_2 DA receptors are probably negatively linked. The D_2 DA receptors have been generally recognized as mediating the action of antipsychotic drugs as well as a variety of behaviors such as rotation and stereotypy. However, until recently, the D_1 DA receptor was regarded as a receptor whose function is unknown and awaiting future discovery. The availability of selective D_1 DA agonists (e.g. SKF 38393) and of D_1 DA antagonists (e.g. SCH 23390) has made it possible to determine some behavioral effects which are associated with D_1 or with both D_1 and D_2 DA receptors. In this presentation we will describe some behavioral responses which might be mediated by D_1 and/or by both D_1 and D_2 DA receptors, and we will discuss their clinical relevance.

CATALEPSY

Catalepsy is generally considered a predictive index for the effectiveness of antipsychotics and for their propensity to develop extrapyramidal side effects. It was of considerable interest to determine whether a selective D_1 DA antagonist, such as SCH 23390, will induce catalepsy and whether this behavior is mediated by D_1, or by both D_1 and D_2 DA receptors.

Catalepsy was measured by the previously described procedures (1). Groups of rats were treated with SCH 23390 (0.05-0.2 mg/kg, s.c.) and the duration of catalepsy was measured up to a maximum of 120 sec. Each rat was given two trials and the mean descent latency was recorded for placement of both paws on the floor. Animals were tested every 15 min for 2 hrs. DA agonists were administered 15 min prior to SCH 23390, and the % inhibition of catalepsy was determined at the time of peak effect (30 min) of SCH 23390.

Table 1. ED_{50} Values of Dopamine Agonists for Blockade
of Catalepsy Produced by SCH 23390 in Rats

Drug	ED_{50} (mg./kg, i.p.)
Apomorphine	0.99
LY 141865	0.37
LY 171555	0.18
RU 24213	0.91

Rats were treated with 3-4 different doses of DA agonists 15
min prior to administration of SCH 23390 (0.1 mg/kg, s.c.).
The ID_{50} values were determined from log-probit plots as
previously described (3).

The administration of SCH 23390 produces catalepsy (2,3)
with an ED_{50} of 0.073 mg/kg, s.c. at the time of the peak
effect. Pretreatment with the selective D_2 agonist LY 141865
(0.1-0.8 mg/kg, i.p.) produced a dose-dependent inhibition of
catalepsy elicited by SCH 23390. The selective D_2 agonist RU
24213, as well as the mixed D_1/D_2 agonists pergolide or apomorphine, also inhibited the SCH 23390-induced catalepsy.
The ED_{50} of various DA agonists to block the SCH 23390-
induced catalepsy is presented in Table 1. Thus, the results
of our study show that the selective D_1 antagonist produces
catalepsy and that this effect is prevented when the rats are
pretreated either with selective D_2 or with mixed D_1/D_2 DA
agonists (3).

Although a number of biochemical studies have demonstrated that SCH 23390 selectively antagonizes the D_1 DA
receptors in vitro, possible interaction of this compound
with D_2 DA receptors in vivo cannot be excluded. However, we
have recently shown that SCH 23390, at doses as high as 3
mg/kg (i.p.) selectively protects D_1 from inactivation by the
irreversible receptor blocking agent N-ethoxycarbonyl-2-
ethoxy-1,2-dihydroquinoline (EEDQ) (4). On the other hand, we
have also found that at higher concentrations, SCH 23390
displaces ^{3}H-spiroperidol (^{3}H-Spi) from striatal binding
sites (Table 2).

SCH 23390 may also interact with S_2 receptors (4), and we
have examined whether the addition of the S_2 antagonist ketanserin affects the displacement of ^{3}H-Spi by SCH 23390. It
is evident from the results presented in Table 2 that in the
presence of ketanserin SCH 23390 displaces ^{3}H-Spi less effectively. These results suggest that SCH 23390, in part,
displaces striatal ^{3}H-Spi binding from S_2 receptors, and at
higher concentrations it might also displace ^{3}H-Spi from D_2 DA
receptors. Furthermore, the displacement of ^{3}H-Spi binding by
SCH 23390 is GTP-sensitive (at a concentration of 5×10^{-4}M GTP
decreases the affinity of SCH 23390), suggesting that SCH
23390 may interact as an agonist with the S_2 receptors. Since
SCH 23390 interacts with the D_2 DA receptors only at very high
concentrations, it seems unlikely that the catalepsy induced
by this drug is related to the blockade of D_2 DA receptors.

Table 2. Displacement of Striatal ^{3}H-Spiroperidol Binding
          by SCH 23390 in Presence and Absence of Ketanserin

Concentrations of SCH 23390	Specific binding*	
	-Ketanserin	+Ketanserin**
10^{-9}M	131	0
10^{-8}M	240	84
10^{-7}M	305	160
10^{-6}M	370	235
10^{-5}M	430	405

* The specific binding is expressed as c.p.m. per incubation
mixture and the results are the means from three experiments
$\pm$ S.E.M. of 3-12%. The binding of ^{3}H-Spi was determined as
described by Howlett and Nahorski (12).

**The concentration of ketanserin was 20 nM.

SELF-MUTILATIVE BITING (SMB) BEHAVIOR

     In a number of studies, we have shown that monkeys with
unilateral ventromedial tegmental (VMT) lesions of the brain
stem serve as a useful model for investigating the anti-
Parkinsonian activity of DA agonists. The administration of
DA agonists results in a relief of the surgically induced
tremor and in the occurrence of abnormal involuntary movements
(AIM) in these monkeys (5). During the course of these
studies, we have observed that in a group of monkeys in which
the surgical lesion was placed 10-14 years ago when the
monkeys were very young (2-3 years of age), the administration
of some DA agonists elicits SMB behavior of the forelimb
digits contralateral to the lesion and spasticity of the
contralateral hindlimb (6,7). The results summarized in Table
3 show that the administration of mixed D_1/D_2 DA agonists
such as L-Dopa (in combination with the peripheral
decarboxylase inhibitor MK-486) or apomorphine (Apo) results
in the occurrence of SMB behavior. The recently described
mixed D_1/D_2 DA agonist aberorphine 201-678 (8) produces SMB
behavior at a lower dose and for a longer duration than Apo
or L-Dopa. However, pergolide, which predominantly exerts D_2
DA agonist activity, and the selective D_2 DA agonist
quinpirole (LY 171555), do not produce SMB behavior.
Interestingly, the D_1 agonist SKF 38393-A, at low doses, does
not produce this behavior, but the combined administration of
SKF 38393-A and quinpirole induces intermittent SMB behavior
for a short period of time (quinpirole alone induces
stereotyped biting behavior of the surrounding cage, but not
SMB behavior). The results presented in Table 3 also show
that the D_1 antagonist SCH 23390 or the D_2 DA antagonist
fluphenazine prevent the DA agonist-induced SMB behavior. On
the other hand, the D_2 DA antagonist ($\pm$)sulpiride does not
prevent the DA agonist-induced SMB behavior.

Table 3. Induction of SMB Behavior in Monkeys with
Unilateral VMT Lesions by DA Agonists and Its
Prevention by DA Antagonists

Drug (mg/kg; i.m.)	Effect on	
	Occurrence of SMB behavior	Blockade of SMB behavior
Apo (0.5)	++	
Apo (0.5) + Flu (1.5) or SCH 23390 (0.3)	0	complete blockade
Abeorphine 201-678 (0.1)	++	
Abeorphine 201-678 (0.1) + ($\pm$)Sulpiride (100)	++	no blockade
Abeorphine 201-678 (1.5) + Flu (1.5) or SCH 23390 (1.5)	0	complete blockade
Quinpirole (0.2)	-	
SKF 38393-A (2.5)	-	
Quinpirole (0.2) + SKF 38393-A (2.5)	+	

The DA antagonists were given 20-30 min prior to the
administration of DA agonists.

++ Persistent SMB behavior for at least 20 min.

+ Intermittent SMB behavior for 30 min or less.

THE POSSIBLE RELATIONSHIPS BETWEEN ABNORMAL GUANINE NUCLEOTIDE
METABOLISM AND DOPAMINERGIC NEURONAL FUNCTION: IMPLICATIONS
IN LESCH-NYHAN SYNDROME AND IN SOME MENTAL DISORDERS

The findings that DA and its metabolites, as well as the
enzyme responsible for DA synthesis, namely tyrosine
hydroxylase (TH), are reduced in post mortem striatum of
Lesch-Nyhan patients (9) were the first indications that the
DA neuronal systems might be involved in the neurological and
mental manifestations of this disorder. This notion is now
further strengthened by our findings that in some monkeys
with supersensitive DA receptors, D_1 or mixed D_1/D_2 DA
agonists induce SMB behavior and spasticity which resemble
the behavior and motor abnormalities observed in Lesch-Nyhan
patients. The question is whether the major biochemical
defect in Lesch-Nyhan syndrome, namely the deficiency in
hypoxanthine- guanine phosphoribosyltransferase (HPRT)
(salvage enzyme) has any relationship to the abnormal
dopaminergic functions. A hypothetical mechanism which might
be the underlying cause of the development of supersensitivity of brain DA receptors in Lesch-Nyhan patients and

which might lead to abnormal DA function is shown in Fig. 1.
We assume that the defective HPRT enzyme in the Lesch-Nyhan
brain leads to reduced levels of striatal GTP which, in turn,
results in the reduced formation of the pteridine cofactor
(10). The pteridine cofactor is required for the activity of
TH, and its reduction will result in decreased TH activity,
leading to a decreased synthesis of DA. The decreased
formation of DA could explain the low levels of this
transmitter in the post mortem striatum of Lesch-Nyhan
patients and could also explain the development of DA
receptor supersensitivity. Furthermore, decreased GTP levels
might affect the conversion of the high to low affinity state
of the DA receptors, and this might also result in the
development of DA receptor supersensitivity. We have shown
that HPRT is localized on intrastriatal neurons which also
contain D_1 and D_2 DA receptors, as well as the DARPP-32
protein which is linked to the D_1 DA receptor (P. Greengard,
unpublished data) (7). These findings indicate that the DA
receptors might be regulated by the nucleotides which are
formed by the salvage enzyme. It is well established that GTP
regulates agonist-receptor interaction in a number of
neurotransmitter receptor systems (11) and it is conceivable
that DA agonist-induced SMB behavior is related to the
abnormal regulation of the affinity states of the DA receptors
by guanine nucleotides. It is noteworthy that automutilation
also occurs in some autistic patients as well as in some
children with mental retardation, and in patients with
infantile muscular hypertrophy associated with brain injury
(De Lange syndrome). It will be of interest to determine
whether different forms of automutilation are associated with
a dysfunction of the DA neuronal systems.

DISCUSSION

Several studies have shown that stimulation or blockade
of D_1 DA receptors leads to opposite biochemical responses
than stimulation or blockade of D_2 DA receptors. However,
stimulation or blockade of D_1 or D_2 DA receptors leads, in
some instances, to the same behavioral responses. These
findings suggest that the behavioral responses do not
necessarily reflect the biochemical changes at the synapse

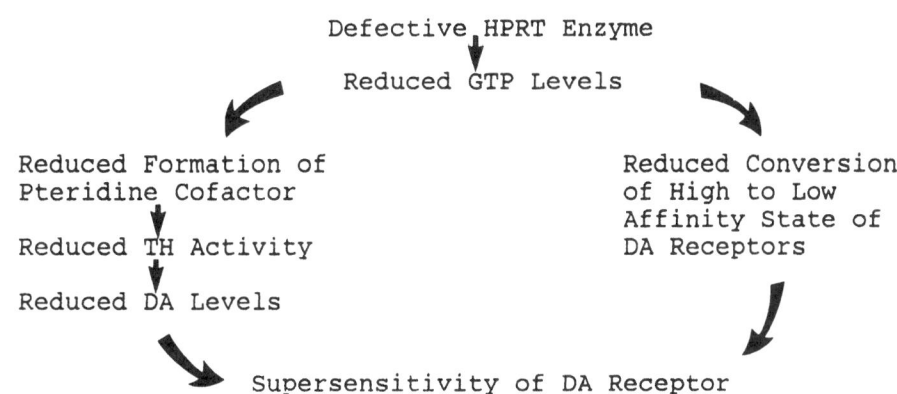

Figure 1. Hypothetical Mechanisms Underlying the Development of Supersensitivity of Dopamine Receptors in the Brain of Lesch-Nyhan Patients

and that D_1 and D_2 DA receptors may influence distinct dopaminergic striatal efferent pathways which, in some instances, reflect convergent neuronal activity of both systems. It is noteworthy that the blockade of D_1 and of D_2 DA receptors produces catalepsy and that the muscarinic antagonist scopolamine reverses this behavior induced by either D_1 or by D_2 DA receptor antagonists (Goldstein et al., unpublished data). It is therefore conceivable that catalepsy elicited either by D_1 or by D_2 DA receptors reflects some postsynaptic neuronal activity associated with cholinergic neuronal systems.

The findings that D_1 and the mixed D_1/D_2 DA agonist induces SMB behavior in some monkeys with supersensitive DA receptors indicates that this motor dysfunction is, in part, mediated by the D_1 DA system. On the other hand, treatment with DA agonists of Parkinsonian patients which are known to have denervated nigro-striatal DA neurons does not induce SMB behavior. However, the monkey model with surgical VMT lesions of the brain stem may not completely replicate the pathology of Parkinson's disease, and it is possible that the neuronal degeneration in the monkeys differs from that which occurs in the brain of Parkinsonian patients. Furthermore, it is noteworthy that not all monkeys with VMT lesions of the brain stem developed SMB behavior upon DA agonist administration, and only monkeys in which the lesion was placed at a relatively young age developed this behavior. It should also be noted that Parkinsonian patients are usually treated with much lower doses of DA agonists than those which produce SMB behavior in the monkeys with VMT lesions of the brain stem.

Among the tested DA agonists, only those which stimulate D_1 or D_1/D_2 DA receptors induced SMB behavior in the monkeys. The recently described DA agonist abeorphine 201-678 induces this behavior at relatively low doses. This agonist predominantly stimulates D_1 DA receptors, but also α_2-adreno-receptors (8). It is conceivable that in addition to the dopaminergic neuronal systems, noradrenergic and other neuronal systems are also involved in the development of SMB behavior.

SUMMARY

1. The administration of the D_1 DA receptor antagonist SCH 23390 produces catalepsy in rat, and this behavior can be abolished by pretreatment with selective D_2 DA receptor agonists.
2. The administration of mixed D_1/D_2 DA agonists, but not of selective D_2 DA agonists, produces SMB behavior in monkeys with surgical unilateral VMT lesions of the brain stem. The DA agonist-induced SMB behavior is abolished by pretreatment of the monkeys with either the D_1 DA antagonist SCH 23390 or with the mixed D_1/D_2 antagonist fluphenazine, but not with the selective D_2 antagonist ($\pm$) sulpiride.
3. A hypothetical relationship between abnormal guanine nucleotide metabolism in Lesch-Nyhan syndrome and the development of DA receptor supersensitivity is presented. The possible role of abnormal guanine nucleotide metabolism in some mental disorders associated with DA dysfunctions is discussed.

REFERENCES

1. C. Ezrin-Waters and P. Seeman, 1977, Tolerance to haloperidol catalepsy, Eur. J. Pharmacol., 41:321-327.
2. E. Meller, J.Y. Lew, S. Kuga and M. Goldstein, 1984, The interaction of SCH 23390 with normosensitive (N) and supersensitive (S) dopamine receptors, The Pharamcologist, 26:163.
3. E. Meller, S. Kuga, A.J. Friedhoff and M. Goldstein, 1985, Selective D_2 dopamine receptor agonists prevent catalepsy induced by SCH 23390, a selective D_1 antagonist, Life Sci., 36:1857-1864.
4. E. Meller, K. Bohmaker, M. Goldstein and A.J. Friedhoff, 1985, Inactivation of D_1 and D_2 dopamine receptors by N-ethoxycarbonyl-2-ethoxy-1,2-dihydroquinoline in vivo, J. Pharmacol. Exp. Ther., 233:656-662.
5. M. Goldstein, A.H. Battista, T. Ohmoto, B. Anagnoste and K. Fuxe, 1973, Tremor and involuntary movements in monkeys: Effect of L-dopa and of a dopamine receptor stimulating agent, Science, 179:816-817.
6. M. Goldstein and S. Kuga, 1984, Dopamine (DA) agonist induced compulsive biting (CB) behavior in monkeys: Animal model for Lesch-Nyhan syndrome, Soc. Neurosci., 10:239.1.
7. M. Goldstein, S. Kuga, N. Kusano, E. Meller, J. Dancis and R. Schwarcz, 1985, Dopamine agonist induced self-mutilative biting behavior in monkeys with unilateral ventromedial tegmental lesions of the brain stem: Possible pharmacological model for Lesch-Nyhan syndrome, Brain Res., in press.
8. R. Markstein, J.L. Jaton, J.M. Vigouret, R. Giger, A. Closse, U. Briner and A. Enz, 1984, Pharmacological properties of 201-678 a new dopamine agonist, Clin. Neuropharmacol., 7:800-801.
9. K.G. Lloyd, O. Hornykiewicz, L. Davidson, K. Shannak, I. Farley, M. Goldstein, M. Shibuya, W.N. Kelly and I.H. Fox, 1981, Biochemical evidence of dysfunction of brain neurotransmitters in the Lesch-Nyhan syndrome, New Engl. J. Med., 305:1106-1111.
10. G. Kapatos, S. Katoh and S.10. G. Kapatos, S. Katoh and S. Kaufman, Biosynthesis of biopterin by rat brain, 1982, J. Neurochem., 39:1152-1162.
11. R.J. Lefkowitz, M.C. Caron and G.L. Stiles, 1984, Mechanisms of membrane-receptor regulation: Biochemical, physiological, and clinical insights derived from studies of the adrenergic receptors, New Engl. J. Med., 310:1570-1579.
12. D.R. Howlett and S.R. Nahorski, 1980, Quantitative assessment of heterogeneous ^3H-spiperone binding to rat neostriatum and frontal cortex, Life Sci., 26:511-517.

NEUROBIOLOGY OF D_1 DOPAMINE RECEPTORS AFTER NEONATAL-6-OHDA

TREATMENT: RELEVANCE TO LESCH-NYHAN DISEASE

George R. Breese, Robert A. Mueller, T. Celeste
Napier and Gary E. Duncan

Biological Sciences Research Center and the
Mental Health Clinical Research Center,
University of North Carolina School of Medicine
Chapel Hill, N.C. 27514

INTRODUCTION

Central administration of 6-hydroxydopamine (6-OHDA) to
adult or neonatal rats destroys dopamine-containing neurons,
produces a variety of behavioral deficits (Breese et al.,1973;
Smith et al., 1973) and enhances behavioral responses to dopamine agonists (Ungerstedt, 1971; Schoenfeld and Uretsky, 1972;
Hollister et al., 1974; 1979; Setler et al. 1978; Kilts et al.
1979). In spite of the common biochemical deficiency observed in neonatally and adult-lesioned rats, Breese et al.
(1984 a,b) reported that certain behavioral responses to L-
DOPA or apomorphine in adult-6-OHDA-treated rats (Breese et
al., 1970) differ from those observed in rats lesioned as neonates and tested with dopamine agonists as adults (Breese et
al., 1972; Smith et al., 1973). For example, neonatally 6-
OHDA-lesioned rats exhibit self-mutilation behavior (SMB)
after treatment with dopamine agonists which do not elicit
this response in adult-6-OHDA treated rats (Breese et al.,
1984b).

Subsequently, cis-flupentixol was found to be more potent
than haloperidol as an antagonist of the self-biting induced
by L-DOPA in neonatally 6-OHDA-lesioned rats (Breese et al.,
1984b). Hyttel (1978) observed that cis-flupentixol is a
potent inhibitor of dopamine-stimulated adenylate cyclase
without a strong action to displace radiolabeled haloperidol.
Based upon such data, Kebabian and Calne (1979) classified
dopamine-stimulated adenylate cyclase as a D_1 site and the
site acted upon by sulpiride as a D_2-dopamine receptor.
Therefore, the differential effects demonstrated by cis-
flupentixol and haloperidol on L-DOPA-induced self-biting
suggest that SMB is likely associated with D_1-dopamine
receptors (Breese et al., 1984b).

Drugs have been developed recently which have relative
specificity for D_1 and D_2-dopamine receptor sites. Setler et
al. (1978) introduced the dopamine agonist, SKF-38393, which

has properties different from those of apomorphine. Studies have demonstrated that this compound stimulates adenylate cyclase and induces turning in rats with unilateral-6-OHDA lesions of the nigrostriatal pathway (Setler et al., 1978; Arnt and Hyttel, 1984; Christensen et al., 1984). Iorio et al. (1983) introduced the compound, SCH 23390, which antagonizes dopamine stimulation of adenylate cyclase and does not displace radiolabelled haloperidol. Furthermore, butyrophenones, phenothiazines, or other types of neuroleptics, with the exception of cis-flupentixol, do not displace ^{3}H-SCH 23390 binding to striatal tissue (Billard et al., 1984). Recently, this antagonist was found to block turning by SKF-38393 in rats with unilateral lesions to the nigrostriatal pathway (Arnt and Hyttel, 1984; Costall et al., 1984). Therefore, SCH 23390 is presumed to be a D_1-dopamine receptor antagonist and SKF-38393 a D_1-receptor agonist. Tsuruta et al. (1981) provided evidence that LY-171555 is a specific D_2-dopamine agonist. Many neuroleptics, including haloperidol, antagonize D_2-dopamine receptors (Seeman, 1980). Thus, the pharmacological tools are available to explore the role of dopamine receptor subtypes in the behavioral differences observed between rats lesioned neonatally and those lesioned as adults with 6-OHDA.

In the present review, experiments with neonatally and adult-6-OHDA-lesioned rats are described which examine the pharmacology of agonists and antagonists with specificity for D_1 and D_2 dopamine receptors. This work permits conclusions concerning the role of D_1-dopamine receptors in behavior, about the interaction of D_1 receptors with D_2-dopamine receptors, and about the importance of D_1-dopamine receptors for the SMB observed in rats treated neonatally with 6-OHDA when challenged with dopamine agonists as adults. Finally, the relationship of these findings to Lesch-Nyhan disease are discussed.

DOPAMINE AGONIST ADMINISTRATION TO 6-OHDA-LESIONED RATS

Administration of apomorphine to mature animals lesioned neonatally with 6-OHDA produce behaviors which are different from those induced in rats lesioned as adults (Breese et al., 1984). For example, administration of apomorphine to adult-6-OHDA-lesioned rats markedly potentiates locomotor activity, whereas apomorphine produces little change in locomotion when administered to rats lesioned as neonates (Fig. 1). Because L-DOPA (10 mg/kg) produced a major increase in locomotion in rats lesioned both as adults or as neonates (Breese et al., 1984b, 1985a), the mechanism for responses to apomorphine with the two 6-OHDA treatment groups was not apparent at the time these experiments were performed.

Because of our hypothesis that D_1-dopamine receptors are involved in the action of L-DOPA to induce SMB in neonatal 6-OHDA-lesioned rats (Breese et al., 1984b), the locomotion induced in 6-OHDA-lesioned rats by the D_1-dopamine receptor agonist, SKF-38393, was compared with this action after administration of LY-171555, a D_2-dopamine agonist (Fig. 2). In adult-6-OHDA-treated rats administration of LY-171555 was found to increase locomotor activity several times greater than observed in control or neonatally 6-OHDA-lesioned rats (Fig. 2). The response to LY-171555 by adult-6-OHDA-treated rats resembles that observed after apomorphine (Breese et al., 1984b, 1985c).

Fig. 2 illustrates the effects of SKF-38393 on locomotion in 6-OHDA-lesioned rats. In keeping with earlier observations (Setler et al., 1978), a major change in locomotor activity is not apparent in control rats after administration of SKF-38393 (Breese et al., 1985c). When SKF-38393 is administered to neonatally-lesioned rats, a dose-related increase in locomotion is observed (Fig. 2). Adult-6-OHDA-treated rats exhibit less response to the D_1-dopamine agonist. Thus, it appears that SKF-38393-induced locomotion can be used as a quantitative measure of the functional supersensitivity of D_1-dopamine receptors in rats with lesions to dopamine-containing neurons (Breese et al., 1985c).

The animals used to evaluate the action of SKF-38393 on locomotion had previously been treated with several doses of dopamine agonists to assess their effects on behavior. However, when SKF-38393 (3 mg/kg) was administered to rats that had no prior exposure to dopamine agonists, the response to the first dose of SKF-38393 (3 mg/kg), although greater than the saline response (Table 1), was considerably less than the response observed in Fig. 2 (Breese et al., 1985c). After three or four doses of SKF 38393, the locomotor response reached a maximal level (Table 1; Breese et al., 1985c). Thus, the magnitude of the supersensitive locomotor response to SKF-38393 appears to depend upon prior exposure to this dopamine agonist. The "priming" action observed after multiple exposure to a D_1-dopamine agonist is consistent with previous data demonstrating that a second challenge with L-DOPA increases the incidence of SMB over that observed after administration of a single dose of L-DOPA to rats lesioned

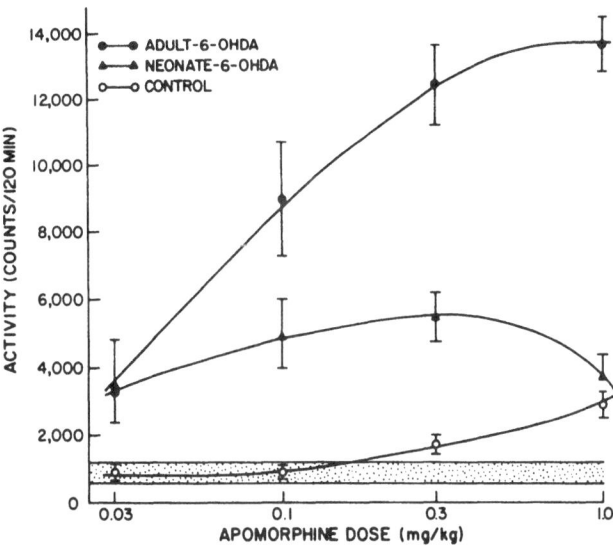

Fig. 1:   Locomotor response of mature rats after apomorphine administration. Rats were treated with 6-OHDA as adults (adult-6-OHDA) or when 3 days of age (neonate 6-OHDA) (From Breese et al., 1985c).

neonatally with 6-OHDA (Breese et al., 1984b). While this increase in supersensitivity appears to be permanent (i.e. supersensitive response present 6 months after last dose) and unrelated to drug accumulation, the neurobiological basis of this "priming" action of SKF-38393 is unknown. Nevertheless, this phenomenon may provide an explanation for the increased behavioral responses reported to occur after multiple treatments with other dopamine agonists (Klawans et al., 1979; Bevan, 1983; Robinson, 1984).

Responses to SKF-38393

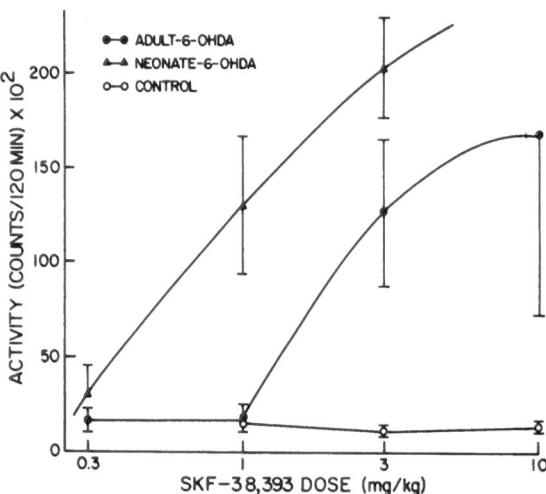

Responses to LY 171555

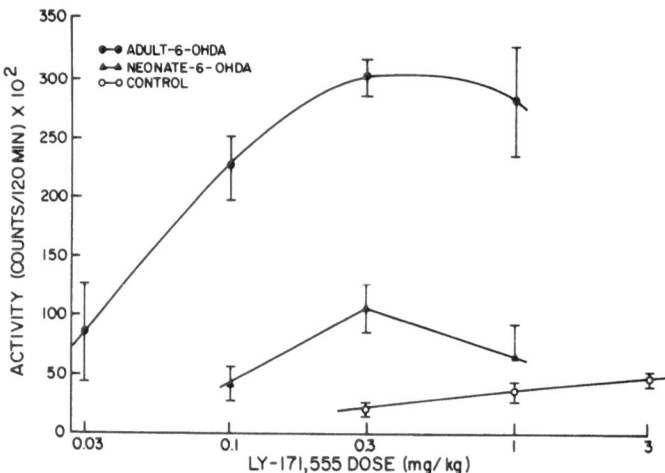

Fig. 2.   Dose-response relationship of SKF-38393 (upper graph) or LY 171555 (lower graph) induced locomotion in rats lesioned when adult (adult-6-OHDA) or as neonates (neonate-6-OHDA).. Animals received several doses of dopamine agonists before the dose-response curves were determined. See Table 1 for "priming" of D_1-dopamine receptors. (From Breese et al., 1985c).

TABLE 1. Responses to Multiple Injections of SKF-38393:
Priming of D_1-Dopamine Receptor Sensitivity

Injection*	Activity (Counts $\pm$ SEM)
Saline	998 $\pm$ 301
Dose 1-SKF-38393	3405 $\pm$ 900 #
Dose 2-SKF-38393	7956 $\pm$ 1643 #
Dose 3-SKF-38393	16946 $\pm$ 2712 #

*Dose of SKF-38393 (3 mg/kg,i.p.) administered at one week
intervals.
# $P < 0.01$ when compared to saline.

SELF-MUTILATION BEHAVIOR AFTER DOPAMINE AGONIST ADMINISTRATION

In addition to the investigations of LY-171555 and SKF-
38383 on locomotor activity, other behaviors induced by these
agonists in neonatally and adult-6-OHDA-lesioned rats were
examined (Breese et al., 1985a). The first question asked was
whether the D_1-dopamine agonist would produce SMB as was observed after L-DOPA administration (Breese et al., 1985a). As
shown in Table 2, it is apparent that SKF-38393 induces SMB in
neonatally-lesioned rats, but to a lesser degree than seen
after L-DOPA administration (Breese et al., 1984). However,
LY-171555 produces no self-mutilation even though self-biting
is observed. Thus, these observations provide evidence that
D_1-dopamine receptors play a critical role in the induction of
SMB.

When SKF-38393 is combined with LY-171555 at doses that
do not elicit SMB after either drug alone, SMB is produced in
the majority of the animals tested (Table 2). This latter
finding provides evidence for a facilitatory interaction
between D_1 and D_2-dopamine receptors and explains the greater
incidence of SMB seen after L-DOPA than after administration
of the D_1-dopamine agonist alone.

ADDITIONAL BEHAVIORS INDUCED BY D_1 AND D_2-DOPAMINE AGONISTS

Not until recently has stimulation of D_1-dopamine
receptors been associated with specific behaviors (Breese et
al., 1984b, 1985ab; Arnt, 1985). Setler et al., (1978)
reported that SKF-38393 increases turning in rats lesioned
unilaterally with 6-OHDA, but produces no other prominent
behaviors in unlesioned rats. Because of the increase in SMB
and locomotion after SKF-38393 and the turning to D_1-dopamine
receptor stimulation in lesioned rats, additional behaviors
were examined in the 6-OHDA-lesioned rats to determine whether
they might also be associated with this dopamine receptor
subtype.

Administration of SKF-38393 and LY-171555 to 6-OHDA-
lesioned rats produced a larger variety, and a greater
incidence, of specific behaviors than observed in unlesioned
rats. In Fig. 3, the incidence over time of selected behaviors
following D_1 and D_2-dopamine agonist administration to adult
and neonatally 6-OHDA-lesioned rats is compared with the

TABLE 2.   Incidence of SMB after LY-171555 and SKF-38393
Administration to Neonatally-Lesioned Rats[*]

Treatment	Dose (mg/kg)	SMB Incidence (No./Total)	%
L-Dopa	100	12/12	100
SKF-38393 (SKF)	1.0	1/12	8
	3.0	2/10#	20
	10.0	4/8#	50
LY-171555 (LY)	0.1	0/4	0
	0.3	0/4	0
	1.0	0/6	0
	3.0	0/6	0
SKF (3) + LY (1)	3+1	4/7#	57
SKF (3) + LY (3)	3+3	4/5#	80

* All rats used were lesioned as neonates with 6-OHDA and had
previously shown SMB when given 100 mg/kg of L-DOPA + RO-4-
4602. Saline does not produce this behavior (From Breese et
al., 1985a).
# $P < 0.05$ when compared to saline.

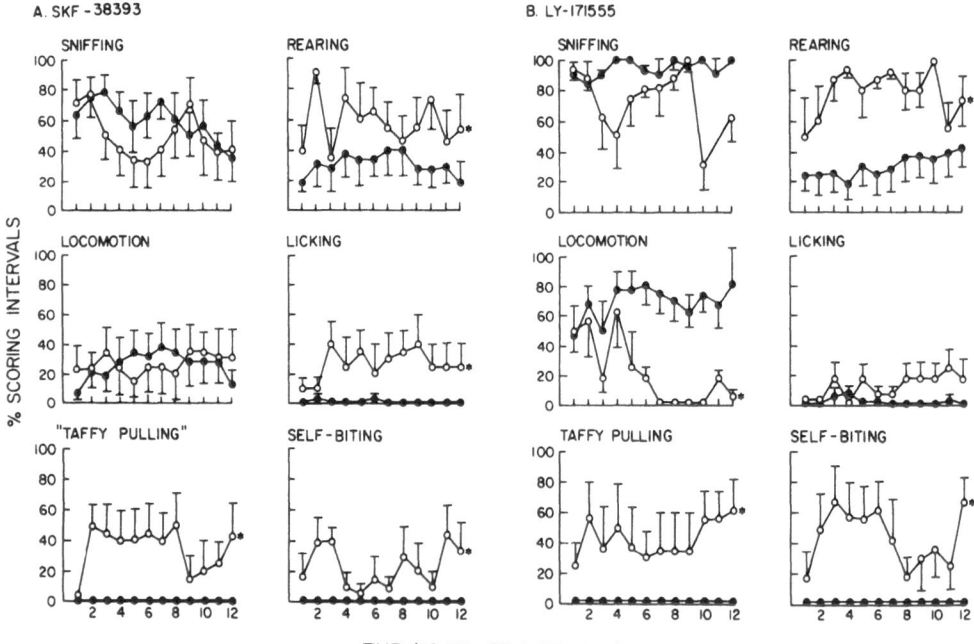

TIME (10 MINUTE INTERVALS)

Fig. 3.   Comparison of behaviors induced by LY-171555
(0.3 mg/kg) (A) and SKF-38393 (3 mg/kg) (B)
in neonatally and adult-6-OHDA-lesioned rats.
The percent scoring interval reflects the
occurrence of a behavior. * $P < 0.05$ when
groups compared. (From Breese et al., 1985a).

TABLE 3. Summary of the Behaviors Associated with D_1 and D_2-Dopamine Receptor Subtypes in Rats Lesioned as Neonates[a]

Response	Dopamine Receptor Involvement	
	D_1	D_2
SMB	Yes[e]	No
Self-biting	Yes[e]	Yes[e]
Taffy-Pulling	Yes[e]	Yes[e]
Licking	Yes[e]	No
Sniffing	Yes[d]	Yes[d]
Rearing	Yes[d]	Yes[d]
Paw Treading	Yes	No[d]
Locomotion	Yes[d]	Yes[bc]
Head Nodding	Yes	No
Digging in wood chips	Yes	No[b]
Grooming	Yes[d]	No

a) Data compiled from responses to D_1 and D_2 agonists and to selected antagonists against SKF-38393 and L-DOPA responses.
b) Significant incidence in adult-6-OHDA-lesioned rats after LY-171555 (D_2 agonist).
c) Locomotion increased only at lowest dose of LY-171555; behavior present in adult-6-OHDA-treated rat.
d) Significant incidence in adult-6-OHDA-lesioned rat after SKF-38393 (D_1 agonist).
e) Behavior not apparent in adult-6-OHDA-lesioned rats. (From Breese et al., 1985a).

incidence in unlesioned rats. Adult-6-OHDA-lesioned rats have a different spectrum of behavioral responses when compared to neonatally 6-OHDA-treated rats. Behaviors absent in the adult-6-OHDA-lesioned rats after treatment with a dopamine agonist include SMB, taffy-pulling (rapid movements of forepaws toward and away from the nose) and self-biting. A complete listing of behaviors associated with administration of these agonists is summarized in Table 3. All behaviors measured are observed after SKF-38393 administration to neonatally-lesioned rats. However, SMB, self-biting, taffy pulling, grooming and head nodding can be attributed only to activation of D_1-dopamine receptors. Malloy and Waddington (1984) have recently observed grooming in unlesioned rats after high doses of SKF-38393.

These data demonstrate that D_1-dopamine receptors contribute to dopaminergic function. The different behavioral pattern observed between adult and neonatally 6-OHDA-lesioned rats is consistent with the behavioral differences observed after L-DOPA administration (Breese et al., 1984b). This observation supports the hypothesis that the age at which dopaminergic neurons are destroyed influences the character of motor responses induced by dopamine agonists (Breese et al., 1984b). Since behavioral supersensitivity is observed following administration of LY-171555 to neonatally 6-OHDA-lesioned rats, the different behavioral responses in neonatally and adult-6-OHDA-lesioned rat, can not be attributed to a selective functional increase in just the D_1-receptor subtype.

EFFECTS OF DOPAMINE ANTAGONISTS ON RESPONSES TO D_1 AND D_2-DOPAMINE AGONISTS

In order to assess the specificity of the dopamine agonists and antagonists used in the various investigations, a
study was undertaken to evaluate the effects of D_1 and D_2-
dopamine antagonists on locomotor activity induced by LY-
171555 or SKF-38393 in 6-OHDA-lesioned rats (Breese et al.,
1985a,c). The antagonist compounds chosen were haloperidol,
fluphenazine, cis-flupentixol and SCH 23390 (Table 4). The
strategy was to determine the lowest dose of these antagonists
which could be administered to antagonize locomotion induced
by one receptor agonist without having an effect on the
response induced by the other agonist. It was found that 0.3
mg/kg of either haloperidol or SCH 23390 met this criteria,
demonstrating the distinctive nature of the dopamine sites
with which these compounds interact. The 1 mg/kg dose of SCH
23390 remained without an effect on the activity induced by
LY-171555, indicating the high degree of in vivo selectivity
of this drug for D_1-dopamine receptors. Both cis-flupentixol
and fluphenazine are potent antagonists of LY-171555, but
antagonize D_1 dopamine receptor activation at higher doses.

In spite of data demonstrating the specificity of SCH
23390 as a D_1-receptor antagonist, several earlier studies
reported that SCH 23390 would also antagonize effects of D_2-
dopamine receptor activation (Iorio, et al., 1983;
Christensen et al., 1984; Mailman et al. 1984; Breese et al.,
1985b). These latter investigations were performed in rats
with intact catecholamine-containing neurons. It became
apparent during the course of our behavioral studies that only
in the 6-OHDA-treated rats could the specificity of SCH 23390
for D_1-dopamine receptors be demonstrated. Such data suggest
that SCH 23390 is not acting directly on D_2-dopamine receptor
sites to antagonize the effects of D_2-dopamine agonists
(Breese et al., 1985 b,c). For this reason, an additional
investigation was undertaken to determine whether destruction
of catecholamine-containing fibers is essential to demonstrate
specificity of SCH 23390 for D_1-receptor sites or whether
disruption of catecholaminergic function by a non-destructive
means (i.e. reserpine + alpha-methyltyrosine) would also
eliminate the ability of SCH 23390 to block D_2 agonists. As
shown in Fig. 4, the ability of SCH 23390 to reduce the
locomotor stimulation induced by LY-171555 is antagonized by a
reserpine + alpha-methyltyrosine regimen. This finding, along
with the previous data collected in 6-OHDA-treated rats,
suggests that D_1-dopamine receptor sites modulate D_2 dopamine
function through a mechanism dependent upon functionally
intact catecholamine-containing neurons.

In the course of performing investigations of D_2-dopa-
mine receptor function, it was observed that the locomotor
response to LY-171555 was drastically reduced in rats treated
with reserpine and alpha-methyltyrosine (Table 5). The dopamine agonists, piribedil and bromocriptine were, similarly influenced by this treatment (Table 5). While this observation
might suggest an indirect mechanism of action for these drugs,
a variety of studies have demonstrated that bromocriptine and
piribedil-induced locomotion and stereotyped behaviors are enhanced after lesions to dopamine-containing fibers (Kilts et
al., 1979), as are responses to LY-171555 in adult-6-OHDA

TABLE 4. Effects of SCH 23390 and Various Neuroleptics on Locomotion Induced by SKF-38393 and LY-171555 in 6-OHDA-Lesioned Rats

Treatment[a]	Antagonist Dose (mg/kg)	SKF-38393 (Activity/180 min)	LY-171555 (Activity/180 min)
Saline	_____	21932 ± 3218	30942 ± 3987
SCH-23390	0.1	4409 ± 1412*	
	0.3	858 ± 421*	25519 ± 1753
	1.0	_____	36280 ± 5061
Haloperidol	0.1	_____	15130 ± 6045*
	0.3	22993 ± 2387	232 ± 67*
	1.0	7877 ± 3382*	_____
Fluphenazine	0.3	19862 ± 3285	472 ± 309*
	1.0	10543 ± 3043*	_____
	3.0	7220 ± 2699	_____
Cis-Flupentixol	0.3	17405 ± 2953	597 ± 233*
	1.0	732 ± 368*	_____

a) Haloperidol, cis-flupentixol and fluphenazine were administered 60 min and SCH 23390 30 min before SKF-38393 (3 mg/kg) or LY-171555 (0.3 mg/kg). SKF-38393 was administered to neonatally-lesioned rats and the LY-171555 was injected into adult-6-OHDA-treated rats (Modified from Breese et al., 1985c and unpublished data).
* $P < 0.01$ when compared to agonist responses after saline.

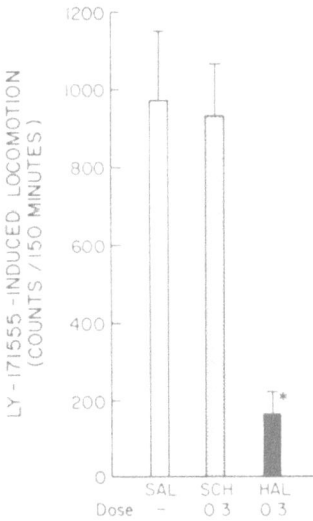

Fig. 4. Effect of reserpine + alpha-methyltyrosine treatment on the action of SCH 23390 (SCH, 0.3 mg/kg) and haloperidol (HAL, 0.3 mg/kg) to antagonize LY-171555 (1 mg/kg). S = Saline. (From Breese and Mueller, 1985).

205

TABLE 5.   Effect of Reserpine + Alpha-Methyltyrosine
on Responses to Dopamine Agonists[a]

Treatment (Dose)	Saline	Reserpine + alpha-methyltryosine[a]
LY-171555 (0.3 mg/kg)	2669 + 349	972 + 178*
Bromocriptine (15 mg/kg)	2892 + 702	301 + 59*
Piribedil (30 mg/kg)	2613 + 832	261 + 187*

a) The alpha-methyltyrosine (40 mg/kg, i.p.) was given just
before a 60 min habituation period and 23 hr after reserpine
(2.5 mg/kg, subcutaneously). Values are mean count + SEM/180
min. (From Breese and Mueller, 1985; unpublished data).
*P < 0.01 when compared to saline.

treated rats. Since the action of d-amphetamine is reduced in
6-OHDA-treated rats (Hollister et al., 1974), an indirect release mechanism does not appear to be a likely explanation for
the findings obtained after administering LY-171555 or other
dopamine agonists.

MICRO-INJECTION OF D_1 AND D_2-DOPAMINE AGONISTS INTO NUCLEUS
ACCUMBENS

Intracerebral administration of dopamine into nucleus
accumbens results in an increase in locomotor activity
(Costall et al., 1975; Jackson et al., 1975; Pijnenburg et
al., 1976). Microinjection of SKF-38393 into nucleus
accumbens of neonatally 6-OHDA-lesioned rats also elevates
locomotion (Table 6; Breese et al., 1986). LY-171555, the D_2-
dopamine agonist, increases locomotion, but is less effective
than the D_1-dopamine agonist in the neonatally-lesioned rats
(Table 6; Breese et al., 1986). These data are consistent
with the lesser efficacy of the D_2 agonist compared to the D_1-
dopamine agonist in neonatally-lesioned rats. Unexpectedly,
the locomotor response to D_1 agonist microinjection into the
nucleus accumbens of adult-6-OHDA-treated rats was also
greater than the response observed after administration of LY-
171555. These latter changes do not parallel locomotor
changes seen in adult-6-OHDA-lesioned rats after peripheral
administration (see Figs 1 and 2).

EFFECT OF 6-OHDA TREATMENTS ON BINDING OF DOPAMINE AGONISTS

It is well documented that a unilateral lesion to
dopamine-containing neurons in adult rats increases [3]H-
spiperone binding in the striatum ipsilateral to the side of
the lesion (Creese et al., 1977; Goldstein et al., 1980;
Heikkila et al., 1981; Neve et al., 1984; Staunton et al.,
1981). This change in ^{3}H-spiperone binding has been suggested
to be responsible for the functional supersensitivity observed
with dopamine agonists after unilateral lesions to dopaminergic fibers (Creese et al., 1977). In spite of such functional
supersensitivity in rats with 6-OHDA lesions, binding of [3]H-
spiperone and ^{3}H-SCH 23390 to striatal tissue is not altered
(Table 7). These findings are in agreement with earlier
reports (Mailman et al., 1981, 1983) and suggest that a change
in receptor number or affinity does not account for the

Table 6. Microinjection of SKF-38393 and LY-171555 Into Nucleus Accumbens of Adult and Neonatally 6-OHDA-Lesioned Rats

Treatment[a]	Activity (Counts/180 min)		
	Control	N-6-OHDA	A-6-OHDA
Saline	1511+344	1621+361	1432+246
LY-171555 (1.0 µg)	1724+864	9131+2290*	11,884+4827*
SKF-38393 (1.0 µg)	1451+491	31,279+4747*	23,581+7840*

a) Drug was dissolved in 0.5 µl of saline and infused over a 5 min period. Locomotor activity was recorded for 180 min. N= neonatal; A = Adult-6-OHDA Treatments.
*P < 0.01 when compared to control or saline.

TABLE 7. Effect of 6-OHDA Lesions on Binding of ^{3}H-SCH 23390 and ^{3}H-Spiperone to Striatal Membranes[a]

TREATMENT	^{3}H-SCH 23390	^{3}H-SPIPERONE
Control	8.9+0.7(6)	22.5+2.3(8)
Neonatal-6-OHDA	8.8+0.5(6)	19.8+2.5(6)
Adult-6-OHDA	8.8+0.5(6)	20.8+1.8(6)

a) Values represent the mean pmoles/g tissue + SEM. Binding was determined with 1.0 nM ^{3}H-spiperone and 0.3 nM ^{3}H-SCH 23390. Values in parentheses indicate the number of determinations made.

functional supersensitivity observed after D_1- and D_2-dopamine agonist administration to neonatally and adult-6-OHDA-treated rats (Breese et al., 1985). Since lesions in the present investigations are not limited to a unilateral nigrostriatal pathway, but destroyed dopaminergic neurons throughout the brain, the type of lesion is a likely explanation for the observed differences in binding characteristics for ^{3}H-spiperone in these studies. The conclusion that behavioral supersensitivity to dopamine agonist challenge is not always accompanied by increased binding of ^{3}H-spiperone has further support by Koller et al., (1985) who found that pergolide, a dopamine agonist, prevents the increase in ^{3}H-spiperone binding, which accompanies chronic administration of haloperidol, but does not reduce the behavioral supersensitivity observed to a dopamine agonist after exposure to such a neuroleptic.

Adult-6-OHDA-treated rats are reported to have an increase in dopamine-stimulated adenylate cyclase (Mailman et al., 1981), whereas activity of the enzyme to dopamine activation is unchanged in neonatally 6-OHDA-treated rats (Mailman et al., 1983). Since binding of ^{3}H-SCH 23390 is not altered by either of these 6-OHDA lesions, it is clear that a simple association does not exist between these two measures. It is not clear whether these findings indicate two distinct

D_1-dopamine receptor sites, an alteration in cyclase activity without a change in receptor number or both. Breese et al. (1975) previously demonstrated that cAMP is not altered in vivo after administration of several dopamine agonists with primary actions on D_2-dopamine receptors. This latter finding would be expected as D_2-dopamine receptor agonists do not activate, but reportedly inhibit dopamine-stimulated adenylate cyclase (Onali et al., 1985). Regardless, it has not yet been determined whether a D_1-dopamine agonist will increase cAMP in vivo.

SPECULATIONS CONCERNING RELATIONSHIP OF D_1-DOPAMINE RECEPTORS TO FUNCTION

Several of the new findings related to dopamine receptor subtypes are summarized in Table 8. The data presented provides overwhelming evidence that D_1-dopamine receptors influence behavior and are functionally distinct from D_2-dopamine receptor sites. These data resolve whether the D_1-dopamine receptors have a function (Laduron, 1983). However, it has not yet been resolved whether the sites associated with behavior are in fact also the same ones linked to adenylate cyclase (see other chapters).

Based on the observation that SCH 23390 blocks the consequences of a D_2-dopamine agonist when catecholaminergic function is intact, we postulate that D_1-dopamine receptors can control D_2-receptor function through a catecholaminergic mechanism (Breese and Mueller, 1985; Breese et al., 1985c). How these latter data may contribute to the observation that reduction of catecholamine synthesis reduces the action of LY-171555 has yet to be determined. Further, it is also presently unclear if dopaminergic or noradrenergic neurons are involved in these changes. We also have observed that SKF-38393 is more effective in the presence of a D_2-agonist and that D_1 and D_2-dopamine receptor agonist responses are facilitated in dopamine-lesioned rats. These observations suggest that the loss of catecholamine-containing neurons "uncouples" critical modulatory circuits and transmitter availability that are responsible for the coordinated function of dopaminergic neurons and their associated D_1 and D_2-receptor sites.

In the case of neonatally-lesioned rats, the response to a D_2-dopamine agonist is limited after peripheral injection compared to the response in adult-lesioned rats. Conversely, in adult-6-OHDA-treated rats, the locomotor response to D_1-dopamine agonists is less vigorously expressed after peripheral administration than in rats lesioned as neonates. These findings suggest that a neural circuit is important for the functional interactions between D_1 and D_2-dopamine receptors, rather than an interaction on the same cell. Perhaps these findings relate to evidence presented by Herrera-Marschitz and Ungerstedt (1984) who proposed that different striatal efferents are associated with different dopamine receptor subtypes. Thus, from these various observations, it can be concluded that destruction of dopamine-containing neurons in the neonate results in adaptive changes in circuits which modulate dopaminergic function that differ from those changes which occur when this lesion is made in the mature rat.

TABLE 8. New Findings Concerning Dopamine Function From
Drugs Acting on Specific Receptor Subtypes

OBSERVATION	CONCLUSION
SCH 23390 does not antagonize LY-171555 after 6-OHDA lesions, but does in unlesioned rats	D_1 receptor controls D_2 receptor by way of a catecholamine link
Combining D_1 and D_2 agonists give a greater response than either alone	Interaction between receptors (Source?)
Potentiation of D_1 and D_2 agonists in 6-OHDA treated rats	Lesion uncouples a dampening mechanism
Absence of change in receptor number in lesioned rats	Mechanisms other than binding responsible for functional super-sensitivity
Priming required for D_1 receptor sensitivity	?

The fact that the receptor number for dopamine antagonist binding is not altered for D_1 and D_2-dopamine sites after 6-OHDA lesions suggests that mechanisms other than receptor number or affinity are responsible for the functional super-sensitivity observed following dopamine agonist administration. Since dopamine agonist binding does not always follow results obtained with a dopamine antagonist, agonist binding for D_1 and D_2-dopamine receptors should be performed in 6-OHDA-lesioned rats. Similarly, because the phosphorylated protein, DARPP-32, is associated with D_1-dopamine receptor function (Walaas et al., 1983), the possible relationship of this protein to functional supersensitivity observed after administration of SKF-38393 to rats lesioned as neonates should be explored. Another phenomenon we have observed is "priming" of D_1-dopamine receptor sensitivity with repeated administration of SKF-38393 to rats lesioned as neonates (Breese et al., 1985c). The physiological basis of this phenomenon also needs further exploration.

RELATIONSHIP OF NEONATAL-6-OHDA-LESIONS TO LESCH-NYHAN SYNDROME

Lloyd et al., (1981) demonstrated that biochemical measures of central dopamine-containing neurons are deficient in Lesch-Nyhan patients. Dopamine content and tyrosine hydroxylase activity are reduced by 80-90 percent in several brain areas associated with dopaminergic fibers, suggesting the absence of these neurons in Lesch-Nyhan patients. Markers for GABA and noradrenergic fibers are not altered. Parkinsonism is an adult syndrome also associated with the loss of dopamine-containing neurons (Hornykiewicz, 1973). Because dopamine-containing fibers are absent in both diseases, one might suppose that their symptoms would be similar. However, the symptoms in these two afflictions are not comparable in spite of their common neurochemical deficiency. Lesch-Nyhan patients have choreoathetoid movements and hypertonicity (Lesch and Nyhan, 1964; Kelley and Wyngaarden, 1983) rather than tremor, bradykinesia and the stooped posture associated with Parkinsonism. Another important difference between Parkinsonism and Lesch-Nyhan disease is the age of onset of the symptoms for these disorders. This latter observation was the original motivation for comparing neonatally and adult-6-OHDA lesioned rats (Breese et al. 1984 ab).

Data collected in neonatally 6-OHDA-lesioned rats suggest that this treatment may serve as a neurochemical model of the deficiency of brain dopamine observed in Lesch-Nyhan disease (Breese et al., 1984 abc; Table 9). In addition to the reduction of dopamine, serotonin is elevated in the striatum of neonatally-lesioned rats (Breese et al., 1984a), just as seen in the Lesch-Nyhan syndrome (Lloyd et al., 1981). Neonatally 6-OHDA-lesioned rats have an increased suscepti- bility for SMB--a cardinal symptom in Lesch-Nyhan disease. Furthermore, several investigations demonstrated that haloperidol does not block SMB in patients with Lesch-Nyhan syndrome. This observation is also consistent with the inability of high doses of haloperidol to prevent SMB induced by L-DOPA in neonatally 6-OHDA-lesioned rats (Breese et al., 1984b, 1985). It should also be noted that neonatally- lesioned rats are aggressive and have a variety of deficits in

Table 9. Relationship of Neonatal-6-OHDA Treatment To Lesch-Nyhan Syndrome

Characteristic	Lesch-Nyhan Syndrome	6-OHDA-Treated Neonates
Dopamine neurons absent	Yes	Yes
Striatal serotonin increased	Yes	Yes
Lesion during brain development	Yes	Yes
Increased susceptibility for self-mutilation (SMB)	Yes	Yes
SMB antagonized by fluphenazine but not haloperidol	Yes	Yes
Aggressive Behaviors	Yes	Yes
Behavioral Deficiencies	Yes	Yes
Choline acetylase reduced in putamen	Yes	?

operant paradigms (Breese et al., 1973; Smith et al., 1973). Aggressiveness and behavioral (mental) deficiencies are commonly seen in Lesch-Nyhan syndrome (Lesch and Nyhan, 1964). Thus, the neurobiology defined in this "model" appears relevant to the clinical disorder.

Goldstein et al. (1985) reported that fluphenazine, not haloperidol, antagonized or attenuated the self-biting in patients with Lesch-Nyhan disease. Since fluphenazine will antagonize both D_1 and D_2-dopamine receptors, these results suggest that D_1-dopamine receptors contribute to the self-mutilation in these patients, as proposed in our original publication (Breese et al., 1984a). Since D_2-dopamine agonists do not produce self-mutilation in neonatally-lesioned rats and are useful in Parkinson's disease (Claveria et al., 1975), such agents would likely alter symptoms in children with Lesch-Nyhan disease. However, it is not known whether administration of the D_2 agonist would be beneficial to motor dysfunction in the Lesch-Nyhan syndrome or exacerbate their choreic symptoms, as observed with L-DOPA in Huntington's chorea (Klawans et al., 1972). Regardless, it would be important to choose an agent that will antagonize D_1-dopamine receptors whenever any dopamine agonist therapy is undertaken in patients with Lesch-Nyhan disease.

ACKNOWLEDGEMENTS

The authors wish to acknowledge the excellent typing assistance of Carolyn Reams. Supported by USPHS grants MH-33127, HD-03110, and HL-31424.

REFERENCES

Arnt, J., 1985, Hyperactivity induced by stimulation of separate D_1 and D_2 receptors in rats with bilateral 6-OHDA lesions, Life Sci., 37:717-723.

Arnt, J., and Hyttel, J., 1984, Differential inhibition by dopamine D_1 and D_2 antagonists of circling behavior induced by dopamine agonists in rats with unilateral 6-hydroxydopamine lesions, Europ. J. Pharmacol., 102:349-354.

Bevan, P., 1983, Repeated apomorphine treatment causes behavioral supersensitivity and dopamine D_2 receptor hyposensitivity, Neurosci. Letter, 35:185-189.

Billard, W., Ruperto, V., Crosby, G., Iorio, L.C., and Barnett, A., 1984, Characterization of the binding of ^{3}H-SCH 23390, a selective D_1 receptor antagonist ligand, in rat striatum, Life Sci., 35:1885-1893.

Breese, G.R. and Traylor, T.D. Effects of 6-hydroxydopamine on brain norepinephrine and dopamine: Evidence for selective degeneration of catecholamine neurons, 1970, J. Pharmacol. Exp. Ther., 174:413-420. .

Breese, G.R., and Traylor, T.D., 1972, Developmental characteristics of brain catecholamines and tyrosine hydroxylase in the rats: Effects of 6-hydroxydopamine, Brit. J. Pharmacol., 44:210-222.

Breese, G.R., Baumeister, A.A., McCown, T.J., Emerick, S.G., Frye, G.D. and Mueller, R.A., 1984a, Neonatal-6-hydroxydopamine: Model of susceptibility for self-mutilation in the Lesch-Nyhan Syndrome, Pharmacol. Biochem. Behav., 21:459-461.

Breese, G.R., Baumeister, A.A., McCown, T.J., Emerick, S.G., Frye, G.D., Crotty, K., and Mueller, R.A., 1984b, Behavioral differences between neonatal and adult-6-hydroxydopamine-treated rats to dopamine agonists: Relevance to neurological symptoms in clinical syndromes with reduced brain dopamine, J. Pharmacol. Exp. Ther., 231:343-354.

Breese, G.R., Baumeister, A., Napier, T.C., Frye, G.D., and Mueller, R.A., 1985a, Evidence that D_1 dopamine receptors contribute to the supersensitive behavioral responses induced by L-dihydroxyphenylalanine in rats treated neonatally with 6-hydroxydopamine, J. Pharmacol. Exp. Ther., 235:287-295.

Breese, G.R., Cooper, B.R. and Smith, R.D., 1973, Biochemical and behavioral alterations following 6-hydroxydopamine administration into brain. In: "Frontiers in Catecholamine Research", Usdin, E. and Snyder, S. (Eds.). Pergamon Press, pp. 701-706.

Breese, G.R. and Mueller, R.A., 1985, SCH 23390 antagonism of a D_2 dopamine agonist depends upon catecholaminergic neurons, Europ. J. Pharmacol., 113:109-114.

Breese, G.R., Mueller, R.A.. and Mailman, R.B., 1979, Effects of dopaminergic agonists and antagonists on in vivo cyclic nucleotide content: Relation of guanosine 3'5'-monophosphate (cGMP) changes in cerebellum to behavior, J. Pharmacol. Exp. Ther., 209:262-270.

Breese, G.R., Napier, T.C., and Mueller, R.A., 1985c, Dopamine agonist-induced locomotor activity in rats treated with 6-hydroxydopamine at differing ages: Functional super-sensitivity of D_1 dopamine receptors in neonatally lesioned rats, J. Pharmacol Exp. Ther., 234:447-455.

Breese, G.R., McCown, T.J., Baumeister, A.A., Emerick, S.G., Frye, G.D. and Mueller, R.A., 1984c, L-DOPA induced self-biting in rats treated with 6-hydroxydopamine as neonates: Model of self-mutilation observed in Lesch-Nyhan syndrome, Fed. Proc., 43:928.

Christensen, A.V., Arnt, J., Hyttel, J., Larson, J.J., and Svendsen, O., 1984, Pharmacological effects of a specific dopamine D_1 antagonist SCH 23390 in comparison with neuroleptics, Life Sci., 34:1529-1540.

Claveria, L.E., Teychenne, P.F., Calne, D.B., Petrie, A. and Bassendine, M.F., 1975, Dopaminergic agonists in Parkinsonism, Adv. Neurol., 9:393-397.

Cooper, B.R., Breese, G.R., Grant, L.D., and Howard, J.J., 1973, Effects of 6-hydroxydopamine treatments on active avoidance responding: Evidence for involvement of brain dopamine, J. Pharmacol. Exp. Ther., 185:358-370.

Costall, B., Kelley, M.E., and Naylor, R.J., 1984, Unilateral striatal denervation: Reduced motor inhibitory effects of dopamine antagonists revealed in models of asymmetric and circling behavior, Nauyn-Schmeideberg's Arch. Pharmacol., 326:29-35.

Costall, B., Naylor, R.J., and Neumeyer, J.L., 1975, Differences in the nature of the stereotyped behavior by apomorphine derivatives in the rat and in their actions in extrapyramidal and mesolimbic brain areas, Europ. J. Pharmacol., 31:1-16.

Creese, I., Burt, D.R., and Snyder, S.H., 1977, Dopamine receptor binding enhancement accompanies lesion-induced behavioral supersensitivity, Science, 197:596-598.

Goldstein, M., Anderson, L.T., Reuben, R. and Dancis, J.,
    1985, Self-mutilation in Lesch-Nyhan disease is caused by
    dopaminergic denervation, <u>Lancet</u>, 1:338-339.
Goldstein, M., Lew, T.Y., Asano, T., and Weta, K., 1980,
    Alterations in dopamine receptors. Effects of lesions and
    haloperidol treatment, <u>Comm. Psychopharm.</u>, 4:21-25.
Heikkila, R.E., Shapiro, B.S., and Duvoisin, R.C., 1981, The
    relationship between loss of dopamine nerve terminals,
    striatal (^{3}H)-spiroperidol binding and rotational
    behavior in unilaterallly 6-hydroxydopamine-lesioned
    rats, <u>Brain Res</u>., 211:285-292.
Herrera-Marschitz, M., and Ungerstedt, U., Evidence that
    striatal efferents relate to different dopamine
    receptors, <u>Brain Res</u>., 323:269-278.
Hollister, A.S., Breese, G.R., and Cooper, B.R., 1974,
    Comparison of tyrosine hydroxylase and dopamine-β-
    hydroxylase inhibition with the effects of various 6-
    hydroxydopamine treatments on d-amphetamine induced motor
    activity, <u>Psychopharmacologia</u>, 36:1-16.
Hollister, A.S., Breese, G.R., and Mueller, R.A., 1979, Role
    of monoamine neural systems in L-dihydroxyphenylalanine
    stimulated activity, <u>J. Pharmacol. Exp. Ther.</u>, 208:37-43.
Hornykiewicz, O., 1973, Parkinson's disease: From brain
    homogenate to treatment, Fed. Proc., <u>32</u>:183-190.
Hyttel, J., 1978, A comparison of the effect of neuroleptic
    drugs on the binding of ^{3}H-haloperidol and ^{3}H-(Z)-
    flupentixol and an adenylate cyclase activity in rat
    striatal tissue <u>in</u> <u>vitro</u>, <u>Prog. Neuro-Psychopharmacol.</u>,
    2:329-335.
Iorio, L.C., Barnett, A., Leitz, F.H., Houser, V.P., and
    Korduba, A., 1983, SCH-23390, a potential benzazepine
    antipsychotic with unique interactions on dopaminergic
    systems, <u>J. Pharmacol. Exp. Ther.</u>, 226:462-468.
Jackson, D.M., Anden, N-E. and Dahlstrom, A., 1975, A
    functional effect of dopamine in the nucleus accumbens
    and in some dopamine-rich areas of the rat brain,
    <u>Psychopharmacologia</u>, 45:139-149.
Kebabian, J.W., and Calne, D.B., 1979, Multiple receptors for
    dopamine, <u>Nature</u> (Lond)., 227:93-96.
Kelley, W.N. and Wyngaarden, T.B., 1983, Clinical syndromes
    associated with hypoxanthine-guanine-phosphoribosyl-
    transferase deficiency. In: "Metabolic Basis of
    Inherited Disease", edited by Stanberry et al. New York:
    McGraw Hill, pp. 1115-1143.
Kilts, C.D., Smith, D.A., Ondrusek, M.G., Mailman, R.B.,
    Mueller, R.A., and Breese, G.R., 1979, Differential
    effects of "Dopaminergic agonists" on measures of
    dopaminergic function, <u>Soc. Neurosci. Abst.</u>, 5:562.
Klawans, W.L., Paulson, G.W., Ringel, S.P. and Barbeau A.,
    1972, Use of L-DOPA in the detection of prof L-DOPA in
    the detection of presymptomatic Hungtington's chorea, <u>N.
    Engl. J. Med.</u>, 286:1332-1334.
Klawans, H.L., Hitri, A., Carvey, P.M., Nausieda, P.A. and
    Weiner, W.J., 1979, Effect of chronic dopaminergic
    agonism on striatal membrane dopamine binding, <u>Adv.
    Neurol.</u>, 24:217-224.
Koller, W.C., Cortin, J.C., and Fields, J.Z., 1984, Pergolide
    down-regulates D_2 dopamine receptors but fails to block
    haloperidol induced behavioral supersensitivity, <u>Society
    Neurosci. Abst.</u>, 10:1136.

Laduron, P.M., 1983, Commentary: Dopamine-sensitive adenylate cyclase as a receptor site, In: "Dopamine Receptors" (ed. C. Kaiser and T.W. Kebabian), Am. Chem. Soc. (Washington, D.C.) pp. 22-28.

Lesch, M. and Nyhan, W.L., 1964, A familial disorder of uric acid metabolism and central nervous system function, Am. J. Med., 36:561-570.

Lloyd, K.G., Hornykiewicz, O., Davidson, L., Shannak, K., Farley, I., Goldstein, M., Shibuya, M., Kelley, W.N., and Fox, I.H., 1981, Biochemical evidence of dysfunction of brain neurotransmitters in the Lesch-Nyhan syndrome, N. Eng. J. Med., 305:1106-1111.

Mailman, R.B., Kilts, C.D., Beaumont, K., and Breese, G.R., 1981, "Supersensitivity" of dopamine systems: Comparisons between haloperidol withdrawal, intracisternal and unilateral 6-hydroxydopamine (6-OHDA) treatments, Fed Proc., 40:291.

Mailman, R.B., Towle, A., Schulz, D.W., Lewis, M.H., Breese, G.R., DeHaven, D.H., and Krigman, M.R., 1983, Neonatal 6-OHDA treatment of rats: Changes in dopamine (DA) receptors, striatal neurochemistry and anatomy, Soc. Neurosci. Abstr., 9:932.

Mailman, R.B., Schulz, D.W., Lewis, M.H., Staples, L. Rollema, H. and DeHaven, D.L., 1984, SCH 23390: A selective D_1 dopamine antagonist with potent D-2 behavioral actions, Europ. J. Pharmacol., 101:159-160.

Molloy, A.G. and Waddington, T.L., 1984, Dopaminergic behavior stereospecifically promoted by the D_1 agonist R- SK & F 38393 and selectively blocked by the D_1 antagonist SCH 23390, Psychopharmacology, 82:409-410.

Neve, K.A., Altar, C.A., Wong, C.A., and Marshall, T.F., 1984, Quantitative analysis of (^{3}H) spiroperidol binding to rat forebrain sections: Plasticity of neostriatal dopamine receptors after nigrostriatal injury, Brain Res., 302:9-18.

Onali, P., Olianas, M. and Gessa, G.L., 1985, Characterization of dopamine receptors mediating inhibition of adenylate cyclase activity in rat striatum, Mol. Pharmacol., 28:138-145.

Pijnenburg, A.J.J., Honig, W.M.M., Van Der Heyden, J.A.M., and Van Rossum, J.M., 1976, Effects of chemical stimulation of the mesolimbic dopamine system upon locomotor activity, Europ. J. Pharmacol., 35:45-58.

Robinson, T.E., 1984, Behavioral sensitization: Characteristics of enduring changes in rotational behavior produced by intermittent injections of amphetamine in male and female rats, Psychopharmacology, 84:466-475.

Schoenfeld, R., and Uretsky, N.,1972, Altered response to apomorphine in 6-hydroxydopamine-treated rats, Europ. J. Pharmacol., 19:115-118.

Seeman, P., 1980, Brain dopamine receptors, Pharmacol. Rev., 32:229-313.

Setler, P.E., Sarau, H.M., Zirkle, C.L., and Saunders, H.L., 1978, The central effects of a novel dopamine agonist, Europ. J. Pharmacol., 50:419-430.

Smith, R.D., Cooper, B.R., and Breese, G.R., 1973, Growth and behavioral changes in developing rats treated intracisternally with 6-hydroxydopamine: Evidence for involvement of brain dopamine, J. Pharmacol. Exp. Ther., 185:609-619.

Staunton, D.A., Wolfe, B.B., Groves, P.M., and Molinoff, P.B., 1981, Dopamine receptor changes following destruction of the nigrostriatal pathway: Lack of a relationship to rotation behavior, Brain Res., 211:315-327.

Tsuruta, K., Frey, E.A., Grewe, C.W., Cote, T.E., Eskay, R.L., and Kebabian, T.W., 1981, Evidence that LY-141865 specifically stimulates the D_2 dopamine receptor, Nature (Lond), 292:463-465.

Ungerstedt, U., 1971, Postsynaptic supersensitivity after 6-hydroxydopamine induced degeneration of the nigro-striatal dopamine system, Acta Physiol. Scand., Supplement 367, pp. 69-93.

Walaas, S.I., Aswad, D.W., and Greengard, P., 1983, A dopamine and cyclic AMP-regulated phosphoprotein enriched in dopamine-innervated brain regions, Nature, 301:69-71.

INDEX